Depression in Parents, Parenting, and Children

Opportunities to Improve Identification, Treatment, and Prevention

Committee on Depression, Parenting Practices, and
the Healthy Development of Children

Board on Children, Youth, and Families
Division of Behavioral and Social Sciences and Education

NATIONAL RESEARCH COUNCIL *AND*
INSTITUTE OF MEDICINE
OF THE NATIONAL ACADEMIES

THE NATIONAL ACADEMIES PRESS
Washington, D.C.
www.nap.edu

THE NATIONAL ACADEMIES PRESS   500 Fifth Street, N.W.   Washington, DC 20001

NOTICE: The project that is the subject of this report was approved by the Governing Board of the National Research Council, whose members are drawn from the councils of the National Academy of Sciences, the National Academy of Engineering, and the Institute of Medicine. The members of the committee responsible for the report were chosen for their special competences and with regard for appropriate balance.

This study was supported by Grant No. 61299 between the National Academy of Sciences and the Robert Wood Johnson Foundation; by Grant No. 20062466 with The California Endowment; by Grant No. 205.0794 with the Annie E. Casey Foundation; by Contract No. HHSH250200446009I with the Health Resources and Services Administration; and by Contract No. 270-03-6002 with the Substance Abuse and Mental Health Services Administration. Any opinions, findings, conclusions, or recommendations expressed in this publication are those of the author(s) and do not necessarily reflect the views of the organizations or agencies that provided support for the project.

Library of Congress Cataloging-in-Publication Data

National Research Council (U.S.). Committee on Depression, Parenting Practices, and the Healthy Development of Children.
   Depression in parents, parenting, and children : opportunities to improve identification, treatment, and prevention / Committee on Depression, Parenting Practices, and the Healthy Development of Children, Board on Children, Youth, and Families, Division of Behavioral and Social Sciences and Education.
       p. cm.
   Includes bibliographical references and index.
   ISBN 978-0-309-12178-1 (hardcover) — ISBN 978-0-309-12179-8 (pdf) 1. Depression, Mental. 2. Depression in children. 3. Parenting—Psychological aspects. I. Title.
   RC537.N375 2009
   362.2'5—dc22
                                 2009023655

Additional copies of this report are available from the National Academies Press, 500 Fifth Street, N.W., Lockbox 285, Washington, DC 20055; (800) 624-6242 or (202) 334-3313 (in the Washington metropolitan area); Internet, http://www.nap.edu.

Suggested citation: National Research Council and Institute of Medicine. (2009). *Depression in Parents, Parenting, and Children: Opportunities to Improve Identification, Treatment, and Prevention.* Committee on Depression, Parenting Practices, and the Healthy Development of Children. Board on Children, Youth, and Families. Division of Behavioral and Social Sciences and Education. Washington, DC: The National Academies Press.

THE NATIONAL ACADEMIES
Advisers to the Nation on Science, Engineering, and Medicine

The **National Academy of Sciences** is a private, nonprofit, self-perpetuating society of distinguished scholars engaged in scientific and engineering research, dedicated to the furtherance of science and technology and to their use for the general welfare. Upon the authority of the charter granted to it by the Congress in 1863, the Academy has a mandate that requires it to advise the federal government on scientific and technical matters. Dr. Ralph J. Cicerone is president of the National Academy of Sciences.

The **National Academy of Engineering** was established in 1964, under the charter of the National Academy of Sciences, as a parallel organization of outstanding engineers. It is autonomous in its administration and in the selection of its members, sharing with the National Academy of Sciences the responsibility for advising the federal government. The National Academy of Engineering also sponsors engineering programs aimed at meeting national needs, encourages education and research, and recognizes the superior achievements of engineers. Dr. Charles M. Vest is president of the National Academy of Engineering.

The **Institute of Medicine** was established in 1970 by the National Academy of Sciences to secure the services of eminent members of appropriate professions in the examination of policy matters pertaining to the health of the public. The Institute acts under the responsibility given to the National Academy of Sciences by its congressional charter to be an adviser to the federal government and, upon its own initiative, to identify issues of medical care, research, and education. Dr. Harvey V. Fineberg is president of the Institute of Medicine.

The **National Research Council** was organized by the National Academy of Sciences in 1916 to associate the broad community of science and technology with the Academy's purposes of furthering knowledge and advising the federal government. Functioning in accordance with general policies determined by the Academy, the Council has become the principal operating agency of both the National Academy of Sciences and the National Academy of Engineering in providing services to the government, the public, and the scientific and engineering communities. The Council is administered jointly by both Academies and the Institute of Medicine. Dr. Ralph J. Cicerone and Dr. Charles M. Vest are chair and vice chair, respectively, of the National Research Council.

www.national-academies.org

v

BRIDGET B. KELLY, *Program Officer*
SARAH JOESTL, *Research Associate* (June–August 2008)
JULIENNE PALBUSA, *Research Assistant* (from December 2008)
REINE Y. HOMAWOO, *Senior Program Assistant*
MATTHEW D. McDONOUGH, *Senior Program Assistant* (until April 2008)
SARA LANGSTON, *Senior Program Assistant* (November 2008–January 2009)

vii

Reviewers

This report has been reviewed in draft form by individuals chosen for their diverse perspectives and technical expertise, in accordance with procedures approved by the National Research Council's Report Review Committee. The purpose of this independent review is to provide candid and critical comments that will assist the institution in making its published report as sound as possible and to ensure that the report meets institutional standards for objectivity, evidence, and responsiveness to the study charge. The review comments and draft manuscript remain confidential to protect the integrity of the deliberative process. We wish to thank the following individuals for their review of this report: Hortensia Amaro, Bouve College of Health Sciences, Institute on Urban Health Research, Northeastern University; Linda Beeber, School of Nursing, University of North Carolina at Chapel Hill; Joseph T. Coyle, McLean Hospital, Harvard Medical School; Deborah A. Gross, Johns Hopkins University; Milton Kotelchuck, Maternal and Child Health Department, School of Public Health, Boston University; Joanne Nicholson, Center for Mental Health Services Research, Department of Psychiatry, University of Massachusetts Medical School; Paul A. Nutting, Research Director's Office, Center for Research Strategies, Denver, CO; Harold Alan Pincus, Department of Psychiatry, College of Physicians and Surgeons, Columbia University and New York State Psychiatry Institute, New York Presbyterian Hospital; Mary Rainwater, Integrated Behavioral Health Project, The Tides Center, Los Angeles, CA; Kenneth B. Wells, Semel Institute Health Services Research Center, University of California, Los Angeles; and Joan Yengo, Programs Division, Mary's Center for Maternal and Child Care, Inc., Washington, DC.

Although the reviewers listed above have provided many constructive comments and suggestions, they were not asked to endorse the conclusions or recommendations nor did they see the final draft of the report before its release. The review of this report was overseen by Floyd E. Bloom, Department of Molecular and Integrative Neuroscience, The Scripps Research Institute and Elena O. Nightingale, Scholar-in-Residence, Institute of Medicine, Washington, DC. Appointed by the National Research Council, they were responsible for making certain that an independent examination of this report was carried out in accordance with institutional procedures and that all review comments were carefully considered. Responsibility for the final content of this report rests entirely with the authoring committee and the institution.

Preface

Today, as science continues to produce new knowledge every day on the myriad ways depression affects parents, parenting, and children in a rapidly changing and stressful social environment, it is extremely important to integrate and apply that new knowledge so we can provide evidence-based identification, treatment, and prevention efforts across a broad spectrum of society. Of particular concern today is the recognition of the increased number of depressed parents whose condition directly affects their families.

To address these issues and develop recommendations for improving services in families with depressed parents, five organizations and federal agencies—the Robert Wood Johnson Foundation, the Annie E. Casey Foundation, The California Endowment, and the Health Resources and Services Administration and the Substance Abuse and Mental Health Services Administration of the U.S. Department of Health and Human Services—provided funding to the National Research Council–Institute of Medicine (NRC–IOM) Board on Children, Youth, and Families. Through the Board, the NRC and IOM formed the Committee on Depression, Parenting Practices, and the Healthy Development of Children in 2008. This report, *Depression in Parents, Parenting, and Children: Opportunities to Improve Identification, Treatment, and Prevention*, is the product of a multidisciplinary collaboration among committee members, NRC–IOM staff, and consultants.

The committee held five meetings and one public workshop. Committee members and staff conducted two site visits to learn firsthand about creative approaches to providing mental health services in substance abuse settings, especially in underserved groups. We participated in vigorous discussion regarding the best approaches to prevent, engage, and treat families with depressed parents, clarifying the underlying approach to this problem, and reconciling different perspectives and priorities. It is our hope that the findings and recommendations presented in this report will help policy makers, service providers and payers, researchers, and government agencies shift the current fragmented approach of depression care in parents from a series of individual services into a family-based system of care.

The committee could not have done its work without the outstanding guidance and support provided by NRC–IOM staff Leslie Sim, study director; Bridget Kelly, program officer; and Kimberly Scott, senior program officer. Reine Homawoo, Wendy Keenan, Sara Langston, Matthew McDonough, and Julienne Palbusa provided highly skilled logistical support. Rosemary Chalk's guidance and counsel were invaluable throughout our deliberations. Finally, health professionals who participated in our workshops and those who shared their stories during our site visits deserve special thanks. Their experience in coping with the current system of care and their aspirations for something better fueled the committee's resolve to make a difference.

Parents today face daunting challenges, but knowledge brought to the heart and applied can help parents, children, and families. That is what this report is about.

Mary Jane England, *Chair*
Committee on Depression, Parenting Practices,
and the Healthy Development of Children

Acknowledgments

Beyond the hard work of the committee and project staff, this report reflects contributions from various other individuals and groups that we want to acknowledge.

The committee greatly benefited from the opportunity for discussion with the individuals who made presentations and attended the committee's workshops and meetings (see Appendix B).

This study was sponsored by the the Robert Wood Johnson Foundation, the Annie E. Casey Foundation, The California Endowment, and the Health Resources and Services Administration and the Substance Abuse and Mental Health Services Administration of the U.S. Department of Health and Human Services. We wish to thank Elaine Cassidy, Patrick Chaulk, Gwen Foster, Lark Huang, Karen Hench, Jane Isaacs Lowe, Robert Phillips, and Linda White-Young for their support.

We appreciate the extensive contributions of Robert Cole, Janice Cooper, Sara Jaffee, Sarah Joestl, Kenneth Kendler, Frances Lynch, and David Racine, who we commissioned to provide technical reviews of various portions of the report. Their insight and expertise added to the quality of the evidence presented. Katherine Elliott and Cristiana Giordano of the UC Davis Center for Reducing Health Disparities as well as Alinne Barrera of University of California, San Francisco, provided outstanding assistance in organizing literature for the committee.

The committee was grateful for the opportunity to conduct site visits to two residential substance abuse treatment programs for women and their children. Committee members and staff toured the facilities and met with program staff to learn about the program history, services offered, sources of funding and support, and partnerships with other service organizations.

Thank you to the leaders of the Entre Familia Program of the Boston Public Health Commission, including Hortensia Amaro, Barbara Ferrer, and Rita Nieves, as well as the other clinical and support staff, current clients, and program graduates who took the time to meet with us and show us the facility. Thank you also to Shela Chapman and Peggy Johnson who joined us from Entre Familia partner organizations.

Thank you to the staff who took the time to meet with us at the PROTOTYPES Women's Center in Pomona, CA, including Rocksy Chenevert, Andrea Heinz, Julie Poirier, Garrett Staley, and April Wilson, as well as staff from other PROTOTYPES partner programs, including Jill McKenzie, Sharmelle Parker, Edith Vega, and Qiana Wallace.

As well, we are indebted to others at the NRC–IOM, including Kirsten Sampson Snyder, DBASSE reports officer, who patiently worked with us through several revisions of this report; Yvonne Wise, DBASSE production editor, who managed the production process through final publication; Christine McShane, who edited several revisions of the report; and Matthew Von Hendy, DBASSE librarian, who performed multiple literature searches throughout the production of this report.

Mary Jane England, *Chair*
Committee on Depression, Parenting Practices,
and the Healthy Development of Children

Contents

APPENDIXES

Tribute to Jane Knitzer

This report is dedicated to Dr. Jane Knitzer, Ed.D., who served as a member of this project's committee until she passed away on March 29, 2009. Dr. Knitzer was a long-time advocate for children's mental health, child welfare, and early childhood, adding tremendous value over her lifetime to the work of The National Center for Children in Poverty at Columbia University's Mailman School of Public Health, Cornell University, New York University, and Bank Street College of Education. Dr. Knitzer influenced many individuals and communities through her advocacy and impact on public policies for America's most vulnerable children, youth, and families.

Dr. Knitzer was an extremely committed activist, scholar, and moral leader. She provided inspiration and guidance through her work, through her extraordinary mentorship of several generations of those who worked in many diverse roles with children, youth, and their families and through her absolute insistence that children and their families deserve justice and fairness above all. Her keen instincts on policy led researchers, policy makers, practitioners, and parents alike to resonate with her message for improving the lives of children and their families based on research-informed strategies and interventions. She particularly brought to our attention the need to attend to those who had the highest risk: children in poverty, children afflicted by violence, those in vulnerable situations, and children whose parents suffered from mental illness and related adversities. She truly helped make invisible children visible and demanded that we attend to their needs. Above all Dr. Knitzer was dedicated to highlighting the need to invest in America's youngest children, demanding that as a nation we give children and their families the best start possible irrespective of their life circumstances.

Jane Knitzer was indomitable in her cause, which was the cause of the most vulnerable among us, and she never wavered in her pursuit of what was best for children and families. Her insights and scholarship guided the deliberations and content of this report, and we dedicate it to her memory.

Members of the Committee on Depression, Parenting
Practices, and the Healthy Development of Children
May 2009

Summary

Depression affects millions of U.S. adults over their lifetime, many of whom are parents with children. In a given year an estimated 7.5 million adults with depression have a child under the age of 18 living with them. It is estimated that at least 15 million children live in households with parents who have major or severe depression. The burden of depression and the barriers to quality of care for depressed adults are increasingly well understood, but the ways in which depression affects parenting, and children's health and psychological functioning, are often ignored.

Many factors are associated with depression, including co-occurring medical and psychiatric disorders (such as substance abuse), economic and social disadvantages, and conflicted or unsupportive relationships. These factors typically amplify stress and erode effective coping. For many adults (30–50 percent), depression becomes a chronic or recurrent disorder in a vicious cycle of stress and poor coping that exacts sustained individual, family, and societal costs.

Effective screening tools and treatments for adult depression are available and offer substantial promise for reducing the negative consequences of the disorder. However, not everyone benefits from even the treatments associated with the strongest evidence base, and individual, provider, and system-level barriers decrease access to these treatments. These institutional and sociocultural barriers both cause and sustain existing disparities in care for depressed adults.

Furthermore, few opportunities exist to identify the vulnerable population of children (i.e., those at risk of adverse health and psychological functioning) living in households with one or more parents experiencing depression or to offer prevention and treatment services that can improve the care of the depressed parent in a framework that also offers services for children. In addition to improving depression care for adults, therefore, is the need to develop and implement an identification, treatment, and prevention strategy that can respond to the parenting and caregiving roles of the affected parents and their children. Although depression has been documented as a major concern in multiple programs that serve families and children (e.g., Head Start; the Special Supplemental Nutrition Program for Women, Infants, and Children; Temporary Assistance for Needy Families), federal and state responses to this problem are diffuse and fragmented across multiple health and human service agencies.

In short, parental depression is prevalent, but a comprehensive strategy to treat the depressed adults and to prevent problems in the children in their care is absent. National leadership, interagency collaboration, state-based linkage efforts, and collaboration with the private sector are what is lacking in the United States at this time to effectively support the development and evaluation of a framework that integrates health, mental health, public health, and parenting in a life-course framework, from pregnancy through adolescence. There is also a lack of support for public and professional education, training, infrastructure development, and implementation efforts to improve the quality of services for affected families and vulnerable children. Likewise, funds rarely exist for research, data collection, or evaluation efforts that might lead to improved prevention and treatment services for this population.

STUDY SCOPE AND APPROACH

Scope

The Committee on Depression, Parenting Practices, and the Healthy Development of Children was charged with reviewing the relevant literature on parental depression, its interaction with parenting practices, and its effects on children and families. In conducting this study, the committee

- clarified what is known about interactions among depression and its co-occurring conditions, parenting practices, and child health and development;
- identified the findings, strengths, and limitations of the evidentiary base that support assessment, treatment, and prevention interventions for depressed parents and their children;
- highlighted disparities in the prevalence, prevention, treatment, and outcomes of parental depression among different sociode-

mographic populations (e.g., racial/ethnic groups, socioeconomic groups);

- examined strategies for widespread implementation of best practice and promising practice programs given the large numbers of depressed parents; and
- identified strategies that can foster the use of effective interventions in different service settings for diverse populations of children and families.

Approach

A variety of sources informed the committee's work, including: five formal committee meetings, expert presentations, and a public workshop; a review of literature from a range of disciplines and sources; technical reviews on selected topics; and analyses of data and research on depression in adults and parents and its consequences for their children. The committee considered research on the causes, comorbidities, and consequences of depression in adults (specifically including parenting and child health outcomes), various health and support services for depression care, the features of interventions and implementation strategies for depression care in diverse populations, and public policies related to implementing promising interventions. The committee also visited two programs that provide a multifaceted approach to mental health services in substance abuse settings to underserved mothers and their families.

Through our review of the literature and discussions with service providers, policy makers, and stakeholder organizations, the committee identified four major issues that are faced in attempting to address the problems associated with the care of depressed parents. These are the *integration* of knowledge regarding the dynamics of parental depression, parenting practices, and child outcomes so that it is transdisciplinary and links research to practice; the need to recognize the *multigenerational dimensions* of the effects of depression in a parent so that the needs of both parent and the child are identified in research and practice; the application of a *developmental* framework in the study and evaluation of the effects of parental depression; and the need to acknowledge the presence of a *constellation* of risk factors, context, and correlates of parental depression. These four themes pervade each area that the committee addressed, and they are essential to improving the quality of care for depressed parents and those who are affected. But many promising strategies identified here for screening, treatment, prevention, and policy interventions have emerged that deserve consideration to engage the large and diverse numbers of families affected by depression.

CONCLUSIONS

The committee's findings are broadly marshaled into the following conclusions that serve as the basis for seven recommendations.

Depression Is a Common Condition and Is Attributed to Multiple Risk Factors and Mechanisms

Depression is a common condition among adults, many of whom are parents. Despite its prevalence, differences exist in rates of depression among particular sociodemographic categories—sex, income level, marital status, race/ethnicity, employment status. Multiple biological mechanisms, genetic factors, environmental risk factors, personal vulnerabilities, and resilience factors for depression—as well as the co-occurrence of other disorders such as substance abuse and trauma—have been identified. Although gaps exist in knowledge of the relationship among multiple contributors to depression, the research clearly implicates stress and adversity, giving important clues about personal vulnerabilities, protection, and resilience—all of which have implications for interventions to identify, treat, and prevent depression.

Multiple Barriers Exist That Decrease the Quality of Depression Care for Adults

Like a variety of other health services, access to care for depression may be influenced by geographic, physical, financial, sociocultural, and temporal barriers. Such barriers include transportation issues, physical disabilities, stigma, language barriers, a history of oppression, racism, discrimination, poverty, immigration status, cultural customs and beliefs, and health insurance coverage. A 2006 Institute of Medicine report entitled *Improving the Quality of Health Care for Mental and Substance-Use Conditions* points out that care for mental health and substance use problems is also distinct from health care generally. The distinctive features they describe include greater stigma associated with diagnoses, a less developed infrastructure for measuring and improving the quality of care, a need for a greater number of linkages among multiple clinicians, organizations and systems providing care to patients with mental health conditions, less widespread use of information technology, a more educationally diverse workforce, and a differently structured marketplace for the purchase of mental health and substance use health care. Although reducing these barriers is essential to improving the quality of care for depressed adults, it is also important to note that these barriers focus on the individual. Additional barriers impose constraints for those depressed adults who are parents and for addressing its effects on parenting and child health and development.

Depression May Interfere with Parenting Quality and Put Children at Risk for Adverse Outcomes

Depression in parents interferes with parenting quality and is associated with poor health and development (e.g., physical, psychological, behavioral, social development and mental health) in their children at all ages. Focusing on symptoms and diagnosis provides important yet incomplete information about the complete picture of depression. A narrow focus on symptoms and diagnosis ignores the larger possible impacts on family development (i.e., individual and social capital, resource allocation). While it is difficult to estimate the true costs of depression in parents, it is essential to consider not only the individual family members but also the family as a whole. Some questions remain regarding conditions that make these interactions stronger or weaker and the specific mechanisms or intermediate steps through which depression in the parent becomes associated with parenting or with outcomes in children; however, the research has clear implications for developing interventions for depressed parents and mitigating its consequences.

Existing Screening and Treatment Interventions Are Safe and Effective for Depressed Adults But Are Rarely Integrated or Consider Their Parental Status or Its Impact on Their Child

Effective screening tools are available to identify adults with depression in a variety of settings. However, current screening programs for depression in adults generally do not consider whether the adult is a parent, and therefore they do not assess parental function or comorbid conditions, do not consider the impact of the parent's mental health status on the health and development of their children, and are rarely integrated with further evaluation and treatment or other existing screening efforts. Community and clinical settings that serve parents at higher risk for depression do not routinely screen for depression.

Safe and effective treatments and strategies to deliver them exist for adults with depression in a range of settings. However, treatment safety, efficacy, and delivery strategies have generally not assessed parental status, the impact of depression on parental functioning, or its effects on child outcomes, except during pregnancy and in mothers postpartum. Models that incorporate multiple interventions (e.g., collaborative care) for adults appear to be a reasonable approach to delivering depression care, although such models have not been tested for their effectiveness in serving parents.

Emerging Preventive Interventions Demonstrate Promise for Improving Outcomes for Families with Depressed Parents

Emerging preventive interventions specifically for families with depressed parents and adaptations of other existing evidence-based parenting and child development interventions demonstrate promise for improving outcomes for these families. However, the data from most of these interventions for families with depression are limited. Broader preventive interventions that support families and the healthy development of children also hold promise for improving parent and child outcomes, although such interventions have not been tested to demonstrate their effects in mitigating the consequences of a *depressed* parent within their families.

Emerging Initiatives Highlight Opportunities and Challenges in Improving the Engagement and Delivery of Care to Diverse Families with a Depressed Parent

The scope and compelling nature of depression in parents and its interaction with parenting and healthy child development supports the need to develop or adopt strategies to meet the needs of a diverse number of families with a depressed parent. Ideally, the identification, treatment, and prevention of depression among adults would integrate mental and physical health services. In addition, for those who are parents, they would strengthen and support parent-child relationships, offer developmentally appropriate treatment and prevention interventions for children, and provide comprehensive resources and referrals for other comorbidities associated with depression (such as substance abuse and trauma). Such services would be available in multiple health care settings, including those that engage children and families. Furthermore, this system of care would use more proactive approaches for prevention or early intervention of depression in parents in the context of a two-generation model that is family-focused, culturally informed, and accessible to vulnerable populations.

Existing health care and social services systems are far from achieving this goal in implementing this system of care for depressed parents and their families. But emerging initiatives at the community, state, and federal level as well as internationally have included key features of a service delivery model for depressed parents and their children and highlight opportunities and challenges to improve, implement, and disseminate more effective, efficient, and equitable service delivery models. A wide range of settings offers opportunities to engage and deliver care to diverse families with a depressed parent. These adult health, child heath, and family support settings often lack linkages with other settings to offer integrated mental health, social support, and parenting interventions for these vulnerable populations.

Multiple Challenges Exist in Implementing and Disseminating Innovative Strategies

Implementing innovative strategies requires addressing existing systemic, workforce, and fiscal barriers. In order for these strategies to be effective they should be flexible, efficient, inexpensive, and, above all, acceptable to the participants by having the ability to engage participants and reduce or overcome barriers to care. Furthermore, numerous opportunities exist to continue to build a knowledge base that can enhance the development of future programs, policies, and professional practice. But overcoming systemic, workforce, and fiscal challenges and developing new knowledge to help in the design of innovative strategies are not sufficient to ensure its use in the routine efforts of service providers and practitioners to identify, treat, and prevent parental depression and to reduce the impact of this disorder on children. The application of evidence-based knowledge requires explicit attention to dissemination, implementation, and the creation of organizational infrastructure and cultures that are intentionally receptive to new research findings. Since the current research base points to no simple path for implementation and dissemination of innovative strategies, both conceptual principles and promising practices should guide large-scale efforts, but large-scale efforts should be undertaken in a staged, sequential fashion with each effort building on the knowledge from the proceeding stage. The ultimate goal should be to have system-wide programs for parental depression that incorporate multiple points of entry, employ flexible strategies, and allow for the types and amounts of services and prevention to be tailored to individual needs and families. Aligning the work that supports the development of innovative strategies with the efforts to implement and disseminate evidence-based programs in specific settings will help to clarify additional work that is needed to deliver care for particular groups and also how to extend these strategies to other populations and systems.

RECOMMENDATIONS

Improve Awareness and Understanding

Sustained commitments will be needed from the federal and state governments to increase the basic knowledge and public awareness about depression in parents and its effects on the healthy development of children. This leadership is central to improve the care of depressed adults who are parents as well as to reduce adverse outcomes in their children.

Recommendation 1: The Office of the U.S. Surgeon General should identify depression in parents and its effects on the healthy develop-

ment of children as part of its public health priorities focused on mental health and eliminating health disparities.

To implement this recommendation, the U.S. Surgeon General should encourage individual agencies, particularly the National Institutes of Health, the Health Resources and Services Administration (HRSA), the Centers for Disease Control and Prevention (CDC), and the Substance Abuse and Mental Health Services Administration (SAMHSA), to support the Healthy People 2020 overarching goal of achieving health equity and eliminating health disparities by including the importance of identification, treatment, and prevention of depression and its potential impact on the healthy development of children of depressed parents. These agencies should pay particular attention to groups and populations that have historically and currently experience barriers in receiving quality health care, including for behavioral health. Efforts should be made to ensure that effective strategies are employed to increase the participation and engagement of these vulnerable populations in critical research studies and clinical trials. New research methods and innovative models that partner with vulnerable communities should be supported. Particular focus should be directed at prevention and early intervention efforts that are community-based and culturally appropriate so that the high burden of disability currently associated with depression in populations experiencing health disparities can be reduced.

> Recommendation 2: The Secretary of the U.S. Department of Health and Human Services, in coordination with state governors, should launch a national effort to further document the magnitude of the problem of depression in adults who are parents, prevent adverse effects on children, and develop activities and materials to foster public education and awareness.

To implement this recommendation the Secretary of the U.S. Department of Health and Human Services (HHS) should encourage individual agencies, particularly the National Institute of Mental Health (NIMH), HRSA, CDC, and the Agency for Healthcare Research and Quality, to identify the parental status of adults and add reliable and valid measures of depression to ongoing longitudinal and cross-sectional studies of parents and children and national health surveys, in ways that will support analyses of prevalence, incidence, disparities, causes, and consequences. Second, CDC should develop guidelines to assist the states in their efforts to collect data on the incidence and prevalence of the number of depressed adults who are parents and the number of children at risk to adverse health and psychological outcomes. Finally, using this information, HHS should encourage agencies, most notably HRSA, to develop a series of public education activities and materials that highlight what is known about the impact of depression in parents. These activities and materials should specifically target the public and individuals who make decisions about care for a diverse population of depressed parents and their children in a variety of settings (e.g., state and county leadership, state health directors, state mental health agencies, and state maternal and child health services).

Support Innovative Strategies

To build on emerging community, state, and federal initiatives to improve the quality of care for depressed parents, further support is necessary to encourage the design and evaluation of innovative services in different settings for diverse populations of children and families.

Recommendation 3: Congress should authorize the creation of a new national demonstration program in the U.S. Department of Health and Human Services that supports innovative efforts to design and evaluate strategies in a wide range of settings and populations to identify, treat, and prevent depression in parents and its adverse outcomes in their children. Such efforts should use a combination of components—including screening and treating the adult, identifying that the adult is a parent, enhancing parenting practices, and preventing adverse outcomes in the children. The results of the new demonstration program should be evaluated and, if warranted, Congress should subsequently fund a coordinated initiative to introduce these strategies in a variety of settings.

To implement this recommendation, agencies in HHS should prepare a request for proposals for community-level demonstration projects. Such demonstration projects

- should test ways to reduce barriers to care by using one or more empirically based strategies to identify, treat, and prevent depression in parents in heterogeneous populations (i.e., race/ethnicity, income level), those in whom depression is typically underidentified, and those with risk factors and co-occurring conditions (e.g., trauma, anxiety disorders, substance use disorders);
- should call attention to effective interventions in which screening and assessment are linked to needed care of parents with depression, that support training in positive parenting, and that encourage strategies to prevent adverse outcomes in their children;
- could identify multiple opportunities to engage parents who are depressed as well as to identify children (at all ages) who are at risk because their parents are depressed;

- could include the Healthy Start Program, the Head Start Program, the Nurse-Family Partnership, home visiting, schools, primary care, mental health and substance abuse treatment settings, and other programs that offer early childhood interventions;
- would ideally use more than one strategy and could use funds to test state-based efforts that experiment with different service strategies and service settings and to strengthen the relationship between mental health services and parental support programs;
- could test ways to reduce the stigma and biases frequently associated with depression, address cultural and racial barriers and disparities in the mental health services system, and explore opportunities to strengthen formal and informal supports for families that are consistent with cultural traditions and resources; and
- should include state mental health agencies and local government (e.g., counties), at least in an advisory capacity.

Finally, SAMHSA should promote interagency collaboration with other HHS agencies—CDC, HRSA, the National Institute on Drug Abuse, the National Institute on Alcohol Abuse and Alcoholism, NIMH, the National Institute on Nursing Research, and the National Institute of Child Health and Human Development—to develop coordinated strategies that support the design and evaluation of these demonstration projects. SAMHSA could identify an interagency committee to pool information about programs that are affected by parents with depression, programs that offer opportunities to engage parents and children in the treatment and prevention of this disorder, and research and evaluation studies that offer insight into effective interventions. SAMHSA could develop opportunities to introduce effective interventions in both community-based systems of care frameworks and in integrated behavioral and mental health services in a variety of settings including primary care and substance abuse treatment settings.

Develop and Implement Systemic, Workforce, and Fiscal Policies

Policies are intended to influence decisions and actions. Some policies provide protections for vulnerable populations, while others create conditions for a desirable future—business, health, or otherwise. Both call for the careful use of policies to foster the delivery of care for depressed parents and their children.

Recommendation 4: State governors, in collaboration with the U.S. Department of Health and Human Services, should support an interagency task force within each state focused on depression in parents. This task force should develop local and regional strategies to support

collaboration and capacity building to prepare for the implementation of evidence-based practices, new service strategies, and promising programs for the identification, treatment, and prevention of depression in parents and its effects in children.

The wide variation in state resources and structures for providing mental health services and family support resources suggests that broad experimentation with different service strategies may be necessary to implement two-generation interventions for the treatment and prevention of depression in parents, to support parenting practices, and to prevent physical, behavioral, and mental health problems in youth. First, state governors should designate a joint task force of state and local agencies to coordinate local efforts (e.g., counties) and to build linkages and the infrastructure that can support a strategic planning process; refine service models and delivery systems through collaboration among diverse agencies; prepare to incorporate an array of programs for different sites, settings, and target populations; prepare model plans that include multiple entry points in a variety of service sectors; and prepare for a stepwise rollout with ongoing or interim evaluation.

Second, the state strategies should include policy protocols and fiscal strategies that offer incentives across multiple systems (including health and education) to expand the state's capacity to respond to parental depression through a family-focused lens. These protocols and strategies could be supported by the efforts funded and coordinated by HHS through agencies that include SAMHSA and HRSA. Third, the state strategies should offer flexible responses that can be adapted to the needs of urban and rural communities. Finally, states should be required to provide a biannual report to a designated office in HHS that describes their strategic plans as well as the challenges and barriers that affect their capacity to address depression in a family context for children of all ages. These reports should be shared to encourage states to learn from each other's initiatives.

Recommendation 5: The Substance Abuse and Mental Health Services Administration and the Health Resources and Services Administration, in collaboration with relevant professional organizations and accrediting bodies, should develop a national collaborative training program for primary, mental health care, and substance abuse treatment providers to improve their capacity and competence to identify, treat, and prevent depression in parents and mitigate its effects on children of all ages.

For this recommendation to be realized, the national collaborative training program should strengthen a workforce that is informed about and prepared to address parenting issues associated with depression and the effects of adult disorders on children in a diverse society. This program should explore opportunities to enhance attention to interactions between depression and parenting in ongoing mental health and primary care training and continuing education programs, such as activities funded by Title VII and Title VIII of section 747 of the Public Health Service Act. Training efforts should include an emphasis on developmental issues, exploring the impact of depression and the combination of depression and its commonly co-occurring disorders (e.g., anxiety disorders, parental substance use disorders) on children of different ages, from pregnancy through adolescent development. Options for such training programs could include cross-disciplinary training with an emphasis on parental depression, parenting, and developmentally based family-focused concerns that arise in the treatment of depression. Such training programs should call attention to identifying children at risk to adverse health and psychological outcomes. Training programs should also include efforts to build a more diverse and culturally competent workforce.

> Recommendation 6: Public and private payers—such as the Centers for Medicare and Medicaid Services, managed care plans, health maintenance organizations, health insurers, and employers—should improve current service coverage and reimbursement strategies to support the implementation of research-informed practices, structures, and settings that improve the quality of care for parents who are depressed and their children.

Public and private payers should consider the following options for implementing this recommendation:

- The Centers for Medicare and Medicaid Services (CMS) could extend services and coverage of mothers to 24 months postpartum, which includes a critical period of early child development when interaction with parental care is especially important. Long-term coverage for parents would be optimal. CMS could remove restrictions on Medicaid's rehabilitation option and other payment options (including targeted case management and home visitation programs) that could reimburse services and supports in nonclinical settings and enhance access to quality care; allow same-day visit reimbursement for mental health and primary care services; reimburse primary care providers for mental health services; and remove prohibitions on serving children without medical diagnoses, thereby covering health promotion services for children at risk before diagnosis.

- States could work with CMS to implement financing mechanisms to support access to treatment and supportive services for depressed parents through clarifying existing coverage, billing codes, or encouraging use of research-informed practices. This would complement local and regional strategies developed by the states. Similarly, private health plans and self-insured employers could cover parental depression screening and treatment and support the implementation of effective models.

Promote and Support Research

Knowledge is the basis of effective action and progress, yet current resources are limited and fragmented to expand the knowledge base and encourage the development, implementation, and dissemination of innovative evidence-based strategies for depressed parents and their families.

Recommendation 7: Federal agencies, including the National Institutes of Health, the Centers for Disease Control and Prevention, the Health Resources and Services Administration, and the Substance Abuse and Mental Health Services Administration, should support a collaborative, multiagency research agenda to increase the understanding of risk and protective factors of depression in adults who are parents and the interaction of depression and its co-occurring conditions, parenting practices, and child outcomes across developmental stages. This research agenda should include the development and evaluation of empirically based strategies for screening, treatment, and prevention of depressed parents and the effects on their children and improve widespread dissemination and implementation of these strategies in different services settings for diverse populations of children and their families.

In carrying out this recommendation, these federal agencies should consider partnerships with private organizations, employers, and payers to support this research agenda.

FINAL THOUGHTS

Depression in adults is a prevalent and impairing problem and rarely occurs alone. The study of depression illustrates a larger set of issues, including other illnesses (e.g., anxiety, substance use disorders) and general stresses and risk factors (e.g., poverty). Screening tools, treatments, and delivery strategies available are effective for many with this disorder, especially if identified early, but it remains underrecognized and undertreated. The problem of depression in adults is compounded when those adults are parents because of its potential impact on parenting as well as the impact on the well-being of their children. Although there is significant and important research literature both about adults who are depressed and about parents facing adversity, there is remarkably little systematic examination of depression in parents. Ultimately depression is a good and effectively identified indicator of problems that could trigger a system of care that intervenes not only in treating depression in the parent, but also in enhancing parenting skills, in alleviating other stresses, co-occurring conditions, and social contexts, and in identifying and intervening with children at risk.

Although little research has been focused on improving care for depressed parents and their children, there are both conceptual principles and promising practices that could guide large-scale efforts in a deliberate sequential approach for family-centered care. Remarkable advances in research continue and need to be supported; it is therefore also important to build mechanisms to incorporate new findings into service settings as they become available. As with other areas in mental health and physical health, there are significant infrastructure, workforce, and fiscal problems that need to be addressed to build a system of family-centered care for depression in parents. It is the committee's hope that this report will inspire policy makers and community leaders and practitioners to consider the value of long-term commitments to reducing parental depression and its effects on children. Only then can the knowledge base highlighted in this report be used well to promote access to appropriate services, reduce stigma, and reduce the costs of depression to adults, the children in their care, and society as a whole.

1

Introduction and Magnitude of the Problem

SUMMARY

Prevalence

- In the United States, 16.2 percent of adults reported major depression in their lifetime, while another 4.1 percent reported meeting a milder but chronic form of depression.
- Certain subpopulations of adults defined by selected population characteristics—such as sex, age, ethnicity, and marital status—indicate disparities in prevalence rates of depression. Female, younger, and divorced adults have higher rates of lifetime depression than their male, older, or married adult counterparts. In general, a positive association has been found between social disadvantage and depression prevalence, except in the case of first generation immigrants.
- Many adults in the United States are parents. Parents (with at least one child under age 18) have similar rates of depression compared to the entire U.S. adult population, including similar disparities in depression rates for selected population characteristics.
- Depression rarely occurs alone; 75 percent of individuals with lifetime or recent major depression also had at least one additional mental health or substance abuse diagnosis.

Impact

- Depression, due to its recurrent nature, leads to sustained individual, family, and societal costs.
- 15.6 million children under 18 years of age are living with an adult who had major depression in the past year.
- Depression in parents can have serious biological, psychological, behavioral, and social consequences especially for children who rely on a parent for caregiving, material support, and nurturance.
- Despite this impact, depression is perhaps one of the most effectively treated psychiatric disorders, if recognized and treated early in its onset.

Barriers

- Individual-, provider-, and system-level barriers exist that decrease the access to and quality of care for depressed adults. These institutional, sociocultural, and linguistic barriers are responsible for causing and maintaining existing disparities. Without a system of care that is culturally and linguistically sensitive and supports a family's environment, economic resources and relationships with family, coworkers, the community, and society, such disparities may increase. Improving provider-patient-family communication is an important component of addressing differences in quality of care that are associated with patient race, ethnicity, culture, and language.
- The current policy environment does not encourage a two-generation (i.e., parent, child) identification, treatment, and prevention strategy for adults with depression.

Depression is a common, universal, and debilitating public health problem. The Global Burden of Disease study by the World Health Organization (WHO) determined that depression accounts for more disability worldwide than any other condition during the middle years of adulthood (Murray and Lopez, 1996). In fact, major depressive disorder is now the leading cause of disability worldwide (World Health Organization, 2001). For some with depressive episodes, periods of depression may resolve in a few weeks or months. However, it has been estimated that, for 30 to 50 percent of adults, depression is recurrent or chronic or fails to resolve completely (e.g., Depue and Monroe, 1986; Judd et al., 1998; Solomon et al., 2000). Ironically, depression is perhaps one of the most effectively treated psychiatric disorders and, if recognized early, it can be prevented.

International surveys attest to the universality of depression across cultures. A WHO-based study (using the Composite International Diagnostic Interview[1]) of 10 countries in North America, Latin America, Europe, and Asia reported a range of lifetime major depression from 3 percent in Japan to 16 percent in the United States (Andrade et al., 2003). More recently, the WHO World Health Surveys, a cross-national study comprised of nearly 250,000 participants in 60 countries across all regions of the world, estimated the overall 1-year prevalence of depressive episode (using criteria of the *International Statistical Classification of Diseases and Related Health Problems*, 10th revision) alone to be 3.2 percent (Moussavi et al., 2007).

Depression can be disabling for anyone, but the extent of its impact goes beyond the affected individual to the broader family context and especially to the depressed person's children, who are dependent on their parent for their care and support of their development. Under these circumstances, depression becomes a multigenerational disorder that can have serious biological, psychological, behavioral, and social consequences, especially for children who rely on a parent for caregiving, material support, and nurturance. Effective treatments aimed at reducing or eliminating depression among parents or caregivers may therefore also constitute a significant preventive intervention for children.

Expressed in purely monetary terms, the economic burden of depression is a serious global public health problem as well (Luppa et al., 2007; Moussavi et al., 2007). Estimated costs related to depression in the United States increased in the past decade from $77.4 billion dollars in 1990 to $83.1 billion in 2000 (Greenberg et al., 2003). Of the estimated total amount in 2000, direct treatment costs were $26.1 billion, workplace costs were $51.5 billion (e.g., absenteeism, reduced productivity), and suicide-related costs were $5.4 billion (Greenberg et al., 2003; Muñoz, 2003). There exists, moreover, a strong association between depression and nonadherence to treatment of such medical conditions as diabetes or coronary heart disease, leading to higher treatment costs for their medical care than patients with medical conditions who are not depressed (DiMatteo, Lepper, and Croghan, 2000).

---

[1]The Composite International Diagnostic Interview is a comprehensive interview designed for the assessment of mental disorders according to the definitions and criteria of the *International Statistical Classification of Diseases and Related Health Problems*, 10th revision, and the *Diagnostic and Statistical Manual of Mental Disorders*, 4th edition.

STUDY CHARGE, APPROACH, AND SCOPE

In May 2006, with support from the Annie E. Casey Foundation, the National Research Council and the Institute of Medicine convened a two-day planning meeting to explore the need for and focus of a future study on maternal depression. Researchers from a variety of disciplines, including pediatrics, policy, and community health, reviewed a small set of studies from the research literature and explored whether the quality of the work was sufficient to support a future comprehensive analysis of the evidence base surrounding maternal depression as well as an exploration of how to improve the application of this knowledge to policy, practice, and program development.

The presentations and discussion resulted in a few key conclusions. The research literature on the treatment and prevention of depression among adults and children is rich with findings about effective interventions. More importantly, there exists a sound knowledge base about the effects of depression in families, the mechanisms of transmission of illness, and the risk and protective factors that either trigger or prevent onset or reduce severity of the disorder. The last 10 years have witnessed an increase in evidence-based prevention in general and the development of promising approaches specific to the identification, treatment, and prevention of depression in families. Aside from presenting and assessing the existing evidence, the meeting also shed light on serious gaps in the synthesis and application of extant findings and interventions in the family setting because of the diffuse and disjointed nature of the prevention, identification, and treatment literatures. Specifically, there exists a need to identify approaches that can highlight ways to translate research knowledge into effective interventions in a broad range of parental support and child health and development strategies.

Study Charge

Concerned about these complex issues, the National Academies' Board on Children, Youth, and Families formed the Committee on Depression, Parenting Practices, and the Healthy Development of Children, with funding from the Robert Wood Johnson Foundation, the Annie E. Casey Foundation, The California Endowment, and the Substance Abuse and Mental Health Services Administration and the Health Resources and Services Administration of the U.S. Department of Health and Human Services. The National Research Council and the Institute of Medicine appointed the 17-member committee in October 2007 to review the relevant research literature on the identification, prevention, and treatment of parental depression, its interaction with parenting practices, and its effects on children and families. The committee was asked to

1. clarify what is known about interactions among depression and its co-occurring conditions, parenting practices, and child health and development;
2. identify the findings, strengths, and limitations of the evidentiary base that support assessment, treatment, and prevention interventions for depressed parents and their children;
3. highlight disparities in the prevalence, prevention, treatment, and outcomes of parental depression among different sociodemographic populations (e.g., race/ethnicity, socioeconomic status);
4. examine strategies for widespread implementation of best practice and promising practice programs, given the large numbers of depressed parents; and
5. identify strategies that can foster the use of effective interventions in different service settings for diverse populations of children and families.

Study Approach

A variety of sources informed the committee's work. Five formal committee meetings and one public workshop were held during the course of the study. The workshop explored innovative strategies and models that integrate mental health services for depression, parenting, and child development services within various settings for diverse populations of children and families; explored strategies that insure interventions are appropriate for diverse populations; and explored existing opportunities for interventions as well as existing barriers to implementation or replication of promising programs or best practices at regional, state, multi-state, or national levels in a variety of settings.

The committee also reviewed literature from a range of disciplines and sources. Technical reviews were commissioned by experts on a variety of topics including: genetics and the environment; integration and implementation of services and models of care; the economic burden of depression; public-health policy; and vulnerable populations. Data and research on depression in adults, specifically parents, were analyzed. The committee considered research on the causes, comorbidities, and consequences of depression in adults (including parenting and child health outcomes), various health and support services for depression care, the features of interventions and implementation strategies for depression care in diverse populations, and public policies related to implementing promising interventions.

Additionally, the committee visited programs focused on providing mental health services in substance abuse settings to underserviced populations. The limited evaluation of these programs and the lack of a standard against which to study them make it impossible to designate any of them as exemplary models of care. However, these visits provided examples of health services being delivered specifically to vulnerable and underserviced parents, and they helped the committee gain insight into various services, partnerships, approaches, and care models that are used. The sites visited were Entre Familia Program of the Boston Public Health Commission and PROTOTYPES Women's Center in Pomona, California. Both visits encompassed a tour of the program site and meetings with leaders of the sponsoring institution and other staff and partnering programs.

Study Scope

The committee was charged broadly with an examination of depression in parents and its effects on parenting practices and child development. However, the charge did not specify what "depression" or "parents" should encompass. Therefore, one of the committee's early tasks was to reach consensus on how to define these terms in reviewing the literature.

Defining Depression

The available literature on depression in adults—and, more specifically, on parents and its effects on parenting practices and children and families—has not measured depression in a consistent manner; it is therefore important to consider these varied approaches. In general, there is continual debate on how to define mental disorders, and specifically for depression there are many tools used in the literature to assess adults for depression.

A review by Frank and Glied (2006) on mental health policy in the United States describes three ways in which epidemiologists generally define who has a mental disorder: (1) those who have *symptoms and signs* of a particular disorder, (2) those who have mental health-related *impairment* in daily life, and (3) those who have sought *treatment* for a mental health condition. A combination of these three is generally preferred over a single one because each selects a distinct subgroup of the population, usually with small overlap. In addition, experts continue to argue about the specific combination of signs and symptoms on which diagnoses should be based.

A variety of methods are used to screen for or diagnose depression, which is reflected in the literature that the committee reviewed. The use of diverse methods for defining depression is a result of restrictions on time and cost, study populations' sociodemographic characteristics (e.g., race/ethnicity, socioeconomic status), and differences in provider training. Research that defines parental depression by symptoms is more common in the literature than a clinical diagnosis. Literature that discusses effects of depression on parenting practices is based mostly on depressive symptoms or "distress." In addition, defining depression using symptoms may be more efficient overall from the provider's perspective but may complicate detection in a person also experiencing conditions resulting from substance use or trauma. For example, substance abuse greatly influences symptoms of mental illness and vice versa. Further, using methods that define depression by symptoms may lead to higher rates among one group over another, for example women compared to men.

The problem with using a clinical definition of parental depression is that it generally identifies only those who are active in the mental health system; people who are isolated or who are disadvantaged are less likely to have access to mental health services and hence are more likely to go undiagnosed. And methods used for clinical diagnosis may vary by type of provider. Generalist physicians provide most of the depression screening and care to the general population, whereas the limited number of available specialty mental health providers (i.e., those with advanced mental health training) may see a more severely ill population.

Given these considerations, in describing this literature on depression in adults who are parents and its effects on parenting practices, children, and families, the committee chose to use both symptoms and a clinical diagnosis of depression whenever the data were available. However, due to the concerns described above, it may be important to distinguish the use of methods that use self-report symptoms compared to clinician-rated depression diagnosis because the method could highlight different outcomes seen across studies of depression, parenting, and child outcomes.

Defining Parents and the Family Unit

Family composition is marked by increased diversity and change. It has been estimated that less than 50 percent of children in the United States live in traditional nuclear families, in which two biological parents are married to each other with full siblings (Brandon and Bumpass, 2001). Instead, children's living arrangements increasingly include unmarried parents, stepfamilies, foster parents, and multigenerational households. For example, the proportion of cohabiting same-sex and opposite-sex couples who have children is increasing (Bengtson et al., 2005). In addition, the number of grandparents who are raising their grandchildren has increased dramatically over the past few decades (Casper and Bryson, 1998). However a family unit is composed, it still holds true that 70 percent of children under the age of 18 live in two-parent households (Federal Interagency Forum on Child and Family Statistics, 2007).

The committee focused its search of the impact and prevalence of depression, interventions, and strategies of implementation on depression in parents on all individuals who take care of a child or children in a variety of family structures. This definition of a parent allows discussion to include a variety of caregivers of children. However, having decided to focus the study on a variety of caregivers in a variety of family structures, we found limited literature specifically on parents with depression and even more limited information regarding specific groups of caregivers, including fathers and grandparents. The little information that is available for these other caregivers is highlighted throughout the report when available.

STUDY CONTEXT

Parents and Their Children

In 2004, it was estimated that approximately 148.8 million parents live in the United States (U.S. Census Bureau, 2005a, 2005b). The Current Population Survey, through its household survey data, helps to track the number of mothers, fathers, and other caregivers who take care of children under the age of 18 in the United States. In 2007, it was estimated that there were 36.5 million married parents, single fathers, and single mothers (i.e., households) who care for their own children under the age of 18—that is, approximately 47 percent of households (U.S. Census Bureau, 2008b). Together, these parents take care of approximately 96 percent of almost 74 million children under age 18 in the United States. The remaining 3 percent of children (2.5 million) do not live with either of their parents, but with a grandparent, other relative, or nonrelative or are in the foster care system (U.S. Census Bureau, 2008a).

Prevalence of Depression

In the United States, the 2001 National Comorbidity Survey-Replication (NCS-R) revealed that the prevalence of major depression (defined by syndrome features, impairment, and duration of at least two weeks) in adults in their lifetime was 16.2 percent (over 3 million adults), while another 4.1 percent met the diagnostic criteria for dysthymic disorder, a milder but chronic form of depression (The ESEMeD/MHEDEA 2000 Investigators, 2004; Kessler et al., 2003). Overall, both international and national data support the universal nature of depression. While many studies do not specifically investigate parental depression or even note parental status among their samples, a few national surveys help give insight into the prevalence of depression among adults who are also parents in the United States. For example, a subsample of the National Comorbidity Survey Replication in 2002 reported that 17 percent of parents (with at least one child) had major or severe depression in their lifetime, a prevalence similar to that of the entire U.S. population of 16.2 percent (see Table 1-1). Examining rates of parental

TABLE 1-1 Prevalence of Major Depressive Disorder with Hierarchy[a] for Adults with at Least One Child Under the Age of 18 Years, 2002

Major Depression	Women (%) (n = 1,301)	Men (%) (n = 942)	Overall (%) (n = 2,243)
Overall			
Lifetime	21.7	12.6	17.3
Past 12 months	10.0	4.3	7.2
With Child ≤ 5 Years of Age			
Lifetime	17.2	11.5	14.8
Past 12 months	10.0	4.4	7.6
With Child 6–12 Years of Age			
Lifetime	22.3	12.9	17.7
Past 12 months	10.0	4.2	7.2
With Child ≥ 13 Years of Age			
Lifetime	24.5	14.2	19.4
Past 12 months	10.5	5.2	7.8

[a]"With hierarchy" refers to a diagnostic criterion in the *Diagnostic and Statistical Manual of Mental Disorders*, 4th edition that specifies that if a disorder is better explained by another mental disorder, that "other" disorder is given hierarchy over the disorder of interest, i.e., a more narrow definition of major depression disorder that does not include those with mania and hypomania.

SOURCE: Tabulations based on the National Comorbidity Survey-Replication (see http://www.icpsr.umich.edu/cpes/).

depression in the past year, the NCS-R found that approximately 7 percent of parents (with at least one child) had major or severe depression in the last 12 months and did not differ by the age of the child (see Table 1-1). The Pregnancy Risk Assessment Monitoring System (PRAMS), another national data set that collects self-reported data, offers further insight on the scope of depression, specifically in postpartum women. The survey found that 11 to 20 percent of new mothers were affected by depressive symptoms following childbirth (Centers for Disease Control and Prevention, 2008). One important longitudinal study in the United Kingdom of parents and child outcomes, the Avon Longitudinal Study of Parents and Children, was used to do secondary analyses of paternal peripartum depression (Ramchandani et al., 2008). Father's depression correlated strongly with maternal depression scores, suggesting that, when fathers are depressed, there may be a high prevalence of both parents being depressed.

Disparities and Vulnerable Populations

Despite its prevalence across cultures, sexes, income strata, and age groups, tremendous differences in depression rates in particular sociodemographic categories is noteworthy. For example, women are about twice as likely to be diagnosed with depression as men in nearly all cultures (Andrade et al., 2003; Kessler, 2003; Riolo et al., 2005). Among adults overall, rates of depression are higher among single or divorced people than among their married counterparts (e.g., The ESEMeD/MHEDEA 2000 Investigators, 2004; Kessler et al., 2003). Stratified by age, depression is more common among teenagers and younger adults than among older adults, with apparently increasing rates in more recently born cohorts (e.g., Cross-National Collaborative Group, 1992; The ESEMeD/MHEDEA 2000 Investigators, 2004; Kessler et al., 2005). Similarly, a subsample of the NCS-R reports significant differences in lifetime and past year major depression prevalence rates among parents by gender, marital status, if English was their primary language while they were growing up, if they were born in the United States, and by race/ethnicity (see Tables 1-2 and 1-3). Mothers have almost double the prevalence of lifetime major depression than fathers. Parents overall and especially mothers who were divorced, widowed, or separated reported higher lifetime prevalence of major depression than those who were married or never married. Also, parents and mothers born in the United States and raised with English as their primary language report lifetime major depression significantly more than those who were not born in the United States or if English was not their primary language. Unlike the general population of parents and mothers, fathers reported significant differences in lifetime depression rates by current work status. Fathers not in the workforce at all have almost double the prevalence of lifetime depression than fathers who are employed or currently unemployed. Among the general population of parents, poverty status, and educational attainment did not significantly affect the prevalence of lifetime major depression. Although differences in rates by gender and marital status were similar as for prevalence of lifetime major depression, reports of major depression in the past year also found additional differences by current work status. Parents, and in particular fathers, who were employed had approximately half of the prevalence of major depression in the past year compared with parents who were unemployed or not in the workforce (see Table 1-3). Finally, similar to the general adult population and specific to the parent population, the Medical Expenditure Panel Survey in 2004 found gender disparities in the prevalence of poor mental health. A total of 4.5 percent of households reported that the mother was the only adult with fair or poor mental health, compared with 2.6 percent of households who reported that the father was the only adult affected. Around 1 percent of households report that both adults (mother and father) had fair or poor mental health (personal communication, Stephen Petterson, Robert Graham Center, February 13, 2008).

It is not clear whether certain subgroups of the population are disproportionately affected by depression. For example, differences in (particularly chronic) depression are reported along the lines of race and ethnicity. However, there seem to be some inconsistencies about whether the prevalence rates for depression in the general adult as well as in the parent population in racial/ethnic minority groups is higher or lower than their white counterparts. Existing national surveys[2] report lower rates in *lifetime* prevalence for adults in these racial/ethnic minority groups (e.g., Asian Americans, African Americans) and similar prevalence rates *in a given year* to that of non-Hispanic whites (Takeuchi et al., 2007; Williams et al., 2007). The limited available evidence suggests the need for research on this topic (Jackson and Williams, 2006). The subsample of the NCS-R specific to parents shows the highest rates of lifetime and past year major depression specifically among parents who are black immigrants from the Caribbean (about 30 percent), followed by non-Hispanic whites (around 20 percent), African Americans (around 12 percent), non-Mexican Hispanics (around 15 percent), and Mexicans (10 percent). Asians report the lowest prevalence (around 9 percent) (see Tables 1-2 and 1-3).

A number of studies have examined depression among groups that are disadvantaged for a variety of reasons, such as poverty. While these studies differ in terms of design, sample size, and specific findings, they all document the same trend: a positive association between depression and *social disadvantage*, except in the case of first generation immigrants. For example, studies of low-income women found depression rates nearly double those in the general population, ranging between 12 and 27 percent for current (Bassuk et al., 1998; Jesse et al., 2005; Lanzi et al., 1999) and 43 percent for lifetime prevalence (Bassuk et al., 1998). A longitudinal population study showed a clear relationship between worsening socioeconomic circumstances and depression, and a meta-analysis of 51 studies found compelling evidence for socioeconomic inequality in depression (Lorant et al., 2003, 2007). Among women participating in state welfare-to-work programs, Siefert and colleagues (2000) recorded current depression among more than a quarter of them. A national survey found homeless women with lifetime prevalence rates of depression around 45 percent and current (i.e., past month) prevalence rates of roughly 10 percent (Bassuk et al., 1998). In their research with incarcerated women, Bloom and colleagues found that 13.7 percent of their sample had been diagnosed with a current episode of depression (Bloom et al., 2003). Research indicates that immigrants from Mexico, the Caribbean, and Africa have lower rates of mental health disorders than their U.S.-born counterparts (Miranda et al., 2005; Vega et al., 1998); however, recent surveys also indicate the mental health

---

[2]For example, the National Survey of American Life and the National Latino and Asian American Study.

TABLE 1-2 Lifetime Prevalence of Major Depression with Hierarchy[a] by Selected Demographic Characteristics for Adults with at Least One Child Under the Age of 18 Years, 2002 (taking into account weighting and complex survey design)

	Women (n = 1,301)		Men (n = 942)		Overall (n = 2,243)	
	Prevalence Rate (%)	P-value	Prevalence Rate (%)	P-value	Prevalence Rate (%)	P-value
Race/Ethnicity						
Non-Hispanic white	25.4	0.007	14.2	0.08	19.6	< 0.0001
African American	14.2		9.3		12.0	
Black immigrants from the Caribbean[b]	28.0		35.9		29.7	
Mexican	11.9		7.8		10.3	
Other Hispanic	18.5		8.2		14.6	
Asian	19.7		1.8		8.8	
Other	27.5		17.6		23.3	
Born in United States						
Yes	22.4	0.009	13.2	0.03	17.9	0.0008
No	15.5		5.9		11.2	
Primary Language While Growing Up						
Not English	14.4	0.0004	8.3	0.04	11.8	< 0.0001
English	23.6		13.5		18.6	
Number of Parents Born Outside United States						
0	17.3	0.30	6.8	0.09	13.0	0.15
1	20.1		17.6		19.0	
2	22.6		12.9		17.8	
Current Work Status						
Employed	23.5	0.14	11.6	0.008	17.0	0.53
Unemployed, in workforce	17.9		11.1		17.3	
Not in workforce	18.5		20.8		19.2	

Poverty Status (categorized income-to-needs ratio using NICHD cutoff)						
Low income (ratio < 2)	22.1	0.12	15.1	0.25	17.5	0.55
Middle income (ratio of 2 to < 4.43)	17.5		11.6		16.3	
Gender						
Male	NA	NA	NA	NA	12.6	< 0.0001
Female	NA	NA	NA	NA	21.7	
Marital Status						
Married/cohabiting	19.8	0.0008	11.0	0.05	15.3	0.0004
Divorced/widowed/separated	31.5		19.1		25.8	
Never married	18.1		15.0		17.2	
Education						
0–11 years	14.7	0.10	16.0	0.44	15.3	0.48
12 years	23.7		13.5		18.7	
13–15 years	23.1		11.7		17.9	
16 years or more	21.9		10.4		16.1	

NOTES: NA = not applicable; NICHD = National Institute of Child Health and Human Development.

TABLE 1-3 12-Month Prevalence of Major Depression with Hierarchy[a] by Selected Demographic Characteristics for Adults with at Least One Child Under the Age of 18 Years, 2002 (taking into account weighting and complex survey design)

	Women (n = 1,301)		Men (n = 942)		Overall (n = 2,243)	
	Prevalence Rate (%)	P-value	Prevalence Rate (%)	P-value	Prevalence Rate (5)	P-value
Race/Ethnicity						
Non-Hispanic white	11.5	NA	4.7	NA	8.0	0.09
African American	7.0		3.3		5.4	
Black immigrants from the Caribbean[b]	0		35.9		7.7	
Mexican	5.3		3.8		4.7	
Other Hispanic	9.3		2.5		6.8	
Asian	9.9		0		3.9	
Other	14.7		7.0		11.4	
Born in United States						
Yes	10.3	0.04	4.5	0.36	7.5	0.08
No	6.7		2.2		4.7	
Primary Language While Growing Up						
Not English	7.3	0.09	3.9	0.76	5.9	0.17
English	10.7		4.4		7.6	
Number of Parents Born Outside United States						
0	7.4	0.41	3.3	0.61	5.7	0.47
1	9.7		6.2		8.1	
2	10.3		4.3		7.4	
Current Work Status						
Employed	9.3	0.28	3.1	<0.0001	5.9	<0.0001
Unemployed, in workforce	10.4		6.3		10.1	
Not in workforce	12.2		15.0		13.0	

Poverty Status (categorized income-to-needs ratio using NICHD cutoff)						
Low income (ratio < 2)	10.9	0.89	5.1	0.91	9.2	0.47
Middle income (ratio of 2 to < 4.43)	10.5		5.3		7.9	
Gender						
Male	NA	NA	NA	NA	4.3	< 0.0001
Female	NA		NA		10.0	
Marital Status						
Married/cohabiting	8.3	0.003	3.5	0.13	5.8	0.0008
Divorced/widowed/separated	16.6		7.0		12.2	
Never married	9.4		7.3		8.7	
Education						
0–11 years	10.8	0.76	7.3	0.24	9.1	0.16
12 years	10.3		4.6		7.5	
13–15 years	10.4		3.7		7.3	
16 years or more	8.4		2.8		5.5	

NOTES: NA = not applicable; NICHD = National Institute of Child Health and Human Development.

[a] "With hierarchy" refers to a diagnostic criterion in the Diagnostic and Statistical Manual of Mental Disorders, 4th edition that specifices that if a disorder is better explained by another mental disorder, that "other" disorder is given hierarchy over the disorder of interest, i.e., a more narrow definition of major depression disorder that does not include mania and hypomania.

status of immigrant populations has been found to deteriorate with the time of tenure in the United States (Grant et al., 2004; Vega et al., 1998).

The scientific literature classifies many of these groups as "vulnerable populations." The notion of vulnerability is based on the epidemiological concept of risk, which is used to quantify the probability that an individual will become ill or suffer adversity in a given period of time. According to this definition, vulnerable populations are comprised of individuals who have a higher probability of experiencing poor physical, psychological, or social health than others at any point in time due to shared sociodemographic or environmental circumstances (Aday, 1994). Social vulnerability affects health in general and depression specifically via several pathways. For example, such factors as limited access to knowledge and resources as well as increased exposure to such social stressors as marginal neighborhoods, community violence, and discrimination directly affect the genesis, progression, and treatment of depression. In addition, the stigma associated with belonging to a disadvantaged group may increase individuals' isolation, thus causing or exacerbating depressive symptoms, and it may affect their treatment-seeking behaviors. More generally, the stigma of having a diagnosis of depression among certain disadvantaged and cultural groups may impede depression-related research endeavors (U.S. Surgeon General, 1999).

The concept of vulnerability has important research and policy implications for two main reasons. First, risks may accumulate additively or multiplicatively, depending on the number of high-risk groups to which an individual or family belongs. Second, compared with their normative counterparts, vulnerable populations may require additional medical and social services to meet their multiple, coinciding physical and mental health needs, as well as their children's developmental needs.

Bearing in mind such vulnerability-related considerations is of particular importance in the context of depression because it is precisely those social environments and characteristics in which depression most commonly occurs—such as poverty, marital status, or disadvantage due to gender, race and ethnicity—that are themselves factors likely to exacerbate or prolong depression. Because of their typically stressful and enduring nature, these conditions may create a constellation of vulnerabilities that overwhelm the person's coping capabilities and diminish the effectiveness of treatments that have proven successful under less challenging circumstances. Moreover, given the disproportionate incidence of depression among women, particularly those who are poor and single, as well as those who are young and in their prime childbearing and child rearing years, depression poses a concern because of its potential for impairing parenting.

The data from the NCS-R specific to parents reveal similar prevalence rates of depression compared with adults in general, including disparities in gender, race/ethnicity, and marital status, and employment status for fathers. Other demographic disparities that are generally considered a contributor to depression, i.e., income level, was not seen to *significantly* contribute to depression in parents in this particular subsample of one study (although a difference is still seen). More longitudinal and cross-sectional data are needed to further document and clarify the prevalence, incidence, disparities, causes, and consequences of depression in adults who are parents.

Comorbidities and Correlates of Depression

According to the National Comorbidity Survey, approximately 75 percent of individuals who had lifetime or recent depression also had at least one additional mental health or substance abuse diagnosis (Kessler et al., 2005), as did 60–65 percent of those with current major depression, as reported in both U.S. and international studies (e.g., De Graaf et al., 2002; Rush et al., 2005). Often the depression occurs in part because of difficulties caused by the other disorders, principally substance abuse, anxiety disorders, and conduct and antisocial disorders. In addition, depression is often comorbid with other chronic medical conditions, such as diabetes, hypertension, and arthritis, and can worsen their associated health outcomes (Ciechanowski, Katon, and Russo, 2000; Katon, 1998, 2003; Moussavi et al., 2007). Individuals who are depressed are more likely to amplify physical symptoms and to develop catastrophic ideas about the causes and consequences of their symptoms (Barsky, 1979; Edwards et al., 2006). The social and physical functioning of depressed individuals often is poor, and they are hospitalized more frequently than people with other major chronic medical problems. Such comorbid conditions may greatly complicate the severity, duration, and recurrence of depression and diminish the effectiveness of treatments for it. The reverse is also true: depression may impede individuals' efforts to find effective treatments or coping strategies for dealing with their co-occurring disorders.

IMPACT OF DEPRESSION

Adding to the problem that depression rarely occurs alone, a further complication is the recurrent nature of depression as well as its impact on individuals, their families, and society. Although depressed mood or sadness are normal human experiences associated with loss of treasured relationships, disappointments, and failures, most people who experience such states recover quickly within hours or a few days. However, clinically significant depression not only persists but also has detrimental effects on intellectual processes and attitudes about the self, the world, and the future; impedes adaptive behaviors and family and social interactions; erodes energy; and disrupts bodily processes—in addition to its effect on mood and emotions.

Individual

The National Institute of Mental Health Collaborative Health Program on the Psychobiology of Depression found that, over a 5-year period, depressed persons had lower educational achievement, lower income levels, fewer periods of employment, and decreased occupational status than nondepressed persons matched for age and gender (Coryell, Endicott, and Keller, 1990). The multisite WHO study on the effects of depression on social functioning found that, after 10 years, 25 percent of depressed patients showed poor functioning and about 40 percent exhibited moderate impairment (Thornicroft and Sartorius, 1993). Even with appropriate treatment, depression has the tendency to be episodic and recurrent; that is, after a person has been depressed once and recovers, he or she is likely to experience one or more subsequent episodes; single episodes of depression are the exception (Andrews, 2001; Solomon et al., 2000). This recurrent pattern of illness leads to sustained individual, family, and societal costs.

Consequently, individuals with depression often cannot function in optimal ways in their close relationships or in work, social, and leisure activities. Thus, depression is associated with decrements in work attendance, work quality, and productivity (Kessler et al., 2006; Wang et al., 2004); with unresponsive, harsh, or rejecting parenting (Cummings and Davies, 1999; Goodman and Gotlib, 1999); with dissatisfaction or conflict in close relationships (Kessler, Walters, and Forthofer, 1998; Whisman, 2001); and with medical problems due both to poor self-care and to the effects of depression on neurobiological and immune functioning (Evans et al., 2005; Katon, 2003). Even depression that is considered "subclinical" in severity may, if sufficiently enduring, predict impaired functioning in important roles or disproportionate use of services (Johnson, Weissman, and Klerman, 1992; Wells et al., 1989).

Family and Society

Addressing the charge to the committee, this report describes a large number of traditional clinical and epidemiological approaches documenting the negative impact of depression in parents on parenting and children's health and development. Using the prevalence data presented above, the number of children under the age of 18 in each household from the NCS-R (i.e., 2.07172), and applying it to U.S. Census data from 2001, the committee estimates that 15.6 million children under 18 years of age are living with an adult who had major depression in the past year (note: the NCS-R public use data does not provide data on depression diagnosis on both parents in a household, so this may be an underestimate of the number of these children). Yet few opportunities currently exist to identify this vulnerable population or to offer prevention and treatment services that can also enhance the parenting practices of a depressed parent in a framework that also offers services for children.

But the focus of the current research literature primarily on symptoms and diagnosis of depression in an adult does not do justice to the larger possible impacts on family development. It is essential to consider both in terms of either difficulties or opportunities for prevention, not just the individuals in the family but the family as a whole. A much broader definition of effects on the family is needed, which the committee introduces here in this report.

This conceptualization considers broadly the environment, economic resources, and relationships with family, coworkers, the community, and society (see Figure 1-1[3]). The community environment may either contribute to the impacts of parental depression in a family or help to mitigate them. Costs to families are much greater than individual economic costs for the depressed person. The burden of suffering is large for the depressed individual and frequently for other family members as well. The community environment is also likely to directly influence child outcomes. And a family's current characteristics and financial resources are likely to affect the economic impact of a depressive episode on the family. Once depressed, parents have an effect on their own potential human capital (i.e., decreased employment, earnings, productivity), social capital (i.e., skills, abilities, knowledge, relationships), and their decisions on allocating their resources (i.e., time, money). These characteristics and decisions affect the well-being of family members in both the short term and the long term. They can include the maintenance and development of their children's physical and mental health (e.g., they cannot take them to the doctor for well-child visits), their development of human capital (e.g., their child dropping out of school, achieving poorer academic performance), and their development of social capital (e.g., their child's impairment in marital and work relationships). Taking a developmental approach that addresses long-term possible negative consequences of parental depression emphasizes both the magnitude of the costs and the need for action.

A parent is central to the family's functioning. His or her impairments can have dramatic effects on their children and the family. These patterns of impairment in depressed parents and the risks to their families offer natural targets for preventive and treatment interventions at various levels, includ-

---

[3]This concept was developed for the committee through commissioned work by Frances Lynch, Ph.D.

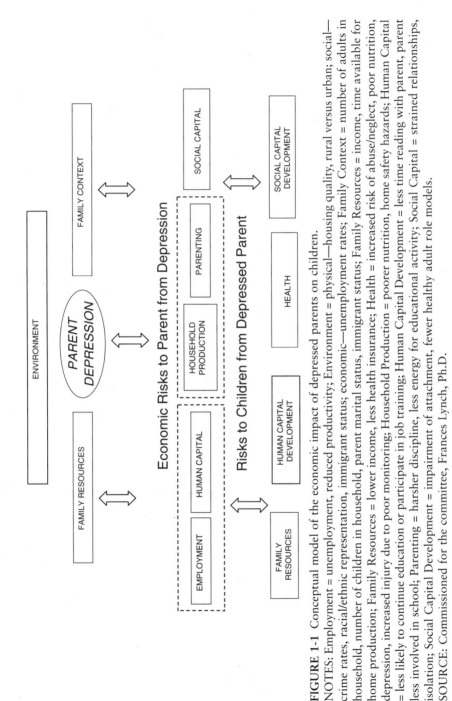

FIGURE 1-1 Conceptual model of the economic impact of depressed parents on children.
NOTES: Employment = unemployment, reduced productivity; Environment = physical—housing quality, rural versus urban; social—crime rates, racial/ethnic representation, immigrant status; economic—unemployment rates; Family Context = number of adults in household, number of children in household, parent marital status, immigrant status; Family Resources = income, time available for home production; Family Resources = lower income, less health insurance; Health = increased risk of abuse/neglect, poor nutrition, depression, increased injury due to poor monitoring; Household Production = poorer nutrition, home safety hazards; Human Capital = less likely to continue education or participate in job training; Human Capital Development = less time reading with parent, parent less involved in school; Parenting = harsher discipline, less energy for educational activity; Social Capital = strained relationships, isolation; Social Capital Development = impairment of attachment, fewer healthy adult role models.
SOURCE: Commissioned for the committee, Frances Lynch, Ph.D.

ing, for example, making sure that families with depression have health insurance or recognizing that, with depression, parents will need additional support to get tasks done.

BARRIERS TO CARE

Like a variety of other health services, access to care for depression may be influenced by geographic, physical, financial, sociocultural, and temporal barriers. Such barriers include transportation issues, physical disabilities, language barriers, cultural customs and beliefs, and health insurance coverage. Furthermore, an individual's ability to access and use care may be affected by demographic characteristics (i.e., age, gender, education level, occupation, race/ethnicity), need (i.e., perceived health) and enabling characteristics (i.e., language, income, convenience, transportation, health system characteristics like infrastructure, linkages to a variety of providers). Stigma is a major barrier to seeking mental health treatment. Both self-stigma (people's own responses to depression and help-seeking) and perceived stigma (perceptions of others' negative responses) partially account for people's reluctance to seek treatment (Barney et al., 2006; Halter, 2004). Many people are not familiar with treatment options, there is stigma associated with mental health treatments, and many providers are not aware of their patients' preferences (Dwight-Johnson et al., 2000; Givens et al., 2007; Jaycox et al., 2006).

A number of institutional and sociocultural barriers are responsible for causing and maintaining existing disparities in access to and quality of mental health services received by minority groups. A succinct summary of the complex constellation of barriers is that "disparities result from ongoing interactions among factors at the levels of the health care environment, health care organization, community, provider, and person throughout the course of the depression development and treatment-seeking process" (Chin et al., 2007; Van Voorhees et al., 2007, p. 1617). Social marginalization, which has played a key role in rendering some populations disproportionately vulnerable to and affected by incidence of depression, extends its adverse impact by limiting the engagement of and treatment in historically underserved communities (Aguilar-Gaxiola et al., 2008). These groups' isolation from mainstream society because of linguistic barriers, geographic isolation, a history of oppression, racism, discrimination, poverty, and immigration status plays a key role in creating and perpetuating many of the barriers to treatment.

In addition to individual and provider barriers to care specific to depression in adults, a body of literature continues to document the system-level limitations in mental health care generally. As described in a 2006 Institute of Medicine report entitled *Improving the Quality of Health Care for Mental and Substance-Use Conditions*, the "inadequacy of [mental health and substance use] health care is a dimension of the poor quality of all health care" (Institute of Medicine, 2006, p. 8). However, it also points out that care for mental health and substance use problems is also distinct from health care generally. The distinctive features they describe include greater stigma associated with diagnoses, a less developed infrastructure for measuring and improving the quality of care, a need for a greater number of linkages among multiple clinicians, organizations and systems providing care to patients with mental health conditions, less widespread use of information technology, a more educationally diverse workforce, and a differently structured marketplace for the purchase of mental health and substance use health care (Institute of Medicine, 2006). With this in mind, the report recommended using the strategy set forth by another Institute of Medicine report (2001), *Crossing the Quality Chasm*, as a basic framework to achieve substantial improvements in quality of care, but to tailor it to the distinctive features of mental health and substance use care.

Depression presents a fundamental paradox: it is one of the most prevalent of psychiatric conditions but also one that is highly amenable to treatment, at least in the acute phase. The U.S. Surgeon General, the National Institutes of Health, the Substance Abuse and Mental Health Services Administration, and many others continue to document advances in the understanding of depression, the identification and assessment of depressed individuals, and the development of efficacious treatments, as well as strategies for delivering these interventions effectively. Yet despite recent scientific advances, in 2007, only 64 percent of adults in the United States who had a major depressive episode in the past year received some form of treatment (Office of Applied Studies, 2008). Only approximately 30 percent of depressed adults in community samples reportedly will receive any treatment (Simon et al., 2004). Further, depression in adults is typically discussed as an isolated problem. The focus is rarely on how depression affects parenting and child outcomes; how often it occurs in combination with other parental risks, like substance abuse and trauma; or what kinds of strategies can help to identify, treat, and prevent these negative consequences for parents and their children (Knitzer, Theberge, and Johnson, 2008). The current policy environment does not encourage an identification and treatment strategy with this kind of two-generation developmental lens, nor does it support the dissemination or implementation of the growing body of knowledge about effective interventions.

CONCLUSION

National surveys exist that describe the rates of depression in adults and indicate disparities as defined by selected population characteristics.

A subsample of one such survey specifically identified the parental status of these adults. Parents (with at least one child under age 18) have similar rates of depression compared to the entire U.S. adult population, including similar disparities in depression rates for selected population characteristics such as sex, age, and marital status. In general, social disadvantage has been positively associated with higher prevalence rates of depression in adults except in the case of newly arrived immigrants. Further, a majority of individuals with major depression also had at least one additional mental health or substance abuse diagnosis. Thus, comorbidity between mental disorders tends to be the norm rather than the exception.

Depression, due to its recurrent nature, leads to sustained individual, family, and societal costs. Furthermore, depression in parents or other caregivers can have serious biological, psychological, behavioral, and social consequences especially for children. More longitudinal and cross-sectional data are needed to further document and clarify the prevalence, incidence, disparities, causes, and consequences of depression in adults who are parents. Individual-, provider-, and system-level barriers exist that decrease the access to and quality of care for depressed adults. These institutional and sociocultural barriers are responsible for causing and maintaining existing disparities. Without a system of care that supports a family's environment, economic resources and relationships with family, coworkers, the community, and society, such disparities may increase.

Ultimately depression is a good and effectively identified indicator of a problem that could trigger a system of care (if it is in place) that intervenes not only by treating depression in the parent but also by enhancing parenting skills and alleviating other stresses, co-occurring conditions, and social contexts, as well as identifying children at risk.

ORGANIZATION OF THE REPORT

Following this introduction, Chapter 2 describes new approaches to tackling parental depression as well as issues and standards in evaluating this literature. Chapter 3 reviews the causes of depression, and Chapter 4 reviews the effects of depression on parenting and child health and psychological functioning. Chapter 5 reviews strategies to identify and assess depression, and Chapter 6 reviews strategies for the treatment of depression in parents and their families. Chapter 7 reviews strategies for preventing depression in parents, with a special emphasis on the prevention or reduction of adverse outcomes in children of parents who are depressed. Chapter 8 describes an ideal vision of a depression care intervention system, highlighting important components of this system that are emerging in selected service settings as well as through state and European initiatives, and reviewing federal-level initiatives that have supported this knowledge base. Chapter 9 describes systemic, workforce, and fiscal policy challenges that have emerged from current initiatives associated with implementing innovative evidence-based strategies in addressing depression in parents and its impact on children. Chapter 10 describes next steps that can be taken to help contribute to the design and implementation of the ideal prevention and depression system for parental depression, which includes knowledge development and the creation of an organizational culture receptive to new research. To aid the reader, the committee's summary of the literature is presented at the beginning of the chapter and the conclusions, research gaps, and committee's recommendations are presented at the end of each chapter, where appropriate. Finally, the role of culture, language, and social determinants of health were identified across the chapters when literature was available when describing vulnerable populations who experience mental health disparities. A list of acronyms is provided in Appendix A. The agenda and participants of the committee's public workshop are listed in Appendix B, and biographical sketches of the committee members and staff are provided in Appendix C.

REFERENCES

Aday, L.A. (1994). Health status of vulnerable populations. *Annual Review of Public Health* 15, 487–509.

Aguilar-Gaxiola, S., Elliott, K., Debb-Sossa, N., King, R.T., Magaña, C.G., Miller, E., Sala, M., Sribney, W.M., and Breslau, J. (2008). *Engaging the Underserved: Personal Accounts of Communities on Mental Health Needs for Prevention and Early Intervention Strategies.* Monograph #1, UC Davis Center for Reducing Health Disparities. Sacramento: UC Davis.

Andrade, L., Caraveo-Anduaga, J.J., Berglund, P., Bijl, R.V., De Graaf, R., Vollebergh, W., Dragomirecka, E., Kohn, R., Keller, M., Kessler, R.C., Kawakami, N., Kilic, C., Offord, D., Ustun, T.B., and Wittchen, H.U. (2003). The epidemiology of major depressive episodes: Results from the International Consortium of Psychiatric Epidemiology (ICPE) Surveys. *International Journal of Methods in Psychiatric Research*, 12, 3–21.

Andrews, G. (2001). Should depression be managed as a chronic disease? *British Medical Journal*, 322, 419–421.

Barney, L.J., Griffiths, K.M., Jorm, A.F., and Christensen, H. (2006). Stigma about depression and its impact on help-seeking intentions. *Australian and New Zealand Journal of Psychiatry*, 40, 51–54.

Barsky, A.J. (1979). Patients who amplify bodily sensations. *Annals of Internal Medicine*, 91, 63–70.

Bassuk, E.L., Buckner, J.C., Perloff, J.N., and Bassuk, S.S. (1998). Prevalence of mental health and substance use disorders among homeless and low-income housed mothers. *American Journal of Psychiatry*, 155, 1561–1564.

Bengtson, V.L., Acock, A.C., Allen, K.R., Dilworth-Anderson, P., and Klein, D.M. (2005). *Sourcebook of Family Theory and Research.* Thousand Oaks, CA: Sage.

Bloom, B., Owen, B., Covington, S., and Raeder, M. (2003). *Gender-Responsive Strategies: Research, Practice, and Guiding Principles for Women Offenders.* Washington, DC: National Institute of Corrections, U.S. Department of Justice.

Brandon, P.D., and Bumpass, L. (2001). Children's living arrangement, coresidence of unmarried fathers, and welfare receipt. *Journal of Family Issues, 22*, 3–26.

Casper, L.M., and Bryson, K.R. (1998). *CoResident Grandparents and Their Grandchildren: Grandparent Maintained Families.* (Current Population Report). Washington, DC: U.S. Bureau of the Census.

Centers for Disease Control and Prevention. (2008). Prevalence of self-reported postpartum depressive symptoms—17 states, 2004–2005. *Morbidity and Mortality Weekly Report, 57*, 361–366.

Chin, M.H., Walters, A.E., Cook, S.C., and Huang, E.S. (2007). Interventions to reduce racial and ethnic disparities in health care. *Medical Care Research and Review, 64*, 7S–28S.

Ciechanowski, P.S., Katon, W.J., and Russo, J.E. (2000). Depression and diabetes: Impact of depressive symptoms on adherence, function, and costs. *Archives of Internal Medicine, 160*, 3278–3285.

Coryell, W., Endicott, J., and Keller, M.B. (1990). Outcome of patients with chronic affective disorder: A five-year follow-up. *American Journal of Psychiatry, 147*, 1627–1633.

Cross-National Collaborative Group. (1992). The changing rate of major depression: Cross-national comparisons. *Journal of the American Medical Association, 268*, 3098–3105.

Cummings, E.M., and Davies, P.T. (1999). Depressed parents and family functioning: Interpersonal effects and children's functioning and development. In T.E. Joiner and J.C. Coyne (Eds.), *The Interactional Nature of Depression: Advances in Interpersonal Approaches* (pp. 299–327). Washington, DC: American Psychological Association.

De Graaf, R., Bijl, R.V., Smith, F., Vollebergh, W.A.M., and Spijker, J. (2002). Risk factors for 12-month comorbidity of mood, anxiety, and substance use disorders: Findings from the Netherlands Mental Health Survey and Incidence Study. *American Journal of Psychiatry, 159*, 620–629.

Depue, R.A., and Monroe, S.M. (1986). Conceptualization and measurement of human disorder and life stress research: The problem of chronic disturbance. *Psychological Bulletin, 99*, 36–51.

DiMatteo, M.R., Lepper, H.S., and Croghan, T.W. (2000). Depression is a risk factor for noncompliance with medical treatment. *Archives of Internal Medicine, 160*, 2101–2107.

Dwight-Johnson, M., Sherbourne, C.D., Liao, D., and Wells, K.B. (2000). Treatment preferences among depressed primary care patients. *Journal of General Internal Medicine, 15*, 527–534.

Edwards, R.R., Bingham, C.O. 3rd, Bathon, J., and Haythornewaite, J.A. (2006). Catastrophizing and pain in arthritis, fibromyalgia, and other rheumatic diseases. *Arthritis and Rheumatism, 55*, 325–332.

The ESEMeD/MHEDEA 2000 Investigators. (2004). Prevalence of mental disorders in Europe: Results from the European Study of the Epidemiology of Mental Disorders (ESEMeD) project. *Acta Psychiatrica Scandinavica, 109*, 21–27.

Evans, D.L., Charney, D.S., Lewis, L., Golden, R.N., Gorman, J.M., Krishnan, K.R.R., Nemeroff, C.B., Bremner, J.D., Carney, R.M., Coyne, J.C., Delong, M.R., Frasure-Smith, N., Glassman, A.H., Gold, P.W., Grant, I., Gwyther, L., Ironson, G., Johnson, R.L., Kanner, A.M., Katon, W.J., Kaufmann, P.G., Keefe, F.J., Ketter, T., Laughren, T.P., Leserman, J., Lyketsos, C.G., McDonald, W.M., McEwen, B.S., Miller, A.H., Mussleman, D., O'Connor, C., Petitto, J.M., Pollock, B.G., Robinson, R.G., Roose, S.P., Rowland, J., Sheline, Y., Sheps, D.S., Simon, G., Spiegel, D., Stunkard, A., Sunderland, T., Tibbits, P., Jr., and Valvo, W.J. (2005). Mood disorders in the medically ill: Scientific review and recommendations. *Biological Psychiatry, 58*, 175–189.

Federal Interagency Forum on Child and Family Statistics. (2007). *America's Children: Key National Indicators of Well-Being, 2007.* Washington, DC: U.S. Government Printing Office.

Frank, R.G., and Glied, S. (2006). The population with mental illness. In R.G. Frank., S. Glied, and R. Carter (Eds.), *Better But Not Well: Mental Health Policy in the United States Since 1950* (pp. 8–25). Baltimore, MD: Johns Hopkins University Press.

Givens, J.L., Katz, I.R., Bellamy, S., and Holmes, W.C. (2007). Stigma and the acceptability of depression treatments among African Americans and whites. *Journal of General Medicine, 22,* 1292–1297.

Goodman, S., and Gotlib, I. (1999). Risk for psychopathology in the children of depressed mothers: A developmental model for understanding mechanisms of transmission. *Psychological Review, 106,* 458–490.

Grant, B.F., Stinson, F.S., Hasin, D.S., Dawson, D.A., Chou, S.P., and Anderson, K. (2004). Immigration and lifetime prevalence of DSM-IV psychiatric disorders among Mexican Americans and non-Hispanic whites in the United States. *Archives of General Psychiatry, 61,* 1226–1233.

Greenberg, P.E., Kessler, R.C., Birnbaum, H.C., Leong, S.A., Lowe, S.W., Berglund, P.A., and Corey-Lisle, P.K. (2003). The economic burden of depression in the United States: How did it change between 1990 and 2000? *Journal of Clinical Psychiatry, 64,* 1465–1475.

Halter, M.J. (2004). The stigma of seeking care and depression. *Archives of Psychiatric Nursing, 18,* 178–184.

Institute of Medicine. (2001). *Crossing the Quality Chasm: A New Health System for the 21st Century.* Washington, DC: National Academy Press.

Institute of Medicine. (2006). *Improving the Quality of Health Care for Mental and Substance-Use Conditions.* Washington, DC: The National Academies Press.

Jackson, P.B., and Williams, D.R. (2006). Culture, race/ethnicity, and depression. In C.L.M. Keyes and S.H. Goodman (Eds.), *Women and Depression: A Handbook for the Social, Behavioral, and Biomedical Sciences* (pp. 328–359). New York: Cambridge University Press.

Jaycox, L.H., Asarnow, J.R., Sherbourne, C.D. Rea, M.M., LaBorde, A.P., and Wells, K.B. (2006). Adolescent primary care patients' preferences for depression treatment. *Administration and Policy in Mental Health, 33,* 198–207.

Jesse, D.E., Walcott-McQuigg, J., Mariella, A., and Swanson, M.S. (2005). Risks and protective factors associated with symptoms of depression in low-income African American and Caucasian women during pregnancy. *Journal of Midwifery and Women's Health, 50,* 405–410.

Johnson, J., Weissman, M.M., and Klerman, G. (1992). Service utilization and social morbidity associated with depressive symptoms in the community. *Journal of the American Medical Association, 267,* 1478–1483.

Judd, L.L., Akiskal, H.S., Maser, J.D., Zeller, P.J., Endicott, J., Coryell, W., Paulus, M.P., Kunovac, J.L., Leon, A.C., Mueller, T.I., Rice, J.A., and Keller, M.B. (1998). A prospective 12-year study of subsyndromal and syndromal depressive symptoms in unipolar major depressive disorders. *Archives of General Psychiatry, 55,* 694–700.

Katon, W. (1998). The effect of major depression on chronic medical illness. *Seminars in Clinical Neuropsychiatry, 3,* 82–86.

Katon, W.J. (2003). Clinical and health services relationships between major depression, depressive symptoms, and general medical illness. *Biological Psychiatry, 54,* 216–226.

Kessler, R.C. (2003). Epidemiology of women and depression. *Journal of Affective Disorders, 74,* 5–13.

Kessler, R.C., Akiskal, H.S., Ames, M., Birnbaum, H., Greenberg, P., Hirschfeld, R.M.A., Jin, R., Merikangas, K.R., Simon, G.E., and Wang, P.S. (2006). Prevalence and effects of mood disorders on work performance in a nationally representative sample of U.S. workers. *American Journal of Psychiatry, 163*(9), 1561–1568.

Kessler, R.C., Berglund, P., Demler, O., Jin, R., Koretz, D., Merikangas, K.R., Rush, A.J., Walters, E.E., and Wang, P.S. (2003). The epidemiology of major depressive disorder: Results from the National Comorbidity Survey Replication (NCS-R). *Journal of the American Medical Association, 289*, 3095–3105.

Kessler, R.C., Berglund, P., Demler, O., Jin, R., Merikangas, K.R., and Walters, E.E. (2005). Lifetime prevalence and age-of-onset distributions of DSM-IV disorders in the National Comorbidity Survey Replication. *Archives of General Psychiatry, 62*, 593–602.

Kessler, R.C., Walters, E.E., and Forthofer, M.S. (1998). The social consequences of psychiatric disorders, III: Probability of marital stability. *American Journal of Psychiatry, 155*, 1092–1096.

Knitzer, J., Theberge, S., and Johnson, K. (2008). *Reducing Maternal Depression and Its Impact on Young Children: Toward a Responsive Early Childhood Policy Framework.* New York: National Center for Children in Poverty.

Lanzi, R.G., Pascoe J.M., Keltner B., and Ramey, S.L. (1999). Correlates of maternal depressive symptoms in a National Head Start Program sample. *Archives of Pediatrics and Adolescent Medicine, 153*(8), 801–807.

Lorant, V., Croux, C., Weich, S., Deliege, D., Mackenbach, J., and Ansseau, M. (2007). Depression and socioeconomic risk factors: 7-year longitudinal population study. *British Journal of Psychiatry, 190*, 293–298.

Lorant, V., Deliege, D., Eaton, W., Robert, A., Philippot, P., and Ansseau, M. (2003). Socioeconomic inequalities in depression: A meta-analysis. *American Journal of Epidemiology, 157*, 98–112.

Luppa, M., Heinrich, S., Angermeyer, M.C., König, H.H., and Riedel-Heller, S.G. (2007). Cost-of-illness studies of depression: A systematic review. *Journal of Affective Disorders, 98*, 29–43.

Miranda, J., Siddique, J., Belin, T.R., and Kohn, L.P. (2005). Depression prevalence in disadvantaged young black women. African and Caribbean immigrants compared to U.S.-born African Americans. *Social Psychiatry and Psychiatric Epidemiology, 40*, 253–258.

Moussavi, S., Chatterji, S., Verdes, E., Tandon, A., Patel, V., and Ustun, B. (2007). Depression, chronic diseases, and decrements in health: Results from the World Health Surveys. *The Lancet, 370*, 851–858.

Muñoz, S.S. (2003). Cost to treat a depression case falls. *The Wall Street Journal*, December 31, p. D2.

Murray, C.J., and Lopez, A.D. (1996). *The Global Burden of Disease.* Cambridge. MA: Harvard University Press.

Office of Applied Studies. (2008). *Results from the 2007 National Survey on Drug Use and Health: National Findings.* (DHHS Pub No. SMA 08-4343). Rockville, MD: Substance Abuse and Mental Health Services Administration.

Ramchandani, P.G., Stein, A., O'Connor, T.G., Heron, J., Murray, L., and Evans, J. (2008). Depression in men in the postnatal period and later child psychopathology: A population cohort study. *Journal of the American Academy of Child and Adolescent Psychiatry, 47*, 390–398.

Riolo, S.A., Nguyen, T.A., Greden, J.F., and King, C.A. (2005). Prevalence of depression by race/ethnicity: Findings from the National Health and Nutrition Examination Survey III. *American Journal of Public Health, 95*, 998–1000.

Rush, A.J., Zimmerman, M., Wisniewski, S.R., Fava, M., Hollon, S.D., Warden, D., Biggs, M.M., Shores-Wilson, K., Shelton, R.C., Luther, J.F., Thomas, B., and Trivedi, M.H. (2005). Comorbid psychiatric disorders in depressed outpatients: Demographic and clinical features. *Journal of Affective Disorders, 87*, 43–55.

Siefert, K., Bowman, P.J., Heflin, C.M., Danzger, S., and Williams, D.R. (2000). Social and environmental predictors of maternal depression in current and recent welfare recipients. *American Journal of Orthopsychiatry, 70*, 510–522.

Simon, G.E., Fleck, M., Lucas, R., Bushnell, D.M., and the LIDO Group. (2004). Prevalence and predictors of depression treatment in an international primary care study. *American Journal of Psychiatry*, 161, 1626–1634.

Solomon, D.A., Keller, M.B., Leon, A.C., Mueller, T.I., Lavori, P.W., Shea, M.T., Coryell, W., Warshaw, M., Turvey, C., Maser, J.D., and Endicott, J. (2000). Multiple recurrences of major depressive disorder. *American Journal of Psychiatry*, 157, 229–233.

Takeuchi, D.T., Zane, N., Hong, S., Chae, D.H., Gong, F., Gee, G.C., Walton, E., Sue, S., and Alegria, M. (2007). Immigration-related factors and mental disorders among Asian Americans. *American Journal of Public Health*, 97, 84–90.

Thornicroft, G., and Sartorius, N. (1993). The course and outcome of depression in different cultures: 10-year follow-up of the WHO Collaborative Study on the Assessment of Depressive Disorders. *Psychological Medicine*, 23, 1023–1032.

U.S. Census Bureau. (2005a). *Facts for Features. Father's Day: June 19, 2005*. Available: http://www.census.gov/Press-Release/www/releases/archives/cb05ff-08.pdf [accessed February 4, 2009].

U.S. Census Bureau. (2005b). *Facts for Features. Mother's Day: May 8, 2005*. Available: http://www.census.gov/Press-Release/www/releases/archives/cb05-ff.05-2.pdf [accessed February 4, 2009].

U.S. Census Bureau. (2008a). *C2. Household Relationship and Living Arrangements of Children/1 Under 18 Years, by Age and Sex: 2007*. Available: http://www.census.gov/population/socdemo/hh-fam/cps2007/tabC2-all.xls [accessed October 29, 2008].

U.S. Census Bureau. (2008b). *Table F1. Family Households/1, by Type, Age of Own Children, Age of Family Members, and Age, Race and Hispanic Origin/2 of Householder: 2007*. Available: http://www.census.gov/population/socdemo/hh-fam/cps2007/tabF1-all.xls [accessed October 29, 2008].

U.S. Surgeon General. (1999). *Mental Health: A Report of the Surgeon General*. Washington, DC: U.S. Department of Health and Human Services.

Van Voorhees, B.W., Walters, A.E., Prochaska, M., and Quinn, M.T. (2007). Reducing health disparities in depressive disorders outcomes between non-Hispanic whites and ethnic minorities: A call for pragmatic strategies over the life course. *Medical Care Research Review*, 64, 157s–194s.

Vega, W.A., Kolody, B., Aguilar-Gaxiola, S., Alderete, E., Catalano, R., and Caraveo-Anduaga, J. (1998). Lifetime prevalence of DSM-III-R psychiatric disorders among urban and rural Mexican Americans in California. *Archives of General Psychiatry*, 55, 771–778.

Wang, P.S., Beck, A.L., Berglund, P., McKenas, D.K., Pronk, N.P., Simon, G.E., and Kessler, R.C. (2004). Effects of major depression on moment-in-time work performance. *American Journal of Psychiatry*, 161, 1885–1891.

Wells, K.B., Stewart, A., Hays, R.D., Burnam, A., Rogers, W., Daniels, M., Berry, S., Greenfield, S., and Ware, J. (1989). The functioning and well-being of depressed patients. *Journal of the American Medical Association*, 262, 914–919.

Whisman, M.A. (2001). The association between depression and marital dissatisfaction. In S.R.H. Beach (Ed.), *Marital and Family Processes in Depression: A Scientific Foundation for Clinical Practice*. Washington, DC: American Psychological Association.

Williams, D.R., Gonzalez, H.M., Neighbors, H., Nesse, R., Abelson, J.M., Sweetman, J., and Jackson, J.S. (2007). Prevalence and distribution of major depressive disorder in African Americans, Caribbean blacks, and non-Hispanic whites: Results from the National Survey of American Life. *Archives of General Psychiatry*, 64, 305–315.

World Health Organization. (2001). *The Global Burden of Disease*. Available: http://files.dcp2.org/pdf/GBD/GBD01.pdf [accessed December 2008].

2

Approach to Research and Its Evaluation

SUMMARY

Research Challenges in Confronting Depression in Parents

- The challenges for researchers, clinicians, and policy makers in attempting to address the problems associated with the care of depression in parents include the integration of knowledge, the application of a developmental framework, conceptualizing the problems in a two-generation nature, and acknowledging the presence of the constellation of risk factors, context, and correlates associated with depression.

Issues Considered in Searching the Literature

- To fully understand the linkages among depression, parenting, and the child health outcomes, researchers should consider issues surrounding (but not limited to) the definition and measurement of depression and parenting, the etiology of depression, timing and use of appropriate screening interventions, the process of risk and resilience in children of depressed parents, correlates of depression, and developmental processes and time points.

Challenges in Evaluating the Literature

- Researchers face multiple methodological challenges studying depression in parents and its effects on parenting practices and child health outcomes that need to be addressed in order to provide recommendations for the development of future research, interventions, and policy—including conceptual frameworks, sampling designs, data analysis, and integration of research findings across literatures.

In this chapter, the committee describes their approach to the literature on the effects of parental depression on parenting practices and child outcomes and its evaluation. The chapter is organized in three sections, relating to the challenges that researchers face in confronting the problem of parental depression, the wide range of issues that we considered relevant, and standards of evidence and methodological issues that are important to keep in mind in reading this report. Some topics are addressed in more than one section, but they are focused on different aspects of the topic. For example, in the section on research challenges, we show that a conceptual framework relating to the effects of parental depression on families should be guided by a developmental psychopathology perspective. Later, in the section on research standards, we mention what the literature has shown in this regard and that research relating to any psychopathology should address questions "across generations and across time" (Hinshaw, 2008).

The type of evidence and criteria used to judge the importance of that evidence vary from area to area. This chapter does not attempt to explicitly summarize the specific criteria used for the evaluation of the evidence in each area, but instead offers a guideline of the general areas of interest and inquiry that the committee used when the committee searched and evaluated the literature. For example, studies of screening for parental depression are different from studies of treatment and intervention, and these are different from studies of prevention programs. These are also different from inquiries relating to changes in policy at the macro level or the available studies on the effects of parental depression. Thus, in this overview on standards of evidence and methodology, we present general guidelines that the reader should apply when appropriate in the subsequent chapters. Recommendations based on the evaluation of the evidence in each area are presented.

RESEARCH CHALLENGES IN CONFRONTING
DEPRESSION IN PARENTS

Four themes emerged from the committee's review of the research literature and discussions with service providers, policy makers, and stakeholder organizations: (1) the integration of knowledge regarding the dynamics of parental depression, parenting practices, and child outcomes; (2) the need to recognize the multigenerational dimensions of the effects of depression in a parent; (3) the application of a developmental framework in the study and evaluation of the effects of parental depression; and (4) the need to acknowledge the presence of the constellation of risk factors, context, and correlates of parental depression. Each of these is discussed in turn.

Integration of Knowledge

Depression is a complex disorder that is affected by biological, psychological, behavioral, interpersonal, and social contextual processes. Examining the effects of depression on parenting and the development of children requires the integration of knowledge from research, practice, and service delivery from multiple scientific, health care, and social service disciplines. Major scientific and integrative advances have emerged that point the way for future research and practice, but the challenges presented by the integration of these widely varied disciplines are enormous. Similarly, addressing parental depression as a public health problem requires multiple points of access for delivery of services and multiple types of intervention and care.

The approach we have taken to the problem of depression, parenting, and the healthy development of children has been interdisciplinary and transdisciplinary from the outset. The composition of the committee reflects multiple disciplines, including pediatrics, psychiatry, psychology, nursing, pharmacology, biostatistics, obstetrics, public health, behavioral health, and community and family medicine. We sought input and information from experts in a wide range of practice and community settings to consider the broad context in which services are delivered to parents with depression and their children.

The range of professionals and settings potentially concerned with depression in parents and their children is vast. Among health care services, it includes mental health professions (psychiatry, psychology, psychiatric nursing, social work), primary care, family practice, obstetrics, and pediatrics. Among family and community support systems, it includes extended families, religious institutions, and formal and informal community supports. Among policy makers, it includes program administrators running home visiting programs, Medicaid officials, mental health administrators, and others with responsibility for fiscal resources that could be reallocated. Much like the divisions that characterize scientific disciplines, we have identified barriers between the delivery (formal or informal) of interventions to parents with depression and delivery of interventions for children and families. Our agenda included the identification of ways to develop new strategies to bridge the different cultures of health care delivery, community and family support services, and policy makers.

Transdisciplinary Approaches to Research, Training, and Service Delivery

Although the need for integration and synthesis across these disciplines is great, the breadth of knowledge and practice that is relevant to understanding and addressing depression and parenting is a double-edged sword. On one hand, depression is a complex disorder that is affected by biological, psychological, behavioral, interpersonal, and social contextual processes. Major scientific advances have been made in all of these areas, and integrative perspectives are emerging to guide the synthesis of current findings and point the way for future research and practice. Similarly, addressing the public health problem of parental depression requires multiple points of access for delivery of services and multiple types of intervention and care. On the other hand, the challenges presented by the integration of these widely varied disciplines are enormous. Much of the work to date has been carried out in separate scientific entities, divided by different methodologies, levels of analysis, terminology, and agendas. The committee has purposefully attempted to break down these barriers in our approach by looking for examples of research that have integrated multiple disciplines and opportunities to move forward with new transdisciplinary work. Over the course of our work, we began to understand that depression in parents is a topic with no home—it is everywhere and nowhere. This is partly a consequence of the many disciplines and fields that are concerned with depression in parents. With this perspective in mind, we undertook the task to begin to build a "home" with this report.

As outlined by the National Institutes of Health, a transdisciplinary approach involves integrative science that spans basic and clinical research from multiple disciplines (e.g., genetics, medicine, behavioral science) and can generate rapid new developments in conceptual models to initiate breakthroughs and speed the translation of findings in basic research into practice and policy. This involves the translation of research from basic science into the development and testing of novel intervention approaches and, conversely, the translation of intervention findings back into basic science studies that can identify and model mechanisms of risk and etiology. Translational and transdisciplinary research is bidirectional in nature, with basic science informing interventions and intervention findings stimulating further basic research inquiry.

A number of recent examples of translational research are relevant to the understanding of depression, parenting, and children. For example, there is growing recognition of the role of multiple biological processes that are relevant to the etiology and course of depression and to the comorbidity of depression and medical conditions, most notably coronary heart disease (Miller and Blackwell, 2006). This work has come from the synthesis of relatively independent lines of research on the role of stress in proinflammatory processes, coronary heart disease, and depression. Similarly, the integration of methodologies and findings from research on genetics and brain structure and function has led to significant advances in knowledge of the underlying neurobiology of depression (Hariri and Brown, 2006). The translation of basic behavioral research on parenting processes and their effects on children's development has provided a foundation for understanding the ways in which parenting may be disrupted by depression and the subsequent impact on children (Bornstein, 2006).

Linking Research and Practice

Throughout this volume we emphasize the importance of the pipeline from the discovery of underlying mechanisms of risk in children of depressed parents to the delivery of services and to the development of policy (Abrams, 2006). This includes, as Abrams notes, "the science of dissemination along with improving the dissemination of evidence-based science" (p. 515). The dissemination of research findings to practitioners and, conversely, the application of the experience and observations of practitioners to research are significant challenges in mental health research and practice (Barlow, 1996; Weisz, Jensen, and McLeod, 2005). This complex process is even more complicated in the case of depression in parents as it spans research and practice with adults (parents), children (from infancy through adolescence), and families. Establishing links between research and practice involves the interactions among the full range of health care services and family and community support systems that may intervene with depressed parents or their children.

A Two-Generation Approach

The evidence of the effects of depression on the parents' parenting skills and on their children's health and development makes a compelling case for fostering this integration through such a two-generation approach (parent and child) at every level, including systems that provide care and services, efforts to more fully understand the epidemiology and effects of parental depression, and future research on intervention approaches. We make reference to this two-generation approach throughout the report.

We also recognized the frequent need for a three-generation perspective, taking into account grandparents who may be thrust into the child rearing role. However, we determined that, despite their importance in understanding and working with parental depression, the three-generation approach as well as concerns about sibling relationships was outside the scope of this report. We were able to glean useful information on the role of marital relationships in the occurrence and treatment of depression (some of which is mentioned later in this chapter) and in the effects of parental depression on children (included in the summaries in Chapter 4).

Developing an explicit focus on the nature and quality of behaviors and relationships between parents and children challenges the traditional division of responsibilities in medicine and mental health practices and in many service settings. Both facilities and professionals traditionally specialize in either adults or children (exceptions to this practice include family medicine and, in some settings, combined medicine and pediatrics). Primary care, mental health, and community service systems that see adults with depression do not routinely consider whether those adults have children, nor do they provide links to services that focus on parenting skills and on the needs of their children. Although increased attention to postpartum depression has led to some changes for women and infant children, most systems that provide care for children are not well equipped to identify parents with depression or at risk for it or to refer them to appropriate services for adequate treatment.

A vast research literature on depression examines its epidemiology, etiology, correlates, and treatments among adults, but, for the most part, this body of work does not identify whether or not these adults are parents. Thus, the literature and national surveys on etiology, prevalence, screening, prevention, and treatment of depression in adults are often not specific to depression in parents and do not include measures of its effects on their children. This limitation makes it difficult to gauge the true extent of the problem.

An extensive body of research on parenting practices and parent and child relationships highlights effective interventions that support positive outcomes for children. Yet with regard to depression in parents, only a few intervention studies have adopted such a two-generation approach, which focuses on the relationships and interactions between parents with depression and their children. In addition, interventions with good evidence for improving child outcomes rarely consider the influence of parental depression on their effectiveness and even more rarely examine the potential effects of including program components that identify and refer or treat parents with depression. When this has been done, improvements in effectiveness have been noted, such as in the work of Kazdin and Sanders and colleagues (Kazdin, 2005; Sanders et al., 2000).

In our work, we noted increasing interest in understanding how and when improvements in parents' depression lead to improvements in parenting and, even further, in child functioning. We include an overview of studies of treatment for depression in parents as a preventive intervention for their children (Chapter 7).

Equally interesting, although less often studied, is how and when interventions designed to improve qualities of parenting or to improve couples' relationship issues also lead to improvements in the parent's depression and potential benefits for their children. We recognized these approaches as reflecting the two-generation perspective, which we judged to be a very promising approach to the problem of depression in parents.

In terms of parenting interventions, a recent review of parenting training interventions noted consistent evidence that depression in parents improves as a secondary benefit of such training, even when the depression per se is not a target of the intervention (Kaminski et al., 2008). Although the authors note that some of the studies' designs did not always allow for ruling out that the depression may have improved even without the intervention, the findings are promising. Other studies targeted mothers with depression and intervened directly in their qualities of parenting (Cicchetti, Rogosch, and Toth, 2000; Gelfand et al., 1996; Lyons-Ruth et al., 1990).

In terms of couples' relationship problems and discord, behavioral approaches to marital therapy have been found to be more effective for the treatment of depression than standard cognitive behavioral therapy targeting the depression per se (Baucom et al., 1998). We also found promising the new generation of marital therapies being designed to treat depression based on knowledge of the associations between depression and marital problems (Beach, Fincham, and Katz, 1998). We also noted a recent meta-analysis that found inconclusive evidence for the efficacy of couple therapy as a treatment for depression yet concluded that couple therapy may still be the treatment of choice when relational distress is predominant (Barbato and D'Avanzo, 2008)

A Developmental Framework

The implementation of a two-generation approach involves many challenges. Childhood is a period of rapid change and development, and the presence or absence of supportive parental behaviors can have lasting effects if they interfere with the children getting their stage-salient needs met. The impact and consequences of depression in parents can vary by both the age of the children in the family as well as the length, severity, and history of exposure to parental depression.

In the course of our work, we recognized the value of a developmental approach. That is, we understood that multiple aspects of concern about depression in parents would vary by the age of the children in the family at any particular point in time of studying these families. We also recognized the importance, and the challenge, of understanding any child's history of exposure to depression in a parent. We expected that the age of the children at the times the parent was depressed would influence the particular risks to their development, the resiliencies that they would be able to bring to bear, the mechanisms by which those risks might be transmitted, the challenges to parenting with depression, the approach to screening for depression, and the nature of the preventive or other intervention that might be found to be effective. Although we reviewed literature that suggests reasons to be concerned and to intervene regardless of the children's ages, we also noted a compelling case for the youngest children. Most important was the understanding that development needs to be taken into account.

A Developmental Psychopathology Perspective

We were also guided by a developmental psychopathology perspective, which conceptualizes risk for the development of psychopathology in terms of processes that extend through time and are considered in the context of normal developmental processes (Cicchetti and Schneider-Rosen, 1984; Sroufe and Rutter, 1984). Understanding the mechanisms of risk in children of depressed parents requires understanding the processes underlying individual patterns of adaptation and the consequences of the individual patterns for the development of depression or other problems. Early in their developmental pathways, children of depressed mothers may develop vulnerabilities for depression, which, in turn, increase the likelihood of developing depression. Given the stage-salient needs of infants, of particular concern have been limits on depressed mothers' abilities to provide the sensitive, responsive care needed for the development of healthy attachment relationships (Egeland and Farber, 1984) and emotional self-regulation (Tronick and Gianino, 1986). We recognized the value of knowledge of children's potential vulnerabilities and developmental needs to inform screening, prevention, treatment, and policy.

Depression and Parenting Children Across Development

Even when one takes a developmental perspective, it is often ignored that, among women with depression, it occurs during pregnancy with at least as high a rate as in the postpartum period (Evans et al., 2001). Antenatal depression may be an early life stress that alters fetal development of stress-related biological systems (especially hypothalamic-pituitary-adrenal functioning), retards fetal growth, constricts the length of gestation, and increases risk of obstetrical complications (Van den Bergh et al., 2005). Concerns about the fetus suggest potential long-term implications for the development of problems in cognitive and social-emotional functioning. We therefore sought to expand on the typical perspective of parenting with depression to include the prenatal period.

Infants and young children are dependent on sensitive, responsive caregiving in order to develop skills in emotion regulation, interpersonal skills, and stress response mechanisms, problems in any of which may disrupt the earliest stages of development, predisposing children to the later development of depression. Consistent with these understandings, a meta-analytic review identified a larger body of research suggesting that depression is even more strongly associated with parenting problems in parents of infants compared with parents of older children (Lovejoy et al., 2000). Another literature shows that brain development continues at a rapid pace at least for several years after birth (Chugani and Phelps, 1986), and its course of development can be strongly influenced by early life stressors, such as might be associated with having a mother with depression. Thus we were particularly concerned about depression in parents of young children.

Despite compelling reasons for concern about pregnancy and infancy and early childhood, we recognized that they are not the only developmental periods of concern in relation to depression in parents. For example, depressive symptoms and depressive disorder interfere with the tasks of parenting in parents of school-age children and adolescents (e.g., Du Rocher, Schudlich, and Cummings, 2007; Gerdes et al., 2007). Disruptions in parenting associated with depression in parents (e.g., parental withdrawal, intrusiveness, and irritability) are related to higher levels of internalizing and externalizing problems in adolescents (e.g., Jaser et al., 2005). Furthermore, certain aspects of brain development, particularly in the prefrontal regions responsible for executive functions and emotion regulation, continue on into young adulthood and are vulnerable to the effects of chronic stress throughout childhood and adolescence (e.g., Nelson et al., 2005; Romeo and McEwen, 2006). These lines of research suggest that the risks associated with depression in a parent extend well beyond early infancy and early childhood.

Depression Does Not Exist in a Vacuum: Bringing Comorbidities, Correlates, and Context to Light

Depression rarely occurs in isolation. Depressed adults often face other health problems and psychopathologies (such as substance use disorders, anxiety disorders) and stressful social environments (such as poverty, bereavement, social isolation). Those risk factors may be essential to understanding the problems in children of depressed parents. The associated features also may be essential in identifying approaches to treating parents' depression and also improving the quality of parenting and children's outcomes. Such recognition might involve, at a minimum, assessing the constellation of risk factors and also evaluating the relative contribution of the multiple disorders to the problems with parenting and with child functioning. These risk factors may also affect how and where services can best be provided.

A long history of research supports the theory that depression is both exacerbated by problems in interpersonal relationships and also contributes to them (Joiner, Coyne, and Blalock, 1999). This includes the finding that living with a parent with depression is stressful, not only in relation to problems with parenting but also in relation to the parent's problems with other relationships (Hammen, 2002), and children struggle to cope with these stressors (Compas et al., 2002). Attention to the context of the lives of women with depression suggests concern for the children in terms of their exposure to a wide range of stressors (Hammen, 2002).

More broadly, the methodological issue this raises is that depression in parents may be an essential marker of risk for problems in children but not necessarily a "main effect." Whereas depression is known to be comorbid with anxiety disorders and substance abuse, in particular, and these are addressed in this report, we also addressed the potential importance of other correlates and contexts, including intrafamily violence, child abuse, and neglect. This report shows that the comorbidities, correlates, and contexts may function as independent risk factors for adverse child outcomes or as modifying factors, which exacerbate the effects of parental depression. Yet research on the effects of parental depression on parenting or child functioning rarely provides adequate tests of the role of co-occurring conditions.

Integrating the Comorbidities, Correlates, and Context into Approaches to Treating or Preventing Depression in Parents

Understanding the dynamics of how parental depression and its comorbidities, correlates, and context impact child outcomes are important to the design and implementation of successful future service delivery models for families affected by parental depression. We recognized the tendency of interventions to focus on depression in the parent as a risk factor for the development of psychopathology in the children without considering that the families might best be characterized by the broader set of risk and protective factors we bring to light here. Moreover, if depression is secondary to other overriding issues in the family, such as poverty, violence, marital or couple distress, issues related to immigration, acculturation, etc., then the implications for screening, prevention, and treatment are quite different than if one were addressing depression as the primary problem. At a minimum, one would need to assess co-occurring conditions and also evaluate the relative contribution of the multiple conditions to the problems with parenting and with child functioning. Once carefully assessed, the associated features are likely to suggest different approaches to treating the parent's depression, improving the quality of parenting, and in preventing negative outcomes in the children, relative to the situation in which depression is the primary problem. We also recognized that comorbidities may affect how and where services can best be provided.

Integrating Services in Different Settings for Diverse Populations

The methodological issues raised by comorbidities, correlates, and context also have implications for where depressed parents might receive services. In our approach to the problem of depression in parents, we recognized that the services for comorbidities, such as substance abuse, or correlates and contextual variables, such as family violence or issues related to immigration, are typically offered in settings other than where mainstream mental health services are offered. We are also aware that many of these problems related to depression in parents first come to light in primary care settings, such as family practice, obstetrics, and pediatrics. Thus, another issue concerns strategies that can bridge service cultures and institutional networks.

Needs of Vulnerable Populations

As this understanding of the context in which depression reveals, certain populations are particularly at risk. The committee thus worked to determine that we were including literature that addresses the needs of a wide range of populations, including vulnerable populations, for example, first- and second-generation immigrants and refugees and others, especially those who are known to be at risk, including those who live in poverty. Learning about correlates of psychiatric disorders among vulnerable populations is of critical importance to inform clinical practice and guide program development. Although current research has not yet covered the specific topic of parental depression among vulnerable populations—with the exception of a few qualitative studies (e.g., Lazear et al., 2008)—for the purpose of this report it is important to point to major studies of mental illness in specific racial and ethnic populations that may provide significant insights into prevalence rate differences, help-seeking behaviors, and patterns of use of mental health services. We identify below some of the largest and most recent psychiatric epidemiological studies that have been used in studies described throughout the report in order to help provide insight into how specific racial and ethnic populations use and need mental health services in Box 2-1.

BOX 2-1
Summary of Large Psychiatric Epidemiological
Studies in Racial and Ethnic Minority Populations

- Mexican American Prevalence and Service Survey
  - U.S.-born Mexican Americans and Mexican immigrants
  - Residents of Fresno, California
  - Ages 18–59
  - National Survey of American Life
  - African Americans, black immigrants from the Caribbean (recent and second-generation), non-Hispanic whites
  - Prevalence of mental health disorders, use of mental health services
- National Latino and Asian American Study
  - Hispanics, Asian Americans, further stratified by ethnic subgroups
  - Ages 18 and older
  - Similarities and differences in mental illness and service use
- National Epidemiologic Survey on Alcohol and Related Conditions
  - U.S.-born Mexican Americans, Mexican immigrants residing in the United States, U.S.-born non-Hispanic whites, and non-Hispanic white immigrants residing in the United States
  - Considers immigration status in conjunction with psychiatric morbidity

---

Doorways into the Domain of Depression in Parents

Research has highlighted two key facts relevant to our task of evaluating how best to approach the problem of depression in parents. First, most adults with depression do not get treated for it (Kessler et al., 1999; Kessler, Merikangas, and Wang, 2007; Narrow et al., 1993; Regier et al., 1993). The large-scale, psychiatric, epidemiological study by Kessler et al. revealed that less than one-third of adults with major depression or dysthymia used either general medical or specialty outpatient mental health services in the previous year. Second, the one-third of adults of parenting age with depression who do get treated uses a wide range of alternative points of contact. Yet given the number and multiplicity of depressive disorders' comorbid mental and physical health problems (e.g., substance abuse, chronic pain), impairment (e.g., problems getting to work), and co-occurring conditions (e.g., poverty), one promising avenue to the identification of parents with depression is to focus on those who are seeking treatment or assistance for those associated conditions.

These alternative avenues to identifying parents with depression include a wide range of formal and informal service settings, which offer important points for screening and identification. Also, the children themselves may be an important avenue for identifying parents with depression. For example, in Finland, a national program involves educating children and adolescents about mental health problems in adults and how children can cope with depression in their parents (Solantaus and Toikka, 2006). More broadly, the committee recognized that children being screened for developmental delays or evaluated or treated for emotional or behavior problems, school behavior problems, or even chronic illnesses or injuries present a typically neglected opportunity to screen for depression in parents.

Finally, in the realm of policy relating to parental depression and its effects, we conducted interviews with states leading initiatives on maternal depression (Illinois, Iowa, New Jersey), seeking evaluation data when they were available, drawing on primary data from two other studies conducted by the National Center for Children in Poverty (Cooper et al., 2008; Knitzer, Theberge, and Johnson, 2008). We also reviewed other literature on program initiatives, as well as the policy literature, to extract, whenever possible, the policy implications. To assess the feasibility of the recommendations, we asked four basic policy-relevant questions (Kingdon, 1995): Will it promote efficiency? Will it promote equity? It is politically feasible? Does it seem doable from a cost perspective? Finally, we relied on our own understanding of how policy processes work and what kinds of recommendations are likely to be persuasive.

ISSUES CONSIDERED IN SEARCHING THE LITERATURE

To fully understand the linkages among depression, parenting, and children's development, we considered a wide range of research. This includes research on but not limited to the definition and measurement of depression and parenting practices, the etiology of depression, timing and use of appropriate screening interventions, the processes of risk and resilience in children of depressed parents, correlates of depression, and developmental processes and time points.

Definition and Measurement of Depression and Parenting

Depression presents a number of challenges in its definition and measurement. Foremost of these is the distinction between depression as a categorical psychiatric diagnosis and dimensional approaches that consider symptoms of depression as a matter of degree along a continuum. Diagnoses of depression are derived from psychiatric interviews, whereas dimensional approaches are assessed through symptom inventories and questionnaires. We have considered both in our review and have offered suggestions for the integration of what are often seen as contrasting, rather than complementary, approaches. Furthermore, depression is a heterogeneous disorder with varying patterns of symptom presentation, chronicity, duration, and severity. Similar issues were encountered in our review of parenting. The central dimensions of parenting (e.g., warmth, structure) are addressed, and we provide consideration of the characteristics of effective versus impaired parenting. However, there is far less consensus regarding the measurement of parenting than the measurement of depression.

At the same time, it is important to recognize that "parental depression," "maternal depression," and even "postpartum depression" are not distinct diagnostic entities from depression as it occurs in any adult. Perinatal depression is not a separate diagnosis according to the *Diagnostic and Statistical Manual of Mental Disorders*, 4th edition (DSM-IV) (American Psychiatric Association, 1994). Typically, clinically significant perinatal depression is operationalized as major depression, a diagnosis that requires meeting a set of symptom, duration, and impairment criteria as defined by the DSM-IV. Under Depressive Disorders in the DSM-IV, pregnancy is not given any special consideration; however, "postpartum" is an added qualifier to refer to the timing of a major depressive episode. It is thus important to recognize that when we refer to parental, maternal, or paternal depression, we refer to depression defined in the same ways as depression that occurs at other times in people's lives.

Etiology of Depression

We have examined the broad literature on the etiology of depression in parents and in their children. This includes genetic, biological, and interpersonal processes that contribute to depression in parents as well as in their children. Recent research has begun to illuminate the complex interactions and combinations of biological and social processes that are associated with increased risk for depression. Examples of integrative research on the etiology of depression include studies of the interaction of stress and genetic liabilities, such as mutations of the genes responsible for serotonin transport in the brain (e.g., Caspi et al., 2003) and research showing that traumatic stress early in development can lead to a cascade of biological processes that increase the risk for depression (Gillespie and Nemeroff, 2007).

Screening for Depression in Parents

The challenge in evaluating the literature is that screening measures are often used without validation by other methods. While very brief and longer symptom checklist measures have been shown to perform similarly as screening tools to detect those at risk of major depression (Whooley et al., 1997), their positive predictive value for a major depressive disorder varies according to the prevalence of depression in that population. Screening measures typically detect 75 percent with any depressive disorder and 25–40 percent with a major depressive disorder (Kroenke, 2006; U.S. Preventive Services Task Force, 2002). Thus, the widespread practice of only using a screening tool to define depression, typically maternal depression, underestimates the prevalence. Similarly, the use of symptom levels without an assessment of functional impact is likely to overestimate the occurrence of maternal depression. The development of a specific screening tool for the postpartum period, the Edinburgh Postpartum Depression Scale, has promoted screening of women in the perinatal period. However, the poor sensitivity of this measure to detect major or minor depression, varying cut scores in different studies, and the infrequent validation with a clinical diagnostic interview (Gaynes et al., 2005) make it difficult to determine the magnitude and severity of postpartum depression and mental health service needs of mothers postpartum. Box 2-2 lists the common tools and approaches available for the screening and diagnosis of depression.

Effective interventions depend on identification of who, when, and what pattern. The type of intervention to use may be affected by the duration of depression and the intensity of its symptoms. Postpartum depression may be limited to the first few months or may persist throughout the first year or beyond. A parent may have chronic unremitting depression, relapsing bouts of depression, or milder depression in which functioning

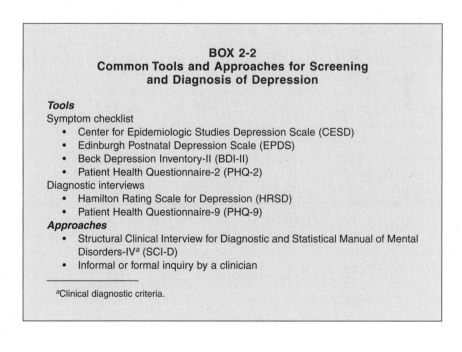

BOX 2-2
Common Tools and Approaches for Screening
and Diagnosis of Depression

Tools
Symptom checklist
  • Center for Epidemiologic Studies Depression Scale (CESD)
  • Edinburgh Postnatal Depression Scale (EPDS)
  • Beck Depression Inventory-II (BDI-II)
  • Patient Health Questionnaire-2 (PHQ-2)
Diagnostic interviews
  • Hamilton Rating Scale for Depression (HRSD)
  • Patient Health Questionnaire-9 (PHQ-9)
Approaches
  • Structural Clinical Interview for Diagnostic and Statistical Manual of Mental Disorders-IV[a] (SCI-D)
  • Informal or formal inquiry by a clinician

---

[a]Clinical diagnostic criteria.

as a parent is maintained; all of these may be considered together in many studies. These complexities of depression are important in determining who is most impacted.

For screening programs, when an adult is identified as suffering from depression, it is important to identify if that adult is a parent, if the spouse/partner is also depressed, or if one or both are at risk for depression, has been diagnosed with depression, if both parents have been diagnosed with depression, or if one or both parents have been diagnosed with other co-morbid conditions (i.e., substance use, trauma). Identification of these issues in both parents is necessary. It is also important to note when depression or symptoms of depression were identified in the parents: prenatal, postpartum, the first year of the child's life, the first 3 years of the child's life, the first 5 years of the child's life, or throughout childhood into adolescence. However, the overriding concern with screening is the lack of available and effective resources and knowledge needed after an adult is identified with depression as a result of a screening procedure.

Processes of Risk and Resilience in Children of Depressed Parents

Closely related to etiology is consideration of factors that are associated with increased risk, as contrasted with resilience, among children of depressed parents. Kraemer and colleagues (1997) refer to risk as a predisposition of an individual or a population to a negative outcome. In the field of mental health, these negative outcomes can be measured in terms of the onset, severity, and duration of a disorder or the frequency and intensity of individual symptoms or clusters of symptoms. Individuals and populations at risk have an increased likelihood of developing symptoms or more severe pathology than the population as a whole (Rutter, 1987). The magnitude, or degree, of risk is measured by the probability of a specific negative outcome in the presence of a risk factor versus the probability when the risk factor is absent. The odds of adolescents developing depression are greater for those who are exposed to a parent with a history of depression compared with those whose parents have no such psychopathology.

A risk factor is a feature of an individual or the environment that increases the probability of the occurrence of a negative outcome. Risk factors, however, do not explain the processes through which these factors influence the likelihood of an undesirable outcome. In contrast, risk mechanisms or processes describe the intervening paths that connect risk conditions with specific dysfunctional outcomes (Garber, 2006). In the case of parental depression, it is not merely the presence of psychopathology in the parent that leads to psychopathology in the children, but the processes that result from the disorder (such as a biological predisposition, including genetic mechanisms, negative parenting, or stressful parent-child interactions) linking the risk factor with unfavorable outcomes.

Even in the face of significant risk, not all individuals do poorly—not all children and adolescents of depressed parents develop psychopathology. Although children and adolescents of affectively ill parents are at an increased risk for depression and other forms of psychopathology, a number of studies have demonstrated that many of them actually do quite well. These individuals identified as "resilient" exhibit the ability to respond positively to significant adversity. Masten and colleagues (1999) conceptualize resilience as "phenomena involving successful adaptation in the context of significant threats to development" (p. 143). Although ambiguity exists in the definition of resilience in the literature, researchers have converged on two critical conditions inherent in this concept: (1) exposure to significant threat or adversity and (2) the achievement of positive adaptation despite challenging life circumstances (Luthar, Cicchetti, and Becker, 2000; Luthar and Zigler, 1991; Masten, Best, and Garmezy, 1990).

Research on risk and resilience related to depression is vast and growing, encompassing biological, environmental, and psychological processes and their interface. Examples include psychobiological processes that are related to resilience to stress (Charney, 2004; Southwick, Vythilingam, and Charney, 2005); the developmental neurobiology of stress hormones, including cortisol, that are related to depression (Gunnar and Quevedo, 2007); the primate model of stress inoculation based on experiences in early development (Parker et al., 2005); and oxytocin and protection from depression (Scantamburlo et al., 2007).

Correlates of Depression

As noted above, depression is characterized by high rates of comorbidity with other psychiatric disorders and with medical illnesses. Adults with depression, including those who are parents, have an increased risk of a number of other medical and psychiatric conditions. This presents a challenge to researchers, as it is difficult to disentangle the effects of parental depression on children from the effects of these other comorbid conditions. However, these comorbidities also offer a number of opportunities for the identification of parents with depression and contexts for the delivery of interventions to prevent adverse outcomes in their children.

Depression in parents is also likely to be accompanied by other problems in families and communities. For example, parents with depression are likely to have spouses with psychiatric disorders that further increase the risk of mental health problems in their children. Some depressed parents and their families live in poverty, with limited access to health and mental health care, further compounding the risk to children in these families.

The criteria for major depressive disorder as outlined in the DSM-IV include significant impairment in social functioning, interpersonal relationships, and work. Significant impairment in multiple domains is also associated with high but subthreshold levels of depressive symptoms. Overall, both depressive disorder and depressive symptoms in parents are accompanied by comorbid disorders, problems in families and communities, and disruptions in work, marital relationships, and parenting.

Developmental Approach

We take an explicitly developmental approach in our perspective on parental depression. The effects of depression may be dramatically different when a parent experiences an episode of depression when pregnant or while a child is in infancy, middle childhood, or adolescence. The different effects of parental depression may be due in part to the different developmental tasks that are central as children move through childhood and adolescence. Moreover, the characteristics of effective parenting change as children develop, and depression may affect different aspects of parenting. For example, the formation of fundamental attachment relationships may be impaired when a parent of an infant experiences an episode of depression. In contrast, depression may interfere with the provision of structure and monitoring when a parent of an adolescent is affected. The effects of depression may be greater when a parent experiences multiple episodes that occur throughout a child's lifetime and disrupts parenting at multiple points in development.

Summary of Our Approach Searching the Literature

The committee reviewed multiple types of research or lines of investigation on depression in parents. First, we examined the literature on the effects of depression in parents on children. In this literature, we looked both at effects on physical health and health-related outcomes, such as use of health services, and also on children's psychological outcomes. The latter included not only evidence of emotional or behavioral problems in association with depression in parents, but also problems in psychological functioning that might be early signs of psychopathology or vulnerabilities to the later development of psychopathology. Such vulnerabilities include behavior, psychophysiology, and neuroendocrine functioning. We took into account the full developmental spectrum of infancy through adolescence and also considered fetal development.

Given the understanding that not all children of depressed parents would be expected to develop problems, we made special note of studies that examined moderators—that is, factors that may affect the strength of the relationship between depression in parents and outcomes in children. Tests of moderators of the associations between depression in parents and outcomes in children reveal the characteristics of parents and children who are more or less likely to have adverse outcomes. Moderators that have been examined include child characteristics (e.g., age, sex), characteristics of the parent with depression (e.g., severity, chronicity), and characteristics of the coparent (e.g., mental health and involvement of fathers when mother is depressed), and broader social context qualities (e.g., poverty).

Second, we reviewed the literature on effects of depression in parents on their parenting practices. This literature was of particular interest for two reasons: the well-known reliance of children on good-quality parenting for healthy child development (Collins et al., 2003) and a long-standing understanding that depression is likely to interfere with good-quality parenting (Weissman and Paykel, 1974). Thus, we were particularly interested in research on the mediational role of parenting in the association between depression in parents and adverse outcomes in children. By mediating role, we mean the extent to which depression has negative influences on parenting and, subsequently, the extent to which those changes in parenting account for associations between parents' depression and the outcomes in the children. In general, a mediating variable is one that at least partly explains the association between one variable and another. Thus, we examined evidence that the associations researchers have found between depression in parents and adverse outcomes in children are at least partially explained by parenting practices.

Third, to take into consideration other possible mediators of associations between parents' depression and child outcomes, in addition to parenting practices, we noted studies of the effects of depression in parents on the children that also considered the potential role of marital relationships. However, it was beyond the scope of this report to review the literature on effects of depression in parents on their relationships with their spouse/partner, extended family relationships, or work, although we acknowledge that these are likely important aspects of a broad model of how depression in parents is related to the outcomes in their children.

Fourth, we reviewed evidence for the effectiveness of screening, prevention, and treatment of depression in the parent. In these literatures, we searched broadly for evidence of effectiveness of a range of interventions designed to address the effects of parental depression on children.

CHALLENGES IN THE EVALUATION OF THE LITERATURE

We now present an overview of the many methodological challenges faced by researchers studying parental depression and its effects on parenting practices and child outcomes. We focus particularly on issues that make recommendations possible for the development of new research, interventions, and policy. Such issues involve all aspects of research, from conceptual frameworks, to study sampling designs, to data analysis and the integration of research findings across literatures. As noted previously, these do not specifically address each area of inquiry but instead provide the reader with a set of issues to consider when reading this report. In each subsequent chapter, the committee considered these issues when evaluating the available literature to help guide their conclusions and recommendations.

Balance Hypothesis-Driven and Real-World Challenges

The integration of the large and growing literature on parental depression has presented a number of problems and challenges. First and foremost is the need to balance hypothesis-driven research with real-world challenges in addressing complex health and behavioral disorders. As noted above, the goal of translational research is to move from basic to applied research, from bench to bedside. However, disparities between research conducted under carefully controlled conditions and research in real-world contexts have been widely noted. For example, Weisz and colleagues have shown that psychological treatments for children can be effective when delivered and evaluated under optimal conditions but often have negligible or no effect in community settings (e.g., Weersing and Weisz, 2002). Theories on which interventions on parental depression are based must be tested in the field and modified, if necessary, to increase the likelihood of success when implemented on a large scale. How parental depression affects parenting and children's outcomes is a question that will be best answered using translational research methods that meet the standards that we now outline.

Integrative Models in Research

Scientific research in general is often incremental in its development, and interrelated factors are not always examined properly in the same study. Research in the area of parental depression and its effects on parenting and child development has rarely been conducted to address hypotheses from an integrative model. The use of theory-based models in the design of studies helps to provide a framework for success in ultimate treatment effectiveness that is replicable across locations and time and that can be sustained over time. For example, not accounting for the effects of parental substance abuse, violence, and depression or other psychiatric distress in families may result in an overestimation of the individual effects of these factors on the development of the child. The relative lack of generalizable, integrative research and interventions on the scope and nature of the problems caused by parental depression has provided the impetus for the work of our committee.

A particular interest of the committee was to identify potential untapped sources of information on the scope and dynamics of parental depression on families available in large-scale databases that have been developed in recent years. As a result of this interest, the committee has undertaken analyses of the National Comorbidity Survey-Replication sample and the Medical Expenditure Panel Survey, two large surveys generalizable to the U.S. population with data on family mental health issues, the results of which are included in this report.

Also of note, studies in families have largely not examined the genetic component and its potential interactions, something that is addressed in a paper prepared for the committee as input into this report. Despite being acknowledged as one of the four primary mechanisms by which depression in parents is related to the development of depression and other problems in children (Goodman and Gotlib, 1999; See Figure 4-1 in Chapter 4), few researchers have used genetically informed designs to address questions related to the effect of parental depression on parenting and on child functioning.

A Developmental Perspective

Studies on the effects of parental depression on parenting and child development would benefit from taking a developmental perspective, although we found such an approach to be rare. As described earlier, a developmental perspective considers developmental processes (e.g., the timing of exposure), takes into account roles of early experience of development, integrates multiple transactional influences on development, and considers the multiple alternative pathways through development. For example, assuming that risk factors have effects or interventions that work the same among families with infants and toddlers, school-age children, adolescents, and young adults ignores the vast evidence in the area of child development. A recent editorial by Hinshaw (2008) notes that this is a concern in general with respect to studies of developmental psychopathology and that studies need to address questions "across generations and across time" (p. 361).

A Shared Framework Across Literature

Compounding the challenge of developing shared integrative models, researchers in these areas often have not used common theoretical frameworks, study designs, or measures or had a common focus on the parent-child relationship as the fundamental dynamic to be addressed. This integration has been described as "methodological pluralism" (Hinshaw, 2008, p. 361). For example, depending on the nature of the outcomes of interest and often the field of expertise of the research team (e.g., social science, medicine), the quantification of effects can be varied. Social scientists often use standardized measures of "effect size" (Cohen, 1988) to allow for comparison from study to study. Cutoffs are used to describe these effects as "small" (0.20), "medium" (0.50), or "large" (0.80). The drawback to these measures is that they are unitless and difficult to interpret from a clinical perspective.

In contrast, medical researchers often prefer to examine unstandardized differences, "effects," which make between-study comparisons difficult if the same measures are not used, or they focus on categorical outcomes, such as "depressed" versus "not depressed" on the basis of established criteria, such as the DSM-IV. The effects in studies employing such outcomes are often summarized in the form of odds ratios or risk ratios, which can vary between 0 and 1 (denoting negative association), 1 (no association), or greater than 1 (to infinity, denoting positive association). The size of such ratio-based measures could be interpreted, for example, with respect to positive associations, as "small" (greater than 1.0 to 1.5), "moderate" (1.5 to 2.0), or "large" (2.0 or greater). These must be interpreted cautiously, however, as their size can be dependent on the scale of the independent variable in question. Moreover, the interpretation of the sizes of effects should also take into consideration what has been previously observed in the relevant field in order to provide proper context.

Choice of Target Population of Study and Its Impact on Generalizability

Another issue that can adversely affect the interpretability of research findings in this area is the lack of generalizability of the samples used. This can result, for example, from a study's being based on a population referred to treatment or a population of parents of children with special needs. Results from such studies clearly cannot be generalized to the population of families at risk because of the varying characteristics of each population. Another way in which generalizability can be reduced is by the inadvertent restriction to a subgroup of the population of interest, which can result in studies with small numbers of subjects. Generalizability is enhanced when random sampling is implemented in a design that samples from all subgroups of interest. Examples of such studies can be found in many so-called complex sample surveys funded by the federal government, such as the National Comorbidity Survey (see http://www.icpsr.umich.edu/CPES/).

Randomized Treatment and Intervention Studies

In comparative intervention studies, which compare a given intervention strategy to another, the lack of randomization to study groups can adversely affect the validity of the study findings. With randomization implemented with large sample sizes, one can minimize the likelihood of the misattribution of effects to the intervention that could otherwise be explained by other factors. In the area of parental depression, the relative lack of randomized studies can be explained by the difficulty of implementation because of ethical issues, such as withholding a potentially effective treatment, or scientific concerns, such as avoiding contamination of intervention groups in behavioral studies. However, randomized clinical trials represent the optimal design for evaluating the efficacy of interventions to prevent adverse outcomes in children of depressed parents.

Sample Size and Its Implications

In general, studies that include small numbers of subjects can produce findings that are suggestive but do not provide evidence that is statistically significant. Such studies are said to lack "statistical power." In these cases, results that are clinically relevant may lack precision and thus confidence in their interpretability is reduced. Researchers often gauge the utility of the sample size of a study by the size of effect that it can minimally detect with 80 percent statistical power and a two-sided alpha (type I error rate) of 0.05. This "size" of effect is often quantified by the standardized effect size (Cohen, 1988) in which an effect of 0.20 is considered "small," 0.50 "medium," and 0.80 "large." To achieve 80 percent power, the 0.20 effect size requires approximately 800 subjects overall, 0.50 requires approximately 120, and 0.80 requires approximately 50. From another view, one can evaluate power for selected sample sizes of interest, for example, 100, 150, 200, 300, and 500, the latter two being in the range of what many would consider large. These sample sizes would require minimal effect size respectively of 0.57, 0.46, 0.40, 0.33, and 0.25.

The sizes of the samples employed in research on the effects of parental depression have often not been large, thus limiting the conclusions that can be drawn from the results and consequently preventing the kind of confident interpretation of results that is required to make policy changes. It is not surprising that large effects of individual risk or protective factors have not been observed given the inherent complexity of the factors at play with respect to the relationship of parental depression, parenting, and child development. Specifically in the context of intervention studies, the difficulty in impacting the multiple functional pathways that define this problem is reflected in the frequently observed small-size intervention effects. As we show in reviewing the literature, many published studies have only been able to detect small effects as statistically significant given the sizes of their samples. And large-scale research projects tied specifically to dissemination and implementation strategies are needed to help motivate changes in policies and systems.

Consideration of Possible Mediation of Effects

Integrative models of parental depression and its effects on parenting and child development need to consider the potential mediation of effects, which hold promise for explaining how depression in parents has its effects on children. Tests of mediation require a more complex analytic approach, such as path analysis, structural equations models, or other causal frameworks than simply adjusting out effects as covariates. The examination of possible mediation effects is an important element in understanding the underlying mechanisms for the effects of parental depression, and thus it has implications for the design and implementation of interventions. Potential problems arise, however, when mediational effects are assessed in solely cross-sectional analyses (Cole and Maxwell, 2003). We show that many studies of the effects of parental depression have not employed longitudinal designs and thus have not properly been able to examine how its effects are mediated through other factors, such as parenting practices on child outcomes.

Assessment of Effect-Modifying Factors

In many studies in the area of parental depression as a risk factor, moderators of effect have not been measured, such as exposure to violence. We would expect that when the constellation of factors associated with depression in a parent are measured, effects for the subgroup with multiple risk factors, such as depression and violence exposure, could be significantly higher than for those who have depression and no other factors. More broadly, a moderator is variable that increases or decreases the strength of association between two other variable. With the effect of depression in parents in their children, we considered the circumstances under which the effects may be stronger or weaker, including characteristics of the depression in the parents, characteristics of the children, and so forth.

Such combinations of risk factors in synergy (i.e., multiplicative) may be what actually result in poorer outcomes and not individual effects operating in a purely additive fashion. Such modifying effects may be present even in a randomized trial. Although the randomization aims to balance across the treatment or intervention groups on all potential confounding variables, measures or unmeasured, this does not eliminate the presence of effect modification. For example, if gender is an effect modifier, it is possible that the intervention could work differently in female compared with male subjects. Genetics is likely to play a moderating role in at least one of several possible patterns (Rutter, 2007). Thus, not recognizing the moderation of effects may prevent the targeting for intervention of subgroups of those who are at particularly increased risk.

Developmental models of psychopathology emphasize the importance of cumulative risk or multiple risk factors (Rutter, 2000; Rutter et al., 2001). The action of risk factors is cumulative in the sense that the presence of more risk factors is related to a higher certainty of negative outcomes (Seifer et al., 1992). Cumulative models reflect the natural covariation of many risk factors. These models assume that the confluence of many risk factors, rather than any single risk, is what leads to dysfunction. This is at least partly explained by the multiple risk factors overwhelming the adaptive capacities of the organism. For example, it has been shown that the magnitude of effect of any one family risk factor associated with psychosocial adjustment of youth is relatively small (Reid and Crisafulli, 1990) and that an increase of adjustment difficulties occurs with an increase in the number of risk factors (Forehand, Biggar, and Kotchick, 1998).

Effect of Measurement Error and Other Measurement Issues

An issue that has not been addressed in the interpretation of findings in this area is the difficulty in measuring depression and depressive symptoms, exposure to violence, and degree of substance use problems (because of the possible illicit nature of the behavior or risk of the loss of the child to state custody that might be imposed by identification of use by the authorities). Either the overestimation or underestimation of risk factor or intervention effects is possible in the presence of measurement error.

Replication of Findings

With a lack of large-scale, generalizable trials, researchers are forced to rely on the replication of findings of quasi-experimental and nonexperimental studies with similar consideration of the multiple, intercorrelated factors suspected to impact family function and child development—that is, an integrated model that links these factors together. Such replication has generally not been found in studies of parental depression, parenting, and child development. We consider strategies to reduce the negative effects on parental depression on parental practices and child outcomes that have been efficacious in two or more peer-reviewed studies. We thus consider such strategies to be ready for wider dissemination and evaluated for their effectiveness. Approaches that have not met this level of evidence are described as "promising" and should be tested in future studies to demonstrate their efficacy.

CONCLUSION

In this chapter, we have presented the committee's approach to the evaluation of the extensive literature on the relationship of parental depression, parenting practices, and child outcomes. Our ultimate aim is to set the bar for level of evidence to show (1) associations between parental depression, parenting practices, and child outcomes and (2) the efficacy of screening, prevention, treatments, and policies on the negative effects of parental depression on children. More generally, our aim is to identify the challenges posed by researchers, clinicians, and policy makers in attempting to address problems caused by parental depression.

Four themes emerge from the committee's approach: (1) the integration of knowledge regarding the dynamics of parental depression, parenting practices, and child outcomes; (2) the application of a developmental framework in the study and evaluation of the effects of parental depression; (3) the need to conceptualize the problem as two generation in nature; and (4) the need to acknowledge the presence of the constellation of risk factors, context, and correlates of parental depression. In the chapters that follow, attention is paid to each of these themes, which is essential to understanding the complexity of the problems associated with parental depression. The report shows that, although much is known, there are still many critical questions needing to be addressed with further research and many promising approaches to screening, prevention, treatment, and policy.

REFERENCES

Abrams, D.B. (2006). Applying transdisciplinary research strategies to understanding and eliminating health disparities. *Health Education and Behavior, 33*, 515–531.

American Psychiatric Association. (1994). *Diagnostic and Statistical Manual of Mental Disorders* (4th ed.). Washington, DC: Author.

Barbato, A., and D'Avanzo, B. (2008). Efficacy of couple therapy as a treatment for depression: A meta-analysis. *Psychiatric Quarterly, 79*, 121–132.

Barlow, D.H. (1996). Health care policy, psychotherapy research, and the future of psychotherapy. *American Psychologist, 51*, 1050–1058.

Baucom, D.H., Shoham, V., Mueser, K.T., Daiuto, A.D., and Stickle, T.R. (1998). Empirically supported couple and family interventions for marital distress and adult mental health problems. *Journal of Consulting and Clinical Psychology, 66*, 53–88.

Beach, S.R.H., Fincham, F.D., and Katz, J. (1998). Marital therapy in the treatment of depression: Toward a third generation of therapy and research. *Clinical Psychology Review, 18*, 635–661.

Bornstein, M.H. (2006). *Parenting Science and Practice*. Hoboken, NJ: John Wiley & Sons.

Caspi, A., Sugden, K., Moffitt, T.E., Taylor, A., Craig, I.W., Harrington, H., McClay, J., Mill, J., Martin, J., Braithwait, A., and Poulton, R. (2003). Influence of life stress on depression: Moderation by a polymorphism in the 5-HTT gene. *Science, 301,* 386–389.

Charney, D.S. (2004). Psychobiological mechanisms of resilience and vulnerability: Implications for successful adaptation to extreme stress. *American Journal of Psychiatry, 161,* 195–216.

Chugani, H.T., and Phelps, M.E. (1986). Maturational changes in cerebral function in infants determined by 18FDG positron emission tomography. *Science, 231,* 840–843.

Cicchetti, D., and Schneider-Rosen, K. (1984). Toward a transactional model of childhood depression. *New Directions for Child Development, 26,* 5–27.

Cicchetti, D., Rogosch, F.A., and Toth, S.L. (2000). The efficacy of toddler-parent psychotherapy for fostering cognitive development in offspring of depressed mothers. *Journal of Abnormal Child Psychology, 28,* 135–148.

Cohen, J. (1988). *Statistical Power Analysis for the Behavioral Sciences* (2nd ed.). Hillsdale, NJ: Lawrence Erlbaum Associates.

Cole, D.A., and Maxwell, S.E. (2003). Testing mediational models with longitudinal data: Questions and tips in the use of structural equation modeling. *Journal of Abnormal Psychology, 112,* 558–577.

Collins, W.A., Maccoby, E.E., Steinberg, L., Hetherington, E.M., and Bornstein, M.H. (2003). Contemporary research on parenting: The case for nature and nurture. In M.E. Hertzig and E.A. Farber (Eds.), *Annual Progress in Child Psychiatry and Child Development: 2000-2001* (pp. 113–140). New York: Brunner-Routledge.

Compas, B.E., Langrock, A.M., Keller, G., Merchant, M.J., and Copeland, M.E. (2002). Children coping with parental depression: Processes of adaptation to family stress. In S.H. Goodman and I.H. Gotlib (Eds.), *Children of Depressed Parents: Mechanisms of Risk and Implications for Treatment* (pp. 227–252). Washington, DC: American Psychological Association.

Cooper, J.L., Aratani, Y., Knitzer, J., Douglas-Hall, A., Masi, R., Banghart, P., and Dababnah, S. (2008). *Unclaimed Children Revisited: The Status of Children's Mental Health Policy in the United States.* New York: National Center for Children in Poverty.

Du Rocher Schudlich, T.D., and Cummings, E.M. (2007). Parental dysphoria and children's adjustment: Marital conflict styles, children's emotional security, and parenting as mediators of risk. *Journal of Abnormal Child Psychology, 35,* 627–639.

Egeland, B., and Farber, E.A. (1984). Infant-mother attachment: Factors related to its development and changes over time. *Child Development, 55,* 753–771.

Evans, J., Heron, J., Francomb, H., Oke, S., Golding, J., and Avon Longitudinal Study of Parents and Children Study Team. (2001). Cohort study of depressed mood during pregnancy and after childbirth. *British Medical Journal, 323,* 257–260.

Forehand, R., Biggar, H., and Kotchick, B.A. (1998). Cumulative risk across family stressors: Short- and long-term effects for adolescents. *Journal of Abnormal Child Psychology, 26,* 119–128.

Garber, J. (2006). Depression in children and adolescents: Linking risk research and prevention. *American Journal of Preventative Medicine, 31,* S104–S125.

Gaynes, B.N., Gavin, N., Meltzer-Brody S., Lohr, K.N., Swinson, T., Gartlehner, G., Brody, S., and Miller, W.C. (2005). *Perinatal Depression: Prevalence, Screening Accuracy, and Screening Outcomes.* (Evidence Report/Technology Assessment No. 119, AHRQ Publication No. 05-E006-2.) Rockville, MD: Agency for Healthcare Research and Quality.

Gelfand, D.M., Teti, D.M., Seiner, S.A., and Jameson, P.B. (1996). Helping mothers fight depression: Evaluation of a home-based intervention for depressed mothers and their infants. *Journal of Clinical Child Psychology, 24,* 406–422.

Gerdes, A.C., Hoza, B., Arnold, L.E., Pelham, W.E., Swanson, J.M., Wigal, T., and Jensen, P.S. (2007). Maternal depressive symptomatology and parenting behavior: Exploration of possible mediators. *Journal of Abnormal Child Psychology, 35*, 705–714.

Gilespie, C.F., and Nemeroff, C.B. (2007). Corticotropin-releasing factor and the psychobiology of early-life stress. *Current Directions in Psychological Science, 16*, 85–89.

Goodman, S.H., and Gotlib, I.H. (1999). Risk for psychopathology in the children of depressed mothers: A developmental model for understanding mechanisms of transmission. *Psychological Review, 106*, 458–490.

Gunnar, M.R., and Quevedo, K. (2007). The neurobiology of stress and development. In S.T. Fiske, A.E. Kazdin, and D.L. Schacter (Eds.), *Annual Review of Psychology, 58*, 145–174.

Hammen, C. (2002). Context of stress in families of children with depressed parents. In S.H. Goodman and I.H. Gotlib (Eds.), *Children of Depressed Parents: Mechanisms of Risk and Implications for Treatment* (pp. 175–202). Washington, DC: American Psychological Association.

Hariri, A.R., and Brown, S.M. (2006). Serotonin. *American Journal of Psychiatry, 163*, 12.

Hinshaw, S.P. (2008). Lessons from research on the developmental psychopathology of girls and women. *Journal of the American Academy of Child and Adolescent Psychiatry, 47*, 359–361.

Jaser, S.S., Langrock A.M., Keller G., Merchant, M.J., Benson, M.A., Reeslund, K., Champion, J.E., and Compas, B.E. (2005). Coping with the stress of parental depression II: Adolescent and parent reports of coping and adjustment. *Journal of Child and Adolescent Psychology, 34*, 193–205.

Joiner, T.E., Coyne, J.C., and Blalock, J. (1999). On the interpersonal nature of depression: Overview and synthesis. In T. Joiner and J.C. Coyne (Eds.), *The Interactional Nature of Depression: Advances in Interpersonal Approaches* (pp. 3–20). Washington, DC: American Psychological Association.

Kaminski, J.W., Valle, L.A., Filene, J.H., and Boyle, C.L. (2008). A meta-analytic review of components associated with parent training effectiveness. *Journal of Abnormal Child Psychology, 36*, 567–589.

Kazdin, A.E. (2005). *Parent Management Training: Treatment for Oppositional, Aggressive, and Antisocial Behavior in Children and Adolescents*. New York: Oxford University Press.

Kessler, R.C., Merikangas, K.R., and Wang, P.S. (2007). Prevalence, comorbidity, and service utilization for mood disorders in the United States at the beginning of the twenty-first century. *Annual Review of Clinical Psychology, 3*, 137–158.

Kessler, R.C., Zhao, S., Katz, S.J., Kouzis, A.C., Frank, R.G., Edlund, M., and Leaf, P. (1999). Past-year use of outpatient services for psychiatric problems in the National Comorbidity Survey. *American Journal of Psychiatry, 156*, 115–123.

Kingdon, J.W. (1995). *Agendas, Alternatives and Public Policies*. New York: Addison-Wesley Educational Publishers.

Knitzer, J., Theberge, S., and Johnson, K. (2008). *Reducing Maternal Depression and its Impact on Young Children: Toward a Responsive Early Childhood Policy Framework*. New York: Columbia University, National Center for Children in Poverty.

Kraemer, H.C., Kazdin, A.E., Offord, D.R., Kessler, R.C., Jensen, P.S., and Kupfer, D.J. (1997). Coming to terms with the terms of risks. *Archives of General Psychiatry, 54*, 337–343.

Kroenke, K. (2006). Minor depression: Midway between major depression and euthymia. *Annals of Internal Medicine, 144*, 528–530.

Lazear, K.J., Pires, S.A., Isaacs, M.R., Chaulk, P., and Huang, L. (2008). Depression among low-income women of color: Qualitative findings from cross-cultural focus groups. *Journal of Immigrant Minority Health, 10*, 127–133.

Lovejoy, M.C., Graczyk, P.A., O'Hare, E., and Neuman, G. (2000). Maternal depression and parenting behavior: A meta-analytic review. *Clinical Psychology Review, 20,* 561–592.

Luthar, S.S., and Zigler, E. (1991). Vulnerability and competence: A review of research on resilience in childhood. *American Journal of Orthopsychiatry, 61,* 6–22.

Luthar, S.S., Cicchetti, D., and Becker, B. (2000). The construct of resilience: A critical evaluation and guidelines for future work. *Child Development, 71,* 543–562.

Lyons-Ruth, K., Connell, D.B., Grunebaum, H.U., and Botein, S. (1990). Infants at social risk: Maternal depression and family support as mediators of infant development and security of attachment. *Child Development, 61,* 85–98.

Masten, A.S., Best, K.M., and Garmezy, N. (1990). Resilience and development: Contributions from the study of children who overcome adversity. *Development and Psychopathology, 2,* 425–444.

Masten, A.S., Hubbard, J.J., Gest, S.D., Tellegen, A., Garmezy, N., and Ramirez, M. (1999). Competence in the context of adversity: Pathways to resilience and maladaptation from childhood to late adolescence. *Development and Psychopathology, 11,* 143–169.

Miller, G.E., and Blackwell, E. (2006) Turning up the heat: Inflammation as a mechanism linking chronic stress, depression, and heart disease. *Current Directions in Psychological Science, 15,* 269–272.

Narrow, W.E., Regier, D.A., Rae, D.S., Manderscheid, R.W., and Locke, B.Z. (1993). Use of services by persons with mental and addictive disorders: Findings from the National Institute of Mental Health Epidemiologic Catchment Area Program. *Archives of General Psychiatry, 50,* 95–107.

Nelson, E.E., Leibenluft, E., McClure, E.B., and Pine, D.S. (2005). The social re-orientation of adolescence: A neuroscience perspective on the process and its relation to psychopathology. *Psychological Medicine, 35,* 163–174.

Parker, K.J., Buckmaster, C.L., Justus, K.R., Schatzberg, A.F., and Lyons, D.M. (2005). Mild early stress enhances prefrontal-dependent response inhibition in monkeys. *Biological Psychiatry, 57,* 848–855.

Regier, D.A., Narrow, W.E., Rae, D.S., Manderscheid, R.W., Locke, B.Z., and Goodwin, F.K. (1993). The de facto U.S. mental and addictive disorders service system: Epidemiologic catchment area prospective 1-year prevalence rates of disorders and services. *Archives of General Psychiatry, 50,* 85–94.

Reid, W.J., and Crisafulli, A. (1990). Marital discord and child behavior problems: A meta-analysis. *Journal of Abnormal Child Psychology, 18,* 105–117.

Romeo, R.D., and McEwen, B.S. (2006). Stress and the adolescent brain. *Annals of the New York Academy of Science, 1094,* 202–214.

Rutter, M. (1987). Psychosocial resilience and protective mechanisms. *American Journal of Orthopsychiatry, 57,* 316–331.

Rutter, M. (2000). Psychosocial influences: Critiques, findings, and research needs. *Development and Psychopathology, 12,* 375–405.

Rutter, M. (2007). Gene-environment interdependence. *Developmental Science, 10,* 12–18.

Rutter, M., Pickles, A., Murray, R., and Eaves, L. (2001). Testing hypotheses on specific environmental causal effects on behavior. *Psychological Bulletin, 127,* 291–324.

Sanders, M.R., Markie-Dadds, C., Tully, L.A., and Bor, W. (2000). The Triple P-Positive Parenting Program: A comparison of enhanced, standard, and self-directed behavioral family intervention for parents of children with early onset conduct problems. *Journal of Consulting and Clinical Psychology, 68,* 624–640.

Scantamburlo, G., Hansenne, M., Fuchs, S., Pitchot, W., Maréchal, P., Pequeux, C., Ansseau, M., and Legros, J.J. (2007). Plasma oxytocin levels and anxiety in patients with major depression. *Psychoneuroendocrinology, 32,* 407–410.

Seifer, R., Sameroff, A.J., Baldwin, C.P., and Baldwin, A. (1992). Child and family factors that ameliorate risk between 4 and 13 years of age. *Journal of the American Academy of Child and Adolescent Psychiatry*, *31*, 893–903.

Solantaus, T., and Toikka, S. (2006). The Effective Family Programme: Preventative services for the children of mentally ill parents in Finland. *International Journal of Mental Health Promotion*, *8*, 37–43.

Southwick, S.M., Vythilingam, M., and Charney D.S. (2005). The psychobiology of depression and resilience to stress: Implications for prevention and treatment. *Annual Review of Clinical Psychology*, *1*, 255–291.

Sroufe, L.A., and Rutter, M. (1984). The domain of developmental psychopathology. *Child Development*, *55*, 17–29.

Tronick, E.Z., and Gianino, A.F. (1986). The transmission of maternal disturbance to the infant. In E.Z. Tronick and T. Field (Eds.), *Maternal Depression and Infant Disturbance* (pp. 5–12). San Francisco: Jossey-Bass.

U.S. Preventive Services Task Force. (2002). Screening for depression: recommendations and rationale. *Annals of Internal Medicine*, *136*, 760–764.

Van den Bergh, B.R., Mulder, E.J.H., Mennes, M., and Glover, V. (2005). Antenatal maternal anxiety and stress and the neurobehavioural development of the fetus and child: Links and possible mechanisms. A review. *Neuroscience and Biobehavioral Reviews*, *29*, 237–258.

Weersing, V.R., and Weisz, J.R. (2002). Community clinic treatment of depressed youth: Benchmarking usual care against CBT clinical trials. *Journal of Consulting and Clinical Psychology*, *70*, 299–310.

Weissman, M.M., and Paykel, E.S. (1974). *The Depressed Woman: A Study of Social Relationships*. Chicago: University of Chicago Press.

Weisz, J.R., Jensen, A.L., and McLeod, B.D. (2005). Milestones and methods in the development and dissemination of child and adolescent psychotherapies: Review, commentary, and a new deployment-focused model. In E.D. Hibbs and P.S. Jensen (Eds.), *Psychosocial Treatments for Child and Adolescent Disorders: Empirically Based Strategies for Clinical Practice* (2nd ed., pp. 9–39). Washington, DC: American Psychological Association.

Whooley, M.A., Avins, A.L., Miranda, J., and Browner, W.S. (1997). Case-finding instruments for depression. Two questions are as good as many. *Journal of General Internal Medicine*, *12*, 439–445.

3

The Etiology of Depression

SUMMARY

Timing and Course of Depression

- Age of onset of major depression may have both clinical and etiological implications. Clinically, earlier age of onset is associated with a worse course of depression with greater chances of recurrence, chronicity, and impairment. Etiologically, first onset of depression at different ages (e.g., childhood, adolescent, adult, and older adult) may reflect somewhat different causal factors.
- Many individuals may experience a single, major depressive episode following an acute stressor and recover with little implication for future vulnerability. However, most (50–80 percent) who have one significant episode will have recurrent episodes and intermittent subclinical symptoms, with the risk of recurrence progressively increasing with each episode of major depression.

Biological Factors

- Genetic, neurological, hormonal, immunological, and neuroendocrinological mechanisms appear to play a role in the development of major depression, and many of these factors center around reactions to stressors and the processing of emotional information. Etiological processes may be modified by gender and developmental factors.

73

Environmental and Personal Vulnerabilities

- Etiological models for depression are largely diathesis-stress models in which stressful experiences trigger depression in those who may be vulnerable due to biological and psychosocial characteristics and circumstances.
- Environmental stressors associated with depression include acute life events, chronic stress, and childhood exposure to adversity. Personal vulnerabilities associated with depression include cognitive, interpersonal, and personality factors.
- Biological, environmental, and personal vulnerabilities interact to contribute to the development of depression and also may be affected by depressive states in a bidirectional process.

Co-Occurring Disorders

- Depression rarely occurs independent of other psychological disorders, including anxiety, substance abuse, behavioral, and personality disorders, as well as other medical illnesses. The presence of co-occurring psychological and medical disorders exacerbates the clinical and social consequences of depression, and makes it more challenging to treat.

Resilience and Protective Factors

- Certain biological, environmental, and personal factors have also been associated with the protection from or the overcoming of risk factors and adverse conditions related to the development of depression.

The purpose of this chapter is to review what is known or suspected about the causes of depression. Fundamentally, such depressive symptoms as sad mood, pessimism, and lethargy, are universal human experiences and are considered normal reactions to the struggles, disappointments, and losses of everyday life. However, for some individuals, the intensity and persistence of depressive symptoms are not typical, and a challenge for researchers has been to understand why some individuals experience marked and enduring depressive reactions and others do not. This chapter discusses some of the characteristics of individuals that may make them vulnerable, as well as the features of environments that are particularly likely to provoke depression. The chapter also emphasizes the interplay between persons and environments—the ways in which, for example, stressors may provoke depression but depression further influences social environments, often a vicious cycle that promotes chronic or recurrent depression. A further aspect of this bidirectional influence is the frequent co-occurrence of depression and other disorders, which may complicate its course and treatment. It is noted that some individuals are remarkably resilient in the face of adversity, and a further challenge to the field is to understand such processes.

The first topic to address is that not all depressions are alike; therefore, different etiological models and perspectives are likely to apply to different expressions of depressive disorder.

TIMING AND COURSE OF DEPRESSIVE DISORDERS

Age of onset of major depressive disorder and lifetime course are two factors that have etiological as well as treatment and outcome implications.

Age of First Onset

First onset can occur at any time. Diagnoses of childhood depression are relatively rare (Birmaher et al., 1996; Egger and Angold, 2006), although many preadolescents including preschoolers have significant internalizing symptoms of dysphoria and distress (e.g., Cole et al., 2002; DuBois et al., 1995; Gross et al., 2006). Most diagnosed depressions first appear in adolescence and early adulthood (Andrade et al., 2003; Burke et al., 1990; Kessler et al., 2005)—especially among those born in more recent decades (e.g., Kessler et al., 2003). For example, in recent community studies up to one-third of adolescents met criteria for major depressive disorder (Kessler and Walters, 1998; Lewinsohn, Rohde, and Seeley, 1998).

Age of first onset has both clinical and etiological implications. Clinically, earlier age of onset of depression is generally thought to be associated with a worse course of depression, with greater chances of recurrence, chronicity, and impairment in role functioning (e.g., Hollon et al., 2006; Zisook et al., 2004). Those with adolescent-onset depression include a significant proportion among both treatment and community samples who go on to have recurrent episodes and significant impairment (e.g., Hammen, Brennan, and Keenan-Miller, 2008; Lewinsohn et al., 1999, 2000; Pine et al., 1998; Weissman et al., 1999a).

Evidence increasingly suggests that childhood, adolescent, adult, and older adult first onsets may reflect different causal factors. Childhood depressions may be a mixture of subgroups: those with true genetically familial early-onset recurrent depression; those exposed to significant psychosocial adversity, such as abuse, parental disorder, criminality, and family disruption who continue to experience social maladjustment and other problem behaviors but not depression into adulthood; and some with eventual bipolar disorder (e.g., Harrington et al., 1990; Weissman et al., 1999b).

Adolescent-onset depressions are noteworthy for several factors. One is that increasing rates of adolescent depression in recent years (e.g., Kessler et al., 2003) imply, among other things, that the etiology is substantially psychosocial, with significant cultural shifts in recent decades that have created stressful experiences and reduced resources and contribute to depressive experiences (e.g., Seligman et al., 1995). Another issue is the enormous divergence in rates of depression for girls and boys beginning in adolescence (e.g., reviewed in Hankin and Abramson, 2001). The dramatic increases in girls' rates of depression compared with boys' rates clearly requires etiological models that can explain such differences. For example, different models emphasize genetic (e.g., Silberg, Rutter, and Eaves, 2001), hormonal (e.g., Angold et al., 1999), stress exposure and stress processes (e.g., Rudolph, 2002; Shih et al., 2006), cultural shaping of values and vulnerabilities (Seligman et al., 1995), and gender-based coping strategies (e.g., Nolen-Hoeksema, 1991).

Perinatal Depression

The childbearing years in general, and those around pregnancy in particular, have attracted special attention with respect to the occurrence of depression and its potential effects on children's development. A large majority of women experience mild "blues" following delivery of an infant, and between 10 and 20 percent of new mothers experience clinical depression lasting anywhere from several weeks to a year. A smaller proportion, less than 0.5 percent, experience acute psychosis associated with the depression. A recent large-scale epidemiological survey that examined rates of diagnoses in nonpregnant women compared with past-year pregnant women found no differences overall in mood disorders (Vesga-Lopez et al., 2008). However, the rates of major depression were higher in postpartum women compared with nonpregnant women. For all women pregnant in the past year, their depression was associated with not being married, exposure to trauma and stressful life events in the past year, and overall poor health.

The dramatic hormonal changes a woman experiences during and after pregnancy have focused much attention on the biological and hormonal etiological factors of postpartum depression. However, there is widespread agreement that postpartum major depression is not distinct in terms of etiology from depression at other times. In addition to biological risk factors, social stressors, family composition, levels of social support, and especially poorer economic circumstances all contribute to the risk of developing postpartum depression (Bloch et al., 2005; Crouch, 1999; Grigoriadis and

Romans, 2006; Hayes, Roberts, and Davare, 2000; Robertson et al., 2004; Segre et al., 2007).

Although relatively little research has focused on paternal postpartum depression, the few studies that have report rates among new fathers as lower but not too dissimilar to that of new mothers. Paulson, Dauber, and Lieferman (2006), reporting on depression among two-parent households in a national random sample of over 5,000 families, found rates of depression at 14 percent for mothers and 10 percent for fathers. Fathers' elevated rates of depressive symptoms and disorders after the birth of a child are associated with stressful adjustments and the quality of their relationship with the mother; mothers' depression is also a significant predictor of increased depression in postpartum fathers (Huang and Warner, 2005; Kim and Swain, 2007).

Course of Depression

The course of depression may shed light on both treatment and prevention concerns and etiological issues. Some individuals may experience a single, major depressive episode in response to an acute stressor, never seek treatment, and, except for impairment associated with the acute episode, recover with little implication for future vulnerability. However, many others, especially those with sufficient distress and impairment who seek (or should seek) treatment, will have recurrent episodes and possibly significant residual symptoms (e.g., Judd, 1997; Judd et al., 1998; Keller, 1985). Judd (1997) found that 80 percent of patients had at least one recurrence (with an average of 4 episodes) over a few years' follow-up, and many others had significant even if nondiagnosable symptoms. In an epidemiological study of first episode of depression, more than 50 percent had a recurrence over the multiyear follow-up (Eaton et al., 2008). Moreover, there is evidence that the risk for recurrence progressively increases with each episode of major depression—and decreases as the period of recovery is longer (Solomon et al., 2000). Episodes come closer together over time (Bockting et al., 2006; Kessing et al., 2004; Solomon et al., 2000). As Judd et al. (1998) have documented, impaired functioning in work, family, social, and marital roles persists to a considerable extent even when the individual does not meet the full criteria for a major depressive episode. Thus, recurrent depressive disorders and continuing symptoms are likely to be disruptive of lives and families.

Early-onset recurrent depression may reflect a genetic etiology (Holmans et al., 2007), but its progressive nature has also been speculated to indicate a neurobiological process in which early and successive episodes of depression alter the brain and neuroregulatory processes (e.g., Post, 1992). The "kindling" model postulates that successive episodes change the brain in ways that reduce the threshold at which stressors may trigger a further episode—possibly to the point of autonomous episodes of depression. A review of studies of stress-depression associations in first and later episodes found some support for the model (Monroe and Harkness, 2005). Truly longitudinal within-person studies to test this hypothesis are quite rare, although one such investigation by Kendler, Thornton, and Gardner (2000) studied nearly 2,400 female twins over 4 waves separated by at least 13 months each. They found evidence of a diminishing association between life events and depression as the person experienced increasing numbers of episodes (up to about 6–8 episodes). They suggested that whether the involved mechanism is biological or psychological, it appears to occur intensively in the first few episodes after initial onset, and then the kindling process slows or stops. The stress-depression relationship not only may vary over time with increasing numbers of episodes but also may differ according to genetic risk for depression (Kendler, Thornton, and Gardner, 2001).

Mild, chronic depression—termed dysthymic disorder—may also be very disruptive and enduring. It may be highly predictive of major depressive episodes, and, especially if its onset is early in life, it is associated with slow recovery and high rates of relapse or continuing symptoms (Klein, Shankman, and Rose, 2006). Early-onset dysthymic patients had relatively high rates of poor-quality early home environments (Lizardi et al., 1995) and a relatively elevated exposure to early adverse conditions, including physical and sexual abuse, as well as ongoing stressful life conditions (Riso, Miyaktake, and Thase, 2002). Chronic depression is also associated with higher rates of familial depression than is episodic major depression (Klein et al., 2004), which suggests an etiological subtype.

Key features of the course of depression have significant implications for families. Most depressions first occur in adolescence and young adulthood, periods during which critical developmental accomplishments may be disrupted, such as academic attainment and job planning, peer integration and acquisition of effective social skills, and romantic relationship formation. Obviously, childbearing years are affected as well. Young people who are depressed may select into, or default into, problematic environments that are stressful and may further overwhelm impaired coping capabilities. Depression may become recurrent for biological as well as social and psychological reasons, and thus it may become harder to manage and treat. All members of the family are affected, and children are the most vulnerable to the negative impact of parental depression. Another important observation that comes from this evidence is that prevention programs may be particularly valuable and are probably best targeted at those most vulnerable to depression: those with extensive family history, those with symptoms of depression, and those with multiple risk factors for depression (e.g., poverty, exposure to violence, social isolation).

BIOLOGICAL PERSPECTIVES ON THE ETIOLOGY OF DEPRESSION

A complex set of biological processes has been implicated in the etiology and course of depression—although such research has not always clarified whether such processes are underlying causal factors, correlates, or consequences of depression. These include interrelated mechanisms of genetic vulnerabilities, brain structure and function, neurotransmitter and neuroendocrine processes, and immune system processes. Discussion of the details and transactions among these processes given the vastly expanding research literature in recent years is beyond the scope of this report (but see Thase, 2008, for a review). Advances have been made in each of these areas as well as in studies of interactions among these biological mechanisms and environmental and personal factors that confer increased risk for depression. In light of the heterogeneity of depression, it is not surprising that the research evidence to date has failed to converge on a single set of biological processes that is related to the onset and course of depression. However, evidence supports the role of several important aspects of functioning in the brain, the central nervous system, and the periphery. A theme throughout these various lines of research is the importance of considering the interaction between biology and exposure to stress, particularly chronic or recurring stress, in the etiology and course of depression.

Genetic Vulnerability

It is well known that depression runs in families, a phenomenon implicating both genetic and environmental processes. A review of twin studies finds that about one-third of the risk for major depression in adults derives from genetic differences between individuals (Kendler et al., 2006; Sullivan, Neale, and Kendler, 2000). This figure is substantially lower than for some other psychological disorders, such as schizophrenia or bipolar disorder (McGuffin et al., 2003; Sullivan, Kendler, and Neale, 2003). Similarly, the risk of developing major depression increases about 2.5–3 times for those who have a first-degree relative with depression, whereas having a highly threatening life event increases risk from 5 to 16 times in a few months after the event (Kendler, Karkowski, and Prescott, 1998; Sullivan, Neale, and Kendler, 2000). Genetic influences appear to be modified by gender and developmental phase, and they may influence not only internal biological and psychological characteristics but also the nature of the person's effects on the environment (Kendler et al., 2001, 2006; Kendler and Karkowski-Shuman, 1997; Kendler, Gardner, and Prescott, 2003; Kendler, Gardner, and Lichtenstein, 2008).

Several genetic polymorphisms have been linked to increased risk of depression in response to stress. Foremost among these are genes of the serotonin system (5-HT). The neurotransmitter serotonin exerts effects on a broad range of physiological functions, such as emotions, sleep, circadian rhythm, thermoregulation, appetite, aggression, sexual behavior, pain sensitivity, and sensorimotor reactivity (e.g., Lucki, 1998; Neumeister, Young, and Strastny, 2004). Deficits in the central 5-HT system, such as reduced 5-HT concentrations, impaired uptake function of the 5-HT transporter, altered 5-HT receptor binding, and tryptophan depletion, have been linked to a number of psychological problems and psychiatric disorders, including depression (Neumeister, Young, and Strastny, 2004).

A number of studies have investigated the role of genetic polymorphisms in the serotonin-related genes in the etiology of depression. Currently, the serotonin transporter (5-HTTLPR) gene is the most promising one. Importantly, Caspi et al. (2003) and Kendler et al. (2005) found that individuals with one or two copies of the short allele of 5-HTTLPR experienced more depressive symptoms and higher rates of major depressive disorder in response to stressful life events than individuals who are homozygous for the long allele. These studies are especially noteworthy for their indication that genetic effects on depression may be observed only under conditions of exposure to stressors (see reviews by Uher and McGuffin, 2008; Zammit and Owen, 2006). The effects of the serotonin transporter polymorphism implicated in depression in response to stressful life events may be manifested behaviorally as dysfunctional emotionality in response to stress.

As an illustration of the complex transactions among brain functions, genes, and neurotransmitter systems, Hariri et al. (2005) used neuroimaging techniques to explore how individuals with different polymorphisms of the 5-HTTLPR gene responded to an amygdala activation task involving perception of fearful and angry faces. They found that normal, never-depressed individuals who had the short allele form of the 5-HTTLPR gene showed amygdala hyperreactivity in response to the emotion-arousing stimuli compared with other groups. The results suggest that the serotonin transporter polymorphism is linked to the brain's processing of emotional threat information. The study is noteworthy for helping to shed further light on neurobiological mechanisms by which stressful environmental experiences eventuate in depression in some people but not others.

In addition to the 5-HTTLPR polymorphisms, numerous other serotonin system genes have been studied as well as those known to affect the functioning of the hypothalamic-pituitary-adrenal (HPA) axis and other brain regions. Meta-analytic studies of candidate genes and molecular genetic genome-wide association studies are increasing throughout the world, but it has been noted by a recent large-sample genome-wide association study of the high heritable human trait of height that they are likely to show what has long been predicted in quantitative genetics: Any relevant

gene will have very small effects, and summing risk across multiple identified genes will yield limited explication of the effects (Weedon et al., 2008).
Thus, in view of relatively modest overall heritability of depression, strong
environmental effects, and tiny effects of individual genes, it is unlikely
that genetic testing will prove to be an effective way to identify those at
risk for depression. It has been speculated that "old-fashioned" methods
of identifying risk through individual differences in a family history of
depression or the personality trait of neuroticism will prove to be superior
to molecular genetics (personal communication, Kenneth Kendler, Medical College of Virginia and Virginia Commonwealth University, August 8,
2008). That said, continuing analysis of genetic correlates of depression will
doubtlessly contribute valuable information to fuller understanding of the
neurobiological mechanisms underlying depression, and it may play a role
in the development of pharmacotherapeutic agents.

A final note about genetic contributions to depression is the important
acknowledgment not only that genetic factors have an impact on internal
depressogenic processes but also that gene-environment correlations contribute to outcomes. For example, genetic factors may influence a depressed
person's parenting styles as well as the offspring's heritable traits, so that
the child's genotype and rearing environment are correlated (D'Onofrio
et al., 2005, 2006, 2007; Rice, Harold, and Thapar, 2005). Similarly,
youth with particular heritable characteristics evoke reactions from others and select or create experiences that are congruent with their heritable
characteristics—processes that might increase the likelihood of depressive
outcomes under relevant conditions. Although critically important to full
understanding of genetic influences there is relatively sparse research on
such mechanisms (personal communication, Sara Jaffe, King's College London, August 4, 2008).

Neuroendocrine Functioning

A dominant model of the neurobiology of depression that has emerged in
recent years emphasizes the underlying dysregulation of the body's response
to stress, involving the neuroendocrine system and brain responses (Thase,
2008). Key components are the HPA axis and the related corticotrophin-
releasing hormone (CRH) and locus coeruleus-norepinephrine (LC-NE)
systems, which include limbic and cortical pathways bidirectionally inter-
connected through various neurotransmitter and hormonal circuits (Boyce
and Ellis, 2005; Meyer, Chrousos, and Gold, 2001). The primary glucocorticoid hormone is cortisol, which triggers a cascade of functions that
are adaptive in the acute phases of response to stress and which normally
resolve quickly through inhibitory feedback processes in the HPA axis.
However, failure to normalize, resulting in sustained high cortisol, has

deleterious effects, giving rise to physiological changes thought to promote a variety of illnesses.

Depression has been linked with elevated cortisol and related neurohormones. Numerous studies have indicated higher levels of cortisol and abnormalities in cortisol regulation among depressed compared with nondepressed individuals (e.g., reviewed in Plotsky, Owens, and Nemeroff, 1998; Ribeiro et al., 1993). Furthermore, depressed patients show slower recovery of cortisol levels in response to psychological stress than controls (see meta-analysis by Burke et al., 2005). Individuals who display evidence of abnormal cortisol regulation even after treatment are more likely to relapse and generally have a poorer clinical prognosis than patients whose cortisol functions returned to normal after treatment (e.g., Ribeiro et al., 1993). It appears that sustained hypercortisolism damages the stress system, including death of cells in the hippocampus (Sapolsky, 1996) with generalized effects on the circuits underlying emotion regulation.

It is hypothesized that both genetic and environmental factors account for individual differences in how individuals respond to (and recover from) HPA system activation. Genetic differences in species of animals and nonhuman primates have been shown to be associated with differences in emotional behavior and glucocorticoid responses to stress (e.g., Boyce and Ellis, 2005; Meyer, Chrousos, and Gold, 2001). Human genetic polymorphisms in the glucocorticoid receptor (GR) have been hypothesized as a source of impaired negative feedback regulation contributing to hyperactivity of the HPA-axis in depression (e.g., Holsboer, 2000). Evidence is emerging of GR polymorphisms associated with increased risk of developing major depression (van Rossum et al., 2006) and differences in response to treatment for depression (e.g., Brouwer et al., 2006; van Rossum et al., 2006).

Adverse environmental factors, especially those associated with early childhood development (or even prenatal exposure), have attracted considerable interest as possible contributors to abnormal biological stress regulation. Gold, Goodwin, and Chrousos (1988) speculated that brain circuits associated with stress reactions may have been sensitized as a result of early, acute exposure to stressors, so that in adulthood, depressive reactions to stress may be readily activated by even mild or symbolic representations of early stress precipitants. Evidence supports the impact of prenatal and postnatal stress, as well as disruptions of the parent-child bond, on abnormalities of HPA functioning in animal and human subjects (reviewed in Heim and Nemeroff, 2001; Kaufman et al., 2000; Meyer, Chrousos, and Gold, 2001; Plotsky, Owens, and Nemeroff, 1998). Meaney, Szyf, and Seckl (2007) also propose epigenetic processes by which maternal adversities affect fetal development mediated by adrenal hormone activity, and glucocorticoid levels program gene expression in the direction of impaired HPA function and health in offspring. While not specific to depression, the effects of environmental effects on gene expression in offspring have important implications for depression.

Limited but increasing evidence draws links between early adversity, abnormalities of the HPA, CRH, and LC-NE systems, and depression. For example, Essex et al. (2002) assessed cortisol levels in 4.5-year-olds and found that children who had been exposed to maternal stress both in infancy and concurrently had significantly higher levels of cortisol than nonstressed children or those exposed to either but not both periods of maternal stress. Moreover, the children with elevated cortisol had higher rates of behavioral and emotional symptoms (especially internalizing symptoms) approximately 2 years later. Although not specifically about depression, the results are consistent with the idea that early stress exposure predicts elevated cortisol when stress occurs later in life, and the pattern is predictive of later symptomatology (see also Heim et al., 2000, on early abuse experiences, depression, and adult HPA axis functioning). Preventing adverse environmental factors in children warrants further attention.

Immune System Processes and Depression

Spurred in part by the evidence of the strong association between depression and coronary heart disease, researchers have begun to examine the potential role of the immune system, and particularly proinflammatory cytokines, in the link between stress and depression (e.g., Danese et al., 2008; Miller and Blackwell, 2006). Recent models have proposed that chronic stress activates the immune system in a way that leads to inflammation, and that chronic inflammation in turn leads to symptoms of depression as well as pathological processes underlying heart disease (Miller and Blackwell, 2006). Cytokines are signaling molecules that coordinate inflammation in response to pathogens and include interleukin-1β, interleukin-6 (IL-6), and tumor necrosis factor-α. Among other functions, they direct white blood cells toward infections, signaling them to divide and activating their killing mechanisms. Downstream products of this process, including C-reactive protein (CRP), a molecule produced by the liver in response to IL-6, are used as an index of the inflammatory response.

Although the directions of these effects are yet to be disentangled, evidence indicates that chronic stress is associated with increased levels of both CRP and depression. Levels of IL-6 and CRP are elevated in individuals exposed to chronic stress (Segerstrom and Miller, 2004). Chronic stressors may prime the immune system to make a heightened response to stress. Alternatively, chronic stress may interfere with the capacity of the immune system to return to baseline after termination of a stressor, perhaps due to dysregulation of the HPA response and the production of glucocorticoids in response to stress (Miller and Blackwell, 2006). The inflammatory response may also contribute to symptoms of depression by triggering sickness behaviors, including disruptions in appetite, sleep, and social activity. These processes may be involved in depression in general, or only in those individuals in which depression is comorbid with a medical condition, such as heart disease. Alternatively, depression may be involved in provoking inflammation. A recent meta-analysis reports some support for three causal models: depression to inflammation, inflammation to depression, and bidirectional associations (Howren, Lamkin, and Suls, 2009). Further research using prospective longitudinal designs is needed to clarify the directions of the relations among stress, depression, and inflammation.

Evidence from one longitudinal study has shed some additional light on the possible role of inflammatory processes in depression. Danese et al. (2008) examined the role of early life stress (childhood maltreatment) and later depression and inflammatory response processes (as measured by levels of CRP) as part of the longitudinal study of a birth cohort in Dunedin, New Zealand, followed into young adulthood. Specifically, they were able to compare young adults with no history of childhood maltreatment and no current depression, those with current depression and no maltreatment history, those with a positive history of maltreatment but no current depression, and those with both current depression and a history of maltreatment. It appeared that depressed individuals with a history of maltreatment were more likely to have high levels of CRP when compared to depressed-only individuals. Thus, maltreatment history seems to be an important modifier of the association between depression and inflammatory markers.

Although in its early stages, research on inflammatory responses suggests an additional biological process that may help to explain the link between stress and depression. And inflammatory processes may be especially important in elucidating important medical comorbidities of depression, most notably coronary heart disease.

ENVIRONMENTAL AND PERSONAL CONTRIBUTORS TO DEPRESSION

Environmental Factors

Depression is commonly construed as a reaction to negative environmental circumstances. Etiological models are largely diathesis-stress perspectives. A diathesis is a risk factor or vulnerability process, such as people's biological, personality, or cognitive characteristics, that accounts for individual differences in how they respond to similar stressful challenges. In order to illustrate key points—as well as to draw attention to circumstances that help to identify populations at particular risk for depression—in this section we focus on three kinds of stressful (environmental) conditions: (1) acute negative life events, (2) chronically stressful life circumstances, and (3) exposure to adversity in childhood.

Acute Life Events

A major risk factor for depression is the experience of undesirable, negative life events. There is ample evidence that most major depressive episodes are triggered by stressful life events (see reviews by Hammen, 2005; Kessler, 1997; Mazure, 1998). According to Mazure (1998) recent stressors were 2.5 times more likely in depressed patients compared with controls, and, in community samples, 80 percent of depressed cases were preceded by major negative life events. Most assessment methods survey the occurrence of stressors within the past 3 to 6 months in relation to depression, but Kendler, Karkowski, and Prescott (1998) found that the great majority of major depression onsets occurred within the first month after a significant negative life event. There is some evidence of a generally linear association between severity and number of negative events and the probability of depression onset (Kendler, Karkowski, and Prescott, 1998). However, the "severity" of the impact of an acute life event depends not only on the actual circumstances of the event but also on its subjective meaning to the individual. Thus, one person might become depressed only under extreme conditions of loss and deprivation, but another might become depressed because his or her personal vulnerabilities lead to exaggeration of the meaning of an acute event that is objectively minor.

It has been generally observed throughout the ages that depression is most likely to occur following the loss of something important to the sense of self, such as the loss of significant others or relationships or of a sense of worth and competence. Interpersonal losses or "exits" have been shown to be more associated with depression than with other forms of disorder (Tennant, 2002; see also Kendler et al., 1995)—perhaps especially for women.

For immigrant and refugee populations, experiences of loss and isolation are pervasive (Heilemann, Coffey-Love, and Frutos, 2004). Many immigrants and refugees experience lengthy or permanent separation from immediate and extended family. Loss of home, property, cultural ties, and customs may be significant for these communities. For many refugees and immigrants, these losses are also experienced in the context of the trauma of migration or the trauma of war. The impact of these experiences on the psychological functioning of individuals in these communities is profound. Rates of depression are reportedly high among these groups (Aguilar-Gaxiola et al., 2008). Owing to both biological and socialization processes, women are likely to be more attuned to and concerned about others' reactions to them, as well as reactive to the needs of others (e.g., Cyranowski et al., 2000). This seems to be particularly the case for immigrant women. For example, Hiott and colleagues (2006) reported that immigrant women may experience significant losses of social support and a sense of isolation on moving to a different country, and this loss may be manifested in a grieving process. The isolation may be related to unfulfilled relationships, or it may result from separation from or loss of family. These findings suggest that conflictual family relationships, unmet expectations in familial relationships, and isolation may be risk factors for depression in immigrant women who reside in the United States (Shatell et al., 2008). Thus, women may be especially likely to be depressed in response to stressful social loss experiences and even to the negative experiences of those in their social networks.

Gender differences in depression may be accounted for in part by women's greater exposure to interpersonal life events, as well as their greater likelihood, compared with men, of reacting to such events with depression. Results of studies of adults have been mixed with regard to whether or not women experience more overall recent stressors (e.g., Kendler, Thornton, and Prescott, 2001; McGonagle and Kessler, 1990; Spangler et al., 1996), but several studies have found that adolescent females have higher levels of exposure to recent stressors than do males (Ge et al., 1994; Shih et al., 2006). Moreover, several studies have shown that at comparable levels of acute stressors, women had higher levels of depressive symptoms than did men (Maciejewski, Prigerson, and Mazure, 2001; Rudolph and Hammen, 1999; Shih et al., 2006; van Os and Jones, 1999). Gender differences in exposure and reactivity may also reflect women's higher levels of certain diatheses, such as neuroticism or ruminative response styles, and meaning attached to interpersonal circumstances. In general, however, the risk factors for depression in men are likely to be very similar to those of women, involving complex interactions among environmental and neurobiological factors at different developmental stages (Kendler, Gardner, and Prescott, 2002, 2006). However, examination of gender differences in mechanisms underlying depressive responses to stress is sparse.

Although acute stress may precipitate depression in vulnerable individuals, the relationship is bidirectional: Those with depression or a history of depression experience significantly more acute stressors than those with no depression. This pattern ("stress generation"; Hammen, 1991b) applies particularly to events that are at least partly caused by the characteristics or behaviors of the person, such as interpersonal conflicts (reviewed in Hammen, 2006). One of the true calamities of depression is the vicious cycle of stress-depression-stress-depression that portends recurring or chronic depression.

Chronic Stress

Acute, episodic life events tell only part of the depression story. Another source of depression—although not as commonly studied—is exposure to enduring, long-term stressful circumstances. Many studies of stress-depression associations have not adequately distinguished between the effects of ongoing and acute stressors (e.g., Brown and Harris, 1978; Caspi et al., 2003), and failure to do so makes it difficult to fully explicate the mechanisms by which stressors have their effects on depression. An important feature of chronic stress, as with acute stress, is the bidirectional effect of stressful chronic conditions and depression on each other. The strains of poverty or unemployment or displacement in the case of immigrants and refugees, for example, may trigger depression, but depression erodes the individual's ability to cope with or change his or her circumstances.

Another notable feature of chronic stress is that for many individuals there are multiple, related areas of chronic stress. Consider, for example, the association of several demographic predictors of major depression. Hasin et al. (2005) found that a major depressive episode was associated with being female, having low income, and being widowed, divorced, or separated. In addition, low educational attainment and being unemployed, disabled, or a homemaker are also associated with major depression (e.g., Kessler et al., 2003). Commonly, many of these conditions co-occur, with low educational attainment, low income, and disadvantaged work status related to each other, and being a widowed, divorced, or separated woman is likely to be associated with lower income.

A specific example of a chronically stressful condition amplified by co-occurring adverse conditions is single-mother status. Single mothers have been found to have higher rates of major depression than married mothers (e.g., Davies, Avison, and McApline, 1997; Wang, 2004), especially for separated or divorced compared with never-married mothers (Afifi, Cox, and Enns, 2006). Two large-scale studies have shown that the association between single-parent status and depression is entirely or largely mediated by higher chronic and acute stress and low social support (Cairney et al., 2003; Targosz et al., 2003). Yet the role of chronic stressors is neither simple nor straightforward. Lone mothers have higher risk of depression not only because of the presence of higher levels of chronic social stressors compared with two-parent families or even single parents residing with extended family but also because of their lower socioeconomic position. Furthermore, socioeconomic position might moderate the relationship between social stress and depression. For example, Barrett and Turner (2005) reported that among those with higher socioeconomic position, the adverse impact of racial discrimination and recent life events were more marked than that seen for those with lower socioeconomic position.

Low socioeconomic position is the source of a host of chronic stressors, including chronic strain and uncertainty surrounding a lack of adequate financial and other instrumental resources necessary to make ends meet (Malik et al., 2007; Muntaner et al., 2004). Given that racial and ethnic minorities are overrepresented among low-income populations, another chronic stressor that has been examined extensively in relation to depression is racial discrimination (Gee et al., 2007). While racial and other forms of discrimination are stressors, and, depending on the type of discrimination, such as racial, gender, age, or even social class, they can be either chronic or acute stressors (Banks and Kohn-Wood, 2007) and can increase risk of depression as such. Discrimination, however, can also impact beliefs, self-concept, and coping in ways that increase risk for mood disorders, including depression (Gee et al., 2007).

A number of institutional and sociocultural barriers are responsible for causing and maintaining existing disparities in access to and quality of mental health services received by minority groups. A succinct summary of the complex constellation of barriers is that "disparities result from ongoing interactions among factors at the levels of the health care environment, health care organization, community, provider, and person throughout the course of the depression development and treatment-seeking process (Chin et al., 2007)" (Van Voorhees et al., 2007, pp. 160S–161S). Social exclusion, which has played a key role in rendering these populations disproportionately vulnerable to and affected by incidence of depression, extends its adverse impact by limiting the engagement of and treatment in these historically unserved and underserved communities (Aguilar-Gaxiola et al., 2008). These groups' isolation from mainstream society because of linguistic barriers, geographic isolation, history of oppression, racism, discrimination, poverty, and immigration status plays a key role in creating and perpetuating their social exclusion and challenges to receiving treatment.

The environment can act as a source of chronic stressors as well. Extensive research has been devoted to the area of residential neighborhoods and mental well-being (Muntaner et al., 2004; O'Campo, Salmon, and Burke, 2009; O'Campo and Yonas, 2005). While not the only context or environment known to influence mental well-being—workplace organization and characteristics, for example, have also been studied in relation to major mental disorders—residential neighborhoods have been shown to be the source of multiple stressors, including physical incivilities (such as trash, graffiti), high levels of noise, traffic, crime, and delinquency, to name a few (O'Campo, Salmon, and Burke, 2009; Rajaratnam et al., 2008). These stressors should be considered to contribute to the risk of depression independently of, and may even interact with, any family or individual stressors that may place individuals at risk, including but not limited to economic strain and family and parenting stress (Cutrona, Wallace, and

Wesner, 2006; Rajaratnam et al., 2008). In a randomized trial in which residents residing in neighborhoods characterized by concentrated poverty were given the opportunity to move to higher income neighborhoods, those who moved experienced declines in mental health problems, including depression, supporting the importance of residential context in shaping mental well-being (Del Conte and Kling, 2001; Goering et al., 1999). Efforts to prevent depression should focus not only on individuals and families but also on those larger structural interventions that can make profound differences (e.g., alleviating poverty, moving to a better neighborhood).

Finally, brief mention should be made of stressful parenting circumstances and their contribution to depression. Many parents are challenged by infants' and children's medical illnesses, developmental disabilities, and psychological disturbances, and the stress associated with such circumstances may result in depression. For example, a meta-analysis of 18 studies of mothers of children with and without developmental disabilities found that the former had higher rates of elevated symptoms of depression, falling above suggested clinical cutoffs compared with mothers of children without disabilities (29 versus 19 percent) (Singer, 2006). A further review of a broad array of samples, including mothers with children with mental retardation, autism, and other forms of developmental delay, found similar rates of elevated depressive symptoms and also noted a limited number of studies that reported on depressive diagnoses (Bailey et al., 2007). While limited in number, the findings suggest that depressive diagnoses were more frequent among mothers with disabled children. The study also noted that higher rates of depression were associated with multiple stressors in the family: higher levels of mother-reported stress, less effective coping styles, poorer health, low family support or cohesion, and presence of more than one child with a disability. Similarly, custodial care of children by grandparents (including both three-generation and "skipped-generation" households) is well-known to be associated with elevated depression symptoms and increased medical problems (e.g., Blustein, Chan, and Guanais, 2004; Hughes et al., 2007). Such chronically stressful circumstances are often compounded by low income, disadvantaged social status, and grandchildren with special needs (Blustein, Chan, and Guanais, 2004). Adolescent mothers are another group known to be at substantial risk for significant depression, often compounded by multiple chronic stressors such as low income, relationship difficulties, and reduced social support (Panzarine, Slater, and Sharps, 1995; Reid and Meadows-Oliver, 2007).

Exposure to Early Adversity

In addition to recent negative events and chronically stressful conditions, increasing evidence focuses on the link between childhood exposure to adversity and the development of depression in adolescence or adulthood. One research strategy studies associations between a single specific experience, such as sexual abuse or physical or emotional maltreatment, and depression. There is ample evidence from mostly retrospective community and clinical studies of a significant association between childhood sexual or physical abuse and adult depression particularly among women (e.g., Brown et al., 1999; Kendler et al., 2000; MacMillan et al., 2001) and similar results from prospective studies (e.g., Bifulco et al., 1998; Brown and Harris, 1993). Some studies suggest that abuse experiences are especially predictive of chronic or recurrent depression (Bifulco et al., 2002a; Lizardi et al., 1995). However, several studies suggest that physical and sexual abuse are related to diverse adult psychological disorders, not specifically to depression. Many of the studies have not distinguished among the specific types of abuse, nor have they controlled for factors in the environment that are correlated with abuse, which could themselves influence the likelihood of depression (such as parental psychopathology). In a large study of psychiatric outpatients, Gibb, Butler, and Beck (2003) found that childhood emotional abuse was most specifically related to depression compared with sexual or physical abuse (see also Alloy et al., 2006).

Using a different research strategy, Kessler and Magee (1993) examined associations among one or more from a diverse list of adverse experiences and depression. Their large-scale retrospective epidemiological study of community residents who met criteria for major depression found that several childhood adversities (parental drinking, parental mental illness, family violence, parental marital problems, death of mother or father, and lack of a close relationship with an adult) were predictive of later onset of depression. Three early adversities—parental mental illness, violence, and parental divorce—were significantly predictive of recurrence of depression. In a later similar study, Kessler, Davis, and Kendler (1997), examining 26 adversities occurring by age 16, found that although many of the events were associated with adult major depressive disorder, the adversities were also related to a broad array of psychological disorders besides depression. The investigators also noted that exposure to one or more adversities is common, occurring to three-fourths of respondents, and that the adversities tend to overlap or cluster with each other. Furthermore, they noted that no claim to causal relationships between adversity and disorders is possible, since there may be unmeasured common variables responsible for both adversity exposure and later disorder. Thus, while childhood traumas and early stressful conditions may contribute to depression, more study of the complex pathways is needed.

The mechanisms by which specific childhood stressors, such as physical or sexual abuse, have their effects on later depression are not known directly. However, such experiences are highly likely to occur in the context of parental lack of care, plus exposure to high levels of chronic and episodic stressors. Such environments contribute to dysfunctional cognitions and coping skills that increase vulnerability to depression. Neurobiological mechanisms may also be implicated, with the speculation that severe stress early in life alters the brain's neuroregulatory processes, which promote susceptibility to depression (e.g., Heim and Nemeroff, 2001). Exposure to adverse conditions in childhood may sensitize the youth to stress, so that it may take minimal exposure to later stressful life events to precipitate depression in them compared with those without childhood adversity (e.g., Hammen, Henry, and Daley, 2000; Harkness, Bruce, and Lumley, 2006).

Personal Vulnerabilities to Depression

As noted earlier, etiological approaches to depression commonly invoke diathesis-stress models, in which stress precipitates depressive reactions among those with particular vulnerabilities. In this section, several nonbiological vulnerabilities are discussed: cognitive, interpersonal, and personality factors. As with biological factors, psychosocial vulnerabilities may contribute to the development of depression and also may be consequences of depressive states in a bidirectional process.

Cognitive Vulnerability to Depression

Considerable research on depression in the past 40 years has focused on three variants of cognitive models of depression—the classical cognitive triad model (negative views of the self, world, and future) of Aaron Beck (e.g., 1967, 1976), the versions of the helplessness/hopelessness cognitive style models of Seligman, Abramson, Alloy, and colleagues (e.g., Abramson, Metalsky, and Alloy, 1989; Abramson, Seligman, and Teasdale, 1978), and information-processing perspectives (e.g., reviewed in Joorman, 2008).

The Beck and cognitive style models emphasize the role of distortion in the content of thinking of depressed people. Those at risk for depression are hypothesized to have characteristic ways of interpreting events and circumstances that are excessively pessimistic and self-critical, with perceptions of helplessness and hopelessness about changing or improving their situations. Such underlying beliefs may be activated in the face of undesirable events, so that life events—even minor or fairly neutral experiences—are seen as reflections on one's underlying lack of worth and competence. Such views lead to the exacerbation and maintenance of symptoms of dysphoria and futility, sometimes to the extent of major depressive episodes and suicidality. Ample evidence has accumulated that verifies that, when experiencing depressed moods or episodes, a person's thinking is considerably more negative than he or she would display when not in a depressed mood (e.g., reviewed in Clark, Beck, and Alford, 1999). Moreover, prospective studies have verified that those considered at risk because of characteristic negative thinking are indeed likely to develop depressive reactions (Alloy et al., 2006; Gibb et al., 2006), especially in the face of stress (Hankin et al., 2004; Scher, Ingram, and Segal, 2005).

The information-processing approach to cognitive vulnerability refers to dysfunctional cognitive processes, such as biases in attention and memory, and overgeneralized thinking style (e.g., reviewed in Joorman, 2008; Mathews and MacLeod, 2005). Such biases may result in selective attention to negative information and reduced access to positive memories, increasing the likelihood of dysphoric reactions to negative events.

An interesting recent development in cognitive theories of depression is the study of the origins of depressogenic cognitive styles. Hypothesizing that they are acquired in childhood, several studies have found that children's negative cognitive styles are associated with parent-child communications characterized by criticism and disconfirmation, poor relationship quality, and modeling and learning of the parent's own negative cognitive style. Studies have also shown that negative cognitions are associated with histories of child abuse and maltreatment (e.g., reviewed in Alloy et al., 2006). The committee's review of the literature on the role of genetic factors in child outcomes notes that there is also evidence of heritability of depressogenic attributional style and other indicators of cognitive vulnerability to depression in youth (e.g., Abramson, Seligman, and Teasdale, 1978; Lau, Rijsdijk, and Eley, 2006; McGuire et al., 1999; Neiderhiser and McGuire, 1994; Neiss, Sedikides, and Stevenson, 2006).

Interpersonal Vulnerabilities to Depression

Depressive disorders are known to be associated with considerable impairment in interpersonal functioning—marital discord, intimate partner violence, parenting difficulties, insecure attachment, and low social support, to mention several specific areas. The symptoms of depression may contribute to difficulties in close relationships. Irritability, loss of energy and enjoyment, sensitivity to criticism, and pessimistic or even suicidal thoughts may initially elicit concern from others, but eventually they may seem burdensome, unreasonable, or even willful—sometimes eroding the support of spouses, friends, and family (Coyne, 1976). There is also increasing evidence that enduring maladaptive characteristics of the person's interpersonal style and cognitions about relationships may be observed when the person is not in a depressive state, and may serve as risk factors for the development of depression—perhaps in part because of their contribution to stressful conflict and loss events (Eberhart and Hammen, 2009; Hammen and Brennan, 2002).

A prominent issue in depression is marital discord. Meta-analyses across multiple studies have indicated significant associations between depression and self-reported poor marital satisfaction (Whisman, 2001). Rates of divorce and never-married status are elevated among those with depression (e.g., Coryell et al., 1993). One informative study found that depression, compared with other disorders, is uniquely associated with marital dissatisfaction. Zlotnick et al. (2000) found that depressed individuals—both men and women—reported significantly fewer positive and more negative interactions with their partners than did the nondisorder and nondepressive disorder groups.

Longitudinal studies show that depression may result from marital difficulties (Whisman and Bruce, 1999). Also, depression may cause marital difficulties. Whisman, Uebelacker, and Weinstock (2004) found that not only did current depressed mood predict marital dissatisfaction for the self, but also the spouse's depressed mood predicted the partner's dissatisfaction. Other studies also show bidirectional effects of depression and marital dissatisfaction (Coyne, Thompson, and Palmer, 2002; Davila et al., 2003). The romantic relationships of young women assessed over a 5-year period indicated that lower quality of the relationships at the end of the follow-up, as well as the boyfriend's dissatisfaction, were significantly correlated with the amount of time the woman had spent in major depressive episodes (Rao, Hammen, and Daley, 1999).

Intimate partner violence is a major risk factor for psychopathology, including depression, among abuse survivors (Campbell, 2002; O'Campo, Ahmad, and Cyriac, 2008). Numerous studies have reported high levels of depression among survivors of abuse. In a meta-analysis by Golding (1999), the weighted mean rate for depression among survivors of partner violence was 47 percent. Not only is partner violence a major stressor that increases the risk of depression, but also experiences of violence affect the victim's trust in others, levels of isolation, and coping styles, which further increase the risk of becoming depressed (Calvete, Corral, and Estevez, 2007). A strong predictor of maternal depression in home visiting samples is a maternal history of trauma, especially a maternal history of child abuse, domestic violence, or both (Boris et al., 2006).

Several mechanisms are likely to underlie the association between depression and difficulties in intimate relationships, including maladaptive cognitions and attachment insecurities leading to dependency, distrust, excessive reassurance-seeking, and other behaviors that provoke conflict. Certainly one general mechanism that is likely to affect marital behaviors is experience in one's own family of origin. Depressed individuals commonly report histories of violence and marital disruption in their early lives, as well as poor quality of care and relationships with their own parents. As a result of their early family histories, for example, insecure attachment representations may develop that make them vulnerable both to development of depression (Bifulco et al., 2002b; Kobak, Sudler, and Gamble, 1991) and to poorer quality of relationships (Carnelley, Pietromonaco, and Jaffe, 1994). Individuals exposed to ineffective parental role models are also likely to fail to acquire the social problem-solving skills needed to resolve conflicts in close relationships.

An additional pathway to discord is that depressed people tend to marry other people with psychological problems, thus increasing the chances of marital disharmony. A review and meta-analysis of several studies of patients with mood disorders confirmed the significant likelihood that individuals with depressive disorders marry others with depression (Mathews and Reus, 2001). Depressed women patients have also been found to have higher rates of marriage to men with antisocial and substance use disorders (e.g., Hammen, 1991a). Research on nonpatient samples also shows spouse similarity for depressive disorders (e.g., Galbaud du Fort et al., 1998; Hammen and Brennan, 2002) and wives' major depression associated with husbands' antisocial personality disorder (Galbaud du Fort et al., 1998). While the possible reasons for "nonrandom mating" are beyond the scope of this report, the implications of such marital patterns are clear: Marriages in which both partners experience symptoms and vulnerabilities to disorder may give rise to marital discord and instability by contributing to stressful home environments and potentially to limited skills for resolving interpersonal disputes.

Parenting problems and conflicts between parents and children are commonly associated with depression. Chapter 4, on the effects of parental depression on children, details the nature, extent, and consequences of dysfunctional parenting. Despite the desire of most depressed parents to provide nurturing, consistent, and responsive parenting, many are significantly likely to be negative, critical, or withdrawn in their interactions with their children (e.g., Lovejoy et al., 2000). Notably, intergenerational patterns of parenting problems are evident, with depressed adults highly likely to report that they had difficulties with their own parents (e.g., reviewed in Parker and Gladstone, 1996).

Related findings have been reported in community samples, in which depressed individuals reported more negative views of their parents (e.g., Blatt et al., 1979; Holmes and Robins, 1987, 1988). Andrews and Brown (1988), for example, found that women who became clinically depressed following occurrence of major life events were more likely to report lack of adequate parental care or hostility from their mothers, compared with those who did not become depressed (see also Brown and Harris, 1993). When dealing with vulnerable populations, it is important to consider that parenting style may differ by ethnicity as well as by views on what constitutes appropriate parenting and parenting values (Pinderhughes et al., 2000).

Intergenerational conflict is common among immigrant parents

(Phinney, Ong, and Madden, 2000). Children tend to acculturate and learn new languages faster (Kwak, 2003). This creates conflict in families and may contribute to parental depression or exacerbate difficulties related to parental depression. In reviewing the extensive literature on depressed individuals' recollections of parents, Gerlsma, Emmelkamp, and Arrindell (1990) and Alloy et al. (2006) concluded that parental child rearing styles that include low affection and more control (overprotection) were most consistently related to depression.

In addition to difficulties in intimate family relationships, depressed people and those at risk for depression report problems with social support. They appear to have problems with the availability—or the perception of availability—of supportive relationships with others, including friends and associates. Perceived support helps to reduce depression and its likelihood of recurrence (Sherbourne, Hays, and Wells, 1995). However, depression is associated with low levels of perceived support (Burton, Stice, and Seeley, 2004; Dalgard et al., 2006; Wade and Kendler, 2000). Research evidence suggests that reduced availability of supportive relations with others may be "real" in terms of actual social isolation due to behaviors and traits that discourage sustained and helpful relations with others, such as introversion and behavioral inhibition (Gladstone and Parker, 2006) or poor social skills (Tse and Bond, 2004). Also, depressive states may result in negative and distorted cognitions about one's worthiness and perceptions of the unlikelihood of receiving effective help from others. Such perceptions may cause failure to seek help and support even if it does exist.

Personality Vulnerabilities

Space prevents the elaboration of the many candidates for personality traits and habits that might constitute vulnerability to depression, but we mention two factors that have received considerable recent attention: neuroticism and ruminative response style.

The construct of neuroticism has had a long history in psychology. Neuroticism is a higher order personality dimension, defined by negative emotionality and high reactivity to real and perceived stress. Neuroticism is a powerful predictor of depressive episodes, according to a review by Enns and Cox (1997; see also Fanous et al., 2002; Schmitz, Kugler, and Rollnik, 2003). Although the level of neuroticism may decline with reductions in depressive symptoms, recent longitudinal studies have supported the idea that relatively higher levels of neuroticism persist independent of depressive states (e.g., Clark et al., 2003; Kendler, Karkowski, and Prescott, 1999; Kendler and Karkowski-Shuman, 1997; Santor, Babgy, and Joffe, 1997). It is suggested that neuroticism may be one of the genetically transmitted traits that predisposes an individual to both stressful life events and depression, and to tendencies to respond to stressors with depression (Kendler et al., 1995; Kendler, Gardner, and Prescott, 2003). Kendler, Gardner, and Prescott (2003), for example, found that neuroticism was a strong predictor of stressful life events, particularly those related to interpersonal relationships. In other analyses, Kendler, Kuhn, and Prescott (2004) found that neuroticism moderated the effects of stress on depression, particularly potentiating its effects at the highest levels of stress exposure.

Neuroticism is highly correlated with trait anxiety (Watson and Clark, 1984), harm avoidance (Zuckerman and Cloninger, 1996), and measures of the behavioral inhibition system. Watson and Clark (1984) suggested that these are interchangeable measures of the same stable and pervasive trait, which they label *negative affectivity*. It is defined as the disposition to experience aversive emotional states, including nervousness, tension, worry, anger, scorn, revulsion, guilt, rejection, self-dissatisfaction, and sadness—especially in response to perceived stress.

A related construct, ruminative response style, refers to a cognitive and behavioral coping strategy, employed mainly by women, for responding to negative emotions, particularly dysphoria. Nolen-Hoeksema (1991) proposed that, when experiencing emotional distress, women display a response style that emphasizes rumination, self-focus, and overanalysis of the problem and excessive focus on their own emotions. In contrast, men use more distraction and problem resolution. When ruminative responses are employed, they tend to intensify negative, self-focused thinking and to interfere with active problem solving, hence deepening or prolonging the symptoms of depression. A series of studies has demonstrated support for these hypotheses, including gender differences in coping style and the association of ruminative coping with depression (e.g., Nolen-Hoeksema, Morrow, and Fredrickson, 1993; reviewed in Nolen-Hoeksema and Girgus, 1994; Nolen-Hoeksema, 2000).

Integrative Research

In view of the multiple biological, environmental, social, and personality risk factors for depression, research on risk for depression will be advanced by integrative, multivariable models that link biological factors with environmental and personal characteristics. To date, however, the field is marked mainly by complex models that have not been empirically evaluated or by empirical tests of fairly limited integrative models. Many of the theoretical models have been focused on a particular subtopic, such as predicting outcomes and their mechanisms in children of depressed parents (e.g., Goodman, 2007; Goodman and Gotlib, 1999) or gender differences in adolescent depression (Alloy and Abramson, 2007; Hankin and Abramson,

2001). Broader models linking stress, HPA axis, and neurocognitive as well as cognitive and interpersonal factors, for example, are urgently needed. Limited integrative empirical approaches that include biological factors are emerging, including complex quantitative genetic, environmental, and personal factors (e.g., Kendler, Gardner, and Prescott, 2002, 2006) and gene-environment analyses (e.g., Caspi et al., 2003). Studies that link neuroendocrine, stress, and social-cognitive factors are particularly needed.

CO-OCCURRING DISORDERS

As this chapter has indicated, depression co-occurs with a host of stressful life events, early adversities, and ongoing strains, and it is also commonly associated with a variety of interpersonal difficulties and problematic traits and behavioral tendencies. A further complexity is introduced by the reality that depression typically does not occur in a "pure" form, independent of the effects of additional psychological disorders. In both the original U.S. National Comorbidity Study and the recent replication, of all the community residents who met the criteria for lifetime or 12-month major depression or both, approximately 75 percent had at least one other diagnosis, with only a minority having pure cases of depression (Kessler et al., 2003). For patients with a diagnosis of current major depression, only 40–45 percent had depression in isolation, and 60–65 percent had at least one comorbid diagnosis; similar rates have been reported in different countries (e.g., Blazer et al., 1994; De Graaf et al., 2002; Rush et al., 2005; Zimmerman, Chelminski, and McDermut, 2002).

Approximately 60 percent of comorbid disorders are anxiety disorders, particularly generalized anxiety disorder, panic disorder, social phobia, and posttraumatic stress disorders (Mineka, Watson, and Clark, 1998). Among patients with anxiety disorders, approximately 30 percent have a comorbid mood disorder (Brown et al., 2001). The onset of anxiety disorders typically precedes the onset of depression, with earlier-onset anxiety disorders (panic, social anxiety, generalized anxiety disorder) predicting the subsequent first onset of depression (Andrade et al., 2003; Kessler et al., 1996; Stein et al., 2001; but see Moffitt et al., 2007). So common is the overlap between depressive and anxiety disorders that some have argued that major depression and generalized anxiety disorder may virtually be the same disorder or closely associated, genetically mediated distress disorders (e.g., Kendler et al., 2007; Moffitt et al., 2007).

Besides anxiety disorders, substance abuse and alcoholism and eating disorders are frequently accompanied by depressive disorders, in both clinical and community samples (Rohde, Lewinsohn, and Seeley, 1991; Sanderson, Beck, and Beck, 1990; Swendsen and Merikangas, 2000). Several recent large epidemiological studies found rates of 25–30 percent for comorbid substance or alcohol abuse (Davis et al., 2005; Melartin et al., 2002). In their analysis of the origins of the comorbidity of substance use disorders, Swendsen and Merikangas (2000) considered whether they share a causal relationship (e.g., alcoholism causes depression or the reverse) or are related because of a shared etiological factor. Their data and review suggest a causal association, rather than shared etiology, for alcohol and depression, with evidence both for depression causing alcohol abuse and abuse causing depression. However, for other substance abuse, the patterns were inconsistent, suggesting that multiple mechanisms may be contributing to the comorbidity.

According to the *Diagnostic and Statistical Manual of Mental Disorders*, not only are Axis I disorders (i.e., clinical disorders, including major mental disorders, as well as developmental and learning disorders) highly likely to co-occur with depression, but also personality disorders are more the rule than the exception with depressed patients. Personality disorders refer to a set of patterns of dysfunctional conduct and attitudes that start early in life, are persistent, and affect all areas of a person's functioning. Depending on the study, rates of personality disorders among depressed people range between 23 and 87 percent (Shea et al., 1990; Shea, Widiger, and Klein, 1992). Most studies have found that personality disorders in the "dramatic/erratic" cluster (such as borderline personality disorder) and in the "anxious/fearful" cluster (such as avoidant personality disorder) predominate (e.g., Alpert et al., 1997; Brieger, Ehrt, and Marneros, 2003; Rossi et al., 2001; Shea et al., 1990).

One of the crucial problems with depression co-occurrence with other disorders is that the combinations may greatly complicate both the clinical course of depression and the efficacy of typical treatments. For example, the presence of a comorbid anxiety disorder predicts a significantly worse course of depression and dysthymia (Brown et al., 1996; Gaynes et al., 1999; Shankman and Klein, 2002). Likewise, a comorbid personality disorder predicts a poorer outcome (Daley et al., 1999; Klein, 2003; Klein and Shih, 1998; see the review by Newton-Howes, Tyrer, and Johnson, 2006).

Depression is also a ubiquitous presence in medical illnesses, and a recent large depression treatment study (Sequence Treatment Alternatives to Relieve Depression: STAR*D) found that 53 percent of depressed patients had significant medical comorbidity (Yates et al., 2004). Serious acute and chronic diseases are highly stressful, and depression may be a reaction to the challenges associated with such problems; it can even result from the pathophysiological processes of certain diseases.

Of particular note is the role that depression may play as a contributor to ill health (Katon, 2003). For example, depression may interfere with healthy lifestyle choices, such as regular exercise, smoking cessation, good nutrition, and compliance with medical treatments; dysfunctional self-care behaviors may play a causal role in the onset of certain diseases or in the course of disease and recovery (e.g., Evans et al., 2005). Furthermore, as noted earlier, depression has been linked with inflammatory processes that underlie several major diseases. Depression is associated with biological abnormalities, such as insulin resistance and secretion of inflammatory cytokines, which might contribute to diabetes onset (Musselman et al., 2003). Depression has been shown to be a predictor of heart disease progression or death in longitudinal studies of both initially healthy patients or in follow-up after first heart attack (Frasure-Smith and Lesperance, 2003; Rugulies, 2002; Suls and Bunde, 2005). Depression with medical illness comorbidity is significantly more common among those with lower income, divorced or widowed, less educated, unemployed, and nonwhite (Yates et al., 2004), and it predicts longer and more frequent episodes of major depression.

RESILIENCE AND PROTECTIVE FACTORS

The rich literature on biological, environmental, and personal risk factors for depression also indicates a striking finding: not all individuals who have been exposed to risk factors for depression develop the disorder. As a result, researchers have attempted to identify possible protective factors that serve as sources of resilience in the face of known risk. A protective factor is a feature of the individual or the environment that is associated with a decreased probability of the development of a disorder among individuals exposed to factors that increase risk for the disorder. Resilience refers to the processes through which individuals overcome risk factors and adverse conditions and achieve positive outcomes. Similar to risk research, the investigation of sources of resilience has included biological, environmental, and psychological processes. One of the challenges for researchers has been to avoid the pitfall of defining protective factors and processes of resilience as merely the absence of risk factors. That is, protective factors and evidence for resilience must be found in the presence of risk, not as a consequence of the absence of exposure to risk.

The resilience research literature has focused largely on children exposed to adverse environmental conditions, with relatively less study devoted to depression specifically. However, two key themes in the broader literature are important to note. One is that, across the range of resilience research over three decades, several variables appear universally to promote positive adaptation in children (Masten, 2007). Among these are secure attachment and connection to competent and caring adults and positive family systems (such as parental supervision), normal cognitive development and IQ, competent self-regulatory systems (including agreeable personality traits, effortful control of attention and impulses, healthy executive functioning), positive outlook and achievement motivation, and peer, school, and community systems that promote positive values and opportunities. The second theme in resilience science is an increasing emphasis on integrative, multilevel research on resilience in developing systems, drawing on biological, personality, cognitive, social, family, and environmental constructs that work together to promote adaptation and self-regulatory processes (Masten, 2007).

As specifically applied to resilience in the face of risk for developing depression, researchers have focused on biological factors, such as neurochemical, neuropeptide, and hormonal processes that mediate and moderate the relation between stress and depression (e.g., Charney, 2004; Davidson, 2003; Robbins, 2005; Southwick, Vythilingam, and Charney, 2005). For example, brain structure, brain function, and neurotransmitters related to the ability to sustain positive affect in the face of stress and adversity may be characteristic of individuals who are exposed to chronic stress but who do not develop depression. Dopamine levels in the prefrontal cortex and the nucleus accumbens; serotonin levels in the prefrontal cortex, amygdala, hippocampus, and dorsal raphe; and levels of neuropeptide-Y in several cortical and subcortical regions have been implicated as protective factors against the risk for depression (Charney, 2004; Southwick, Vythilingham, and Charney, 2005). Davidson et al. (2003) have shown that the relative activation of the left versus the right prefrontal cortex is related to the ability to not only dampen negative emotions but also to upregulate positive emotions.

In an interesting animal model of the role of controllable and uncontrollable stress, Amat et al. (2006) found that experience with controllable stressors early in development may have an effect on subsequent responses to uncontrollable stressors that have been implicated in learned helplessness and depression. These researchers found that initial experience with controllable stress blocks intense activation of serotonergic cells in the dorsal raphe nucleus that would typically be produced by uncontrollable stress. Furthermore, activity in the ventral medial prefrontal cortex (PFC) during initial controllable stress was required for the later protective effect to occur. This suggests that the ventral medial PFC is needed to process information about the controllability of stressors and to use such information to regulate responses to subsequent stressors. This finding is consistent with work by Davidson (2000) suggesting that the ventral medial PFC is involved in the representation of positive and negative affective states in the absence of immediately present incentives.

Research on biological processes related to resilience has been complemented by evidence for psychological and behavioral features of resilience— that is, research concerned with what resilient individuals think and do in response to exposure to risk factors that reduce the likelihood that they will develop depression. Research has examined the psychological processes that are linked to these underlying neurobiological processes. Resilient individuals are not passive respondents to stress and adversity. Rather, those who are resilient are able to bring into action a set of skills to regulate thoughts and emotions and engage in behaviors that can resolve controllable sources of stress. Active forms of coping are associated with resilience in response to controllable stressors. In contrast, accommodative or secondary control coping, including emotion regulation skills, are related to better outcomes in response to uncontrollable stress (Compas et al., 2001).

Cognitive reappraisal, or the ability to view a stressful or threatening situation in a more positive light, is an example of an emotion-regulation or coping process that is related to resilience to stress in adolescents and adults (e.g., Compas, Jaser, and Benson, 2008; Gross, 2001). The ability to use cognitive reappraisal to manage stress and emotions develops during adolescence along with the development of basic cognitive executive function skills. Cognitive reappraisal and other forms of secondary control coping skills, including acceptance and the ability to use positive activities as a form of distraction, are a source of resilience in adolescents of parents with a history of depression (Jaser et al., 2005).

In a further study of adolescents whose parents have a history of depression, good-quality parenting despite depression and having a nondepressed parent or other adult to turn to were found to predict resilient outcomes (Brennan, LeBrocque, and Hammen, 2003). Although limited, the research on resilience in the face of risk factors for depression points in the direction of early interventions to improve parenting and children's emotion regulation, and stress management as ways to reduce the negative impact of parental depression and other adverse conditions. Further integrative research on resilience mechanisms—as well as on interventions—is needed to support efforts to break the chain of intergenerational transmission of disorder and impairment.

RESEARCH GAPS

Much is known about risk factors for depression, but further research is needed to test models of how multiple biological and psychosocial factors work together and to clarify the mechanisms by which stressful experiences lead to depressive reactions in individuals and in the family context. Similarly, the processes by which resilient outcomes occur despite exposure to parental depression and other adverse conditions are vastly complex, and research will benefit from developmentally sensitive and integrative models that can be tested over a longitudinal course. We need to know more about optimal timing and methods of intervention to prevent the development and escalation of depression in those at greatest risk—especially young people during their formative family and career years.

CONCLUSION

Depression is highly prevalent and, for many, a chronic or recurring problem that interferes with work and family. It erodes the motivation, energy, and enjoyment needed to nurture and sustain marital, parenting, and social relationships. It is a disorder with many faces—starting at different ages, possibly chronic or waxing and waning, and typically mixed with a variety of other complicating problems, such as anxiety disorders, substance abuse, and behavioral disorders. It frequently occurs as a causal factor or contributor to medical illnesses. There is considerable information on depression prevalence and manifestations in the general population, but less information specifically about depression in adults who are parents and caregivers. However, it is clear that depression's negative and enduring effects on personal functioning also have adverse effects on those living with a depressed person. Children of depressed parents are at great risk for depression and maladjustment in academic, social, and intimate roles, and depressed parents have difficulty functioning effectively in their parenting and marital roles.

Risk factors and causal mechanisms involved in depression have implicated a wide range of biological (genetic, neurological, hormonal, and endocrinological) factors that may play a role in underlying vulnerability or in the processes by which stressors trigger depression in some people. Fundamentally, etiological models are diathesis-stress models, in which stressful experiences—whether early childhood trauma, acute recent life events, or ongoing chronic strains—trigger depression. Finding depression "genes"—or another simple chemical marker—is an illusory goal, and it is not likely to be of practical help in identifying those at risk. Depression will most commonly be found among those facing chronically stressful conditions, such as social disadvantage and distressed relationships or lack of supportive and intimate relationships. There are numerous individual characteristics that moderate or mediate the effects of stress on depression, including personality traits that reflect emotional reactivity and negativity, as well as styles of thinking about self and the world that emphasize beliefs about worthlessness, helplessness, and futility. Skills for coping with adversity that are passive, avoidant, and ineffective may perpetuate depression. Unraveling the complex and interlocking contributors to depression requires more integrative and long-term study than has yet been conducted or supported. Substantial gaps occur in the application of knowledge about etiology to the detection and early treatment of depression.

Because of depression's varying clinical manifestations and co-occurring mental health and medical conditions, its different symptom and course profiles, and its likelihood of recurrence, depression is very difficult to treat effectively in a universal way and over long periods of time. What may help a depressed teenage mother could be very different from what is needed by an adult depressed father—or by the same young woman after several bouts of major depression. Treatments or preventive interventions that are effective for reducing depressive symptoms may not resolve the underlying family or economic difficulties that erode sustained mental health. Thus, no simple prescriptions for treatment or prevention are realistic, and different individuals and settings will need different but multifaceted, flexible, and long-term care that recognizes that depression affects the whole family and that supports recovery rather than cure.

REFERENCES

Abramson, L.Y., Metalsky, G.I., and Alloy, L.B. (1989). Hopelessness depression: A theory-based subtype of depression. *Psychological Review*, 96, 358–372.

Abramson, L.Y., Seligman, M.E.P., and Teasdale, J.D. (1978). Learned helplessness in humans: Critique and reformulation. *Journal of Abnormal Psychology*, 87, 49–74.

Afifi, T.O., Cox, B.J., and Enns, M.W. (2006). Mental health profiles among married, never-married, and separated/divorced mothers in a nationally representative sample. *Social Psychiatry and Psychiatric Epidemiology*, 41, 122–129.

Aguilar-Gaxiola, S., Elliott, K., Deeb-Sossa, N., King, R.T., Magaña, C.G., Miller, E., Sala, M., Sribney, W.M., and Breslau, J. (2008). *Engaging the Underserved: Personal Accounts of Communities on Mental Health Needs for Prevention and Early Intervention Strategies.* Monograph No. 1, Center for Reducing Health Disparities. Sacramento: University of California, Davis.

Alloy, L.B., and Abramson, L.Y. (2007). The adolescent surge in depression and emergence of gender differences: A biocognitive vulnerability-stress model in developmental context. In D. Romer and E.F. Walker (Eds.), *Adolescent Psychopathology and the Developing Brain: Integrating Brain and Prevention Science* (pp. 284–312). New York: Oxford University Press.

Alloy, L.B., Abramson, L.Y., Smith, J.M., Gibb, B.E., and Neeren, A.M. (2006). Role of parenting and maltreatment histories in unipolar and bipolar mood disorders: Mediation by cognitive vulnerability to depression. *Clinical Child and Family Psychology Review*, 9, 23–64.

Alpert, J.E., Uebelacker, L.A., Mclean, N.E., Nierenberg, A.A., Pava, J.A., Worthington, J.J., Tedlow, J.R., Rosenbaum, J.F., and Fava, M. (1997). Social phobia, avoidant personality disorder and atypical depression: Co-occurrence and clinical implications. *Psychological Medicine*, 27, 627–633.

Amat, J., Paul, E., Zarza, C., Watkins, L.R., and Maier, S.F. (2006). Previous experience with behavioral control over stress blocks the behavioral and dorsal raphe nucleus activating effects of later uncontrollable stress: Role of the ventral medial prefrontal cortex. *Journal of Neuroscience*, 26, 13264–13272.

Andrade, L., Caraveo-Anduaga, J.J., Berglund, P., Bijl, R.V., De Graaf, R., Vollebergh, W. Dragomirecka, E., Kohn, R., Keller, M., Kessler, R.C., Kawakami, N., Kilic, C., Offord, D., Ustun, T.B., and Wittchen, H.U. (2003). The epidemiology of major depressive episodes: Results from the International Consortium of Psychiatric Epidemiology (ICPE) Surveys. *International Journal of Methods in Psychiatric Research*, 12, 3–21.

Andrews, B., and Brown, G.W. (1988). Social support, onset of depression and personality: An exploratory analysis. *Social Psychiatry and Psychiatric Epidemiology*, 23, 99–108.

Angold, A., Costello, E.J., Erkanli, A., and Worthman, C.M. (1999). Pubertal changes in hormone levels and depression in girls. *Psychological Medicine*, 29, 1043–1053.

Bailey, D.B., Jr., Golden, R.N., Roberts, J., and Ford, A. (2007). Maternal depression and developmental disability: Research critique. *Mental Retardation and Developmental Disabilities Research Reviews*, *13*, 321–329.

Banks, K.H., and Kohn-Wood, L.P. (2007). The influence of racial identity profiles on the relationship between racial discrimination and depressive symptoms. *Journal of Black Psychology*, *33*, 331–354.

Barrett, A.E., and Turner, R.J. (2005). Family structure and mental health: The mediating effects of socioeconomic status, family process, and social stress. *Journal of Health and Social Behavior*, *46*, 156–169.

Beck, A.T. (1967). *Depression: Clinical, Experimental, and Theoretical Aspects*. New York: Harper and Row.

Beck, A.T. (1976). *Cognitive Therapy and the Emotional Disorders*. New York: International Universities Press.

Bifulco, A., Brown, G.W., Moran, P., Ball, C., and Campbell, C. (1998). Predicting depression in women: The role of past and present vulnerability. *Psychological Medicine*, *28*, 39–50.

Bifulco, A., Moran, P., Baines, R., Bunn, A., and Stanford, K. (2002a). Exploring psychological abuse in childhood: II. Association with other abuse and adult clinical depression. *Bulletin of the Menninger Clinic*, *66*, 241–258.

Bifulco, A., Moran, P., Ball, C., and Bernazzani, O. (2002b). Adult attachment style. I: Its relationship to clinical depression. *Social Psychiatry and Psychiatric Epidemiology*, *37*, 50–59.

Birmaher, B., Ryan, N., Williamson, D., Brent, D., Kaufman, J., Dahl, R., Perel, J., and Nelson, B. (1996). Childhood and adolescent depression: A review of the past 10 years: Part I. *Journal of the Academy of Child and Adolescent Psychiatry*, *35*, 1427–1439.

Blatt, S.J., Wein, S.J., Chevron, E.S., and Quinlan, D.M. (1979). Parental representations and depression in normal young adults. *Journal of Abnormal Psychology*, *88*, 388–397.

Blazer, D.G., Kessler, R.C., McGonagle, K.A., and Swartz, M.S. (1994). The prevalence and distribution of major depression in a national community sample—the National Comorbidity Survey. *American Journal of Psychiatry*, *151*, 979–986.

Bloch, M., Rotenberg, N., Koren, D., and Klein, E. (2005). Risk factors associated with the development of postpartum mood disorders. *Journal of Affective Disorders*, *88*, 9–18.

Blustein, J., Chan, S., and Guanais, F. (2004). Elevated depressive symptoms among caregiving grandparents. *Health Services Research*, *39*, 1671–1689.

Bockting, C.L., Spinhoven, P., Koeter, M.W., Wouters, L.F., Schene, A.H., and the Depression Evaluation Longitudinal Therapy Assessment Study Group. (2006). Prediction of recurrence in recurrent depression and the influence of consecutive episode on vulnerability for depression: A 2-year prospective study. *Journal of Clinical Psychiatry*, *67*, 747–755.

Boris, N.W., Larrieu, J.A., Zeanah, P.D., Nagle, G.A., Steier, A., and McNeill, P. (2006). The process and promise of mental health augmentation of nurse home-visiting programs: Data from the Louisiana Nurse-Family Partnership. *Infant Mental Health Journal*, *27*, 26–40.

Boyce, W.T., and Ellis, B.J. (2005). Biological sensitivity to context: I. An evolutionary-developmental theory of the origins and functions of stress reactivity. *Development and Psychopathology*, *17*, 271–301.

Brennan, P.A., Le Brocque, R., and Hammen, C. (2003). Maternal depression, parent-child relationships and resilient outcomes in adolescence. *Journal of the American Academy of Child and Adolescent Psychiatry*, *42*, 1469–1477.

Brieger, P., Ehrt, U., and Marneros, A. (2003). Frequency of comorbid personality disorders in bipolar and unipolar affective disorders. *Comprehensive Psychiatry*, *44*, 28–34.

Brouwer, J.P., Appelhof, B.C., van Rossum, E.F.C., Koper, J.W., Fliers, E., Huyser, J., Schene, A.H., Tijssen, J.G.P., Van Dyck, R., Lamberts, S.W.J., Wiersinga, W.M., and Hoogendijk, W.J.G. (2006). Prediction of treatment response by HPA-axis and glucocorticoid receptor polymorphisms in major depression. *Psychoneuroendocrinology, 31*, 1154–1163.

Brown, C., Schulberg, H.C., Madonia, M.J., Shear, M.K., and Houck, P.R. (1996). Treatment outcomes for primary care patients with major depression and lifetime anxiety disorders. *American Journal of Psychiatry, 153*, 1293–1300.

Brown, G.W., and Harris, T.O. (1978). *Social Origins of Depression.* New York: Free Press.

Brown, G.W., and Harris, T.O. (1993). Aetiology of anxiety and depressive disorders in an inner-city population: 1. Early adversity. *Psychological Medicine, 23*, 143–154.

Brown, J., Cohen, P., Johnson, J.G., and Smailes, E.M. (1999). Childhood abuse and neglect: Specificity of effects on adolescent and young adult depression and suicidality. *Journal of the American Academy of Child Adolescent Psychiatry, 38*, 1490–1496.

Brown, T.A., Campbell, L.A., Lehman, C.L., Grisham, J.R., and Mancill, R.B. (2001). Current and lifetime comorbidity of the DSM-IV anxiety and mood disorders in a large clinical sample. *Journal of Abnormal Psychology, 110*, 585–599.

Burke, H.M., Davis, M.C., Otte, C., and Mohr, D.C. (2005). Depression and cortisol responses to psychological stress: A meta-analysis. *Psychoneuroendocrinology, 30*, 846–856.

Burke, K.C., Burke, J.D., Regier, D.A., and Rae, D.S. (1990). Age at onset of selected mental disorders in five community populations. *Archives of General Psychiatry, 47*, 511–518.

Burton, E., Stice, E., and Seeley, J.R. (2004). A prospective test of the Stress-Buffering Model of Depression in adolescent girls: No support once again. *Journal of Consulting and Clinical Psychology, 72*, 689–697.

Cairney, J., Boyle, M., Offord, D.R., and Racine, Y. (2003). Stress, social support and depression in single and married mothers. *Social Psychiatry and Psychiatric Epidemiology, 38*, 442–449.

Calvete, E., Corral, S., and Estevez, A. (2007). Cognitive and coping mechanisms in the interplay between intimate partner violence and depression. *Anxiety, Stress and Coping, 20*, 369–382.

Campbell, J.C. (2002). Health consequences of intimate partner violence. *The Lancet, 359*, 1331–1336.

Carnelley, K.B., Pietromonaco, P.R., and Jaffe, K. (1994). Depression, working models of others, and relationship functioning. *Journal of Personality and Social Psychology, 66*, 127–140.

Caspi, A., Sugden, K., Moffitt, T.E., Taylor, A., Craig, I.W., Harington, H., McClay, J., Mill, J., Martin, J., Braithwaite, A., and Poulton, R. (2003). Influence of life stress on depression: Moderation by a polymorphism in the 5-HTT gene. *Science, 301*, 386–389.

Charney, D.S. (2004). Psychobiological mechanisms of resilience and vulnerability: Implications for successful adaptation to extreme stress. *American Journal of Psychiatry, 161*, 195–216.

Chin, M.H., Walters, A.E., Cook, S.C., and Huang, E.S. (2007). Interventions to reduce racial and ethnic disparities in health care. *Medical Care Research and Review, 64*, 7S–28S.

Clark, D.A., Beck, A.T., and Alford, B.A. (1999). *Scientific Foundations of Cognitive Theory and Therapy of Depression.* New York: Wiley.

Clark, L.A., Vittengl, J., Kraft, D., and Jarret, R.B. (2003). Separate personality traits from states to predict depression. *Journal of Personality Disorders, 17*, 152–172.

Cole, D., Tram, J., Martin, J., Hoffman, K., Ruiz, M., Jacquez, F., and Maschman, T. (2002). Individual differences in the emergence of depressive symptoms in children and adolescents: A longitudinal investigation of parent and child reports. *Journal of Abnormal Psychology, 111*, 156–165.

Compas, B.E., Connor-Smith, J.K., Saltzman, H., Thomsen, A.H., and Wadsworth, M.E. (2001). Coping with stress during childhood and adolescence: Problems, progress, and potential in theory and research. *Psychological Bulletin, 127,* 87–127.

Compas, B.E., Jaser, S.S., and Benson, M. (2008). Coping and emotion regulation: Implications for understanding depression during adolescence. In S. Nolen-Hoeksema and L. Hilt (Eds.), *Handbook of Depression in Adolescents* (pp. 419–439). New York: Routledge.

Coryell, W., Scheftner, W., Keller, M., Endicott, J., Maser, J., and Klerman, G.L. (1993). The enduring psychosocial consequences of mania and depression. *American Journal of Psychiatry, 150,* 720–727.

Coyne, J.C. (1976). Depression and the response of others. *Journal of Abnormal Psychology, 85,* 186–193.

Coyne, J.C., Thompson, R., and Palmer, S.C. (2002). Marital quality, coping with conflict, marital complaints, and affection in couples with a depressed wife. *Journal of Family Psychology, 16,* 26–37.

Crouch, M. (1999). The evolutionary context of postnatal depression. *Human Nature, 10,* 163–182.

Cutrona, C.E., Wallace, G., and Wesner, K.A. (2006). Neighborhood characteristics and depression: An examination of stress processes. *Current Directions in Psychological Science, 15,* 188–192.

Cyranowski, J.M., Frank, E., Young, E., and Shear, M.K. (2000). Adolescent onset of the gender difference in lifetime rates of major depression: A theoretical model. *Archives of General Psychiatry, 57,* 21–27.

Daley, S.E., Hammen, C., Burge, D., Davila, J., Paley, B., Lindberg, N., and Herzberg, D.S. (1999). Depression and Axis II symptomatology in an adolescent community sample: Concurrent and longitudinal associations. *Journal of Personality Disorders, 13,* 47–59.

Dalgard, O.S., Dowrick, C., Lehtinen, V., Vazquez-Barquero, J.L., Casey, P., Wilkinson, G., Ayuso-Mateos, J.L., Page, H., Dunn, G., and the ODIN Group. (2006). Negative life events, social support and gender difference in depression. *Social Psychiatry and Psychiatric Epidemiology, 41,* 444–451.

Danese, A., Moffitt, T.E., Pariante, C.M., Ambler, A., Poulton, R., and Caspi, A. (2008). Elevated inflammation levels in depressed adults with a history of childhood maltreatment. *Archives of General Psychiatry, 65,* 409–415.

Davidson, R.J. (2000). Affective style, psychopathology, and resilience: Brain mechanisms and plasticity. *American Psychologist, 55,* 1196–1214.

Davidson, R.J. (2003). Affective neuroscience and psychophysiology: Toward a synthesis. *Psychophysiology, 40,* 655–665.

Davidson, R.J., Kabat-Zinn, J., Schumacher, J., Rosenkranz, M., Muller, D., Santorelli, S.F., Urbanowski, F., Harrington, A., Bonus, K., and Seridan, J.F. (2003). Alterations in brain and immune function produced by mindfulness mediation. *Psychosomatic Medicine, 65,* 564–570.

Davies, L., Avison, W.R., and McAlpine, D.D. (1997). Significant life experiences and depression among single and married mothers. *Journal of Marriage and the Family, 59,* 294–308.

Davila, J., Karney, B.R., Hall, T.W., and Bradbury, T.N. (2003). Depressive symptoms and marital satisfaction: Within-subject associations and the moderating effects of gender and neuroticism. *Journal of Family Psychology, 17,* 557–570.

Davis, L.L., Rush, J.A., Wisniewski, S.R., Rice, K., Cassano, P., Jewell, M.E., Biggs, M.M., Shores-Wilson, K., Balasubramani, G.K., Husain, M.M., Quitkin, F.M., and McGrath P.J. (2005). Substance use disorder comorbidity in major depressive disorder: An exploratory analysis of the Sequenced Treatment Alternatives to Relieve Depression cohort. *Comprehensive Psychiatry, 46,* 81–89.

De Graaf, R., Bijl, R.V., Smith, F., Vollebergh, W.A.M., and Spijker, J. (2002). Risk factors for 12-month comorbidity of mood, anxiety, and substance use disorders: Findings from the Netherlands Mental Health Survey and Incidence Study. *American Journal of Psychiatry, 159*, 620–629.

Del Conte, A., and Kling, J. (2001, January–February). A synthesis of MTO research on self, sufficiency, safety and health, and behavior and delinquency. *Poverty Research News, 5*, 3–6.

D'Onofrio, B.M., Turkheimer, E., Emery, R.E., Maes, H.H., Silberg, J., and Eaves, L.J. (2007). A Children of Twins study of parental divorce and offspring psychopathology. *Journal of Child Psychology and Psychiatry, 48*, 667–675.

D'Onofrio, B.M., Turkheimer, E., Emery, R.E., Slutske, W.S., Heath, A.C., Madden, P.A., and Martin, N.G. (2005). A genetically informed study of marital instability and its association with offspring psychopathology. *Journal of Abnormal Psychology, 114*, 570–586.

D'Onofrio, B.M., Turkheimer, E., Emery, R.E., Slutske, W.S., Heath, A.C., Madden, P.A., and Martin, N.G. (2006). A genetically informed study of the processes underlying the association between parental marital instability and offspring adjustment. *Developmental Psychology, 42*, 486–499.

Dubois, D., Felner, R., Bartels, C., and Silverman, M. (1995). Stability of self-reported depressive symptoms in a community sample of children and adolescents. *Journal of Clinical Child Psychology, 24*, 386–396.

Eaton, W.W., Shao, H., Nestadt, G., Lee, B.H., Bienvenu, O.J., and Zandi, P. (2008). Population-based study of first onset and chronicity in major depressive disorder. *Archives of General Psychiatry, 65*, 513–520.

Eberhart, N., and Hammen, C. (2009). Interpersonal predictors of stress generation. *Personality and Social Psychology Bulletin.* [E pub].

Egger, H.L., and Angold, A. (2006). Common emotional and behavioral disorders in preschool children: Presentation, nosology, and epidemiology. *Journal of Child Psychology and Psychiatry, 47*, 313–337.

Enns, M.W., and Cox, B.J. (1997). Personality dimensions and depression: Review and commentary. *Canadian Journal of Psychiatry, 42*, 274–284.

Essex, M.J., Klein, M.H., Cho, E., and Kalin, N.H. (2002). Maternal stress beginning in infancy may sensitize children to later stress exposure: Effects on cortisol and behavior. *Biological Psychiatry, 52*, 776–784.

Evans, D.L., Charney, D.S., Lewis, L., Golden, R.N., Gorman, J.M., Krishnan, K.R.R., Nemeroff, C.B., Bremner, J.D., Carney, R.M., Coyne, J.C., Delong, M.R., Frasure-Smith, N., Glassman, A.H., Gold, P.W., Grant, I., Gwyther, L., Ironson, G., Johnson, R.L., Kanner, A.M., Katon, W.J., Kaufman, P.G., Keefe, F.J., Ketter, T., Laughren, T.P., Leserman, J., Lyketsos, C.G., McDonald, W.M., McEwen, B.S., Miller, A.H., Musselman, D., O'Connor, C., Petitto, J.M., Pollock, B.G., Robinson, R.G., Roose, S.P., Rowland, J., Sheline, Y., Sheps, D.S., Simon, G., Spiegel, D., Stunkard, A., Sunderland, T., Tibbits, P., Jr., and Valvo, W.J. (2005). Mood disorders in the medically ill: Scientific review and recommendations. *Biological Psychiatry, 58*, 175–189.

Fanous, A., Gardner, C.O., Prescott, C.A., Cancro, R., and Kendler, K.S. (2002). Neuroticism, major depression and gender: A population-based twin study. *Psychological Medicine, 32*, 719–728.

Frasure-Smith, N., and Lesperance, F. (2003). Depression and other psychological risks following myocardial infarction. *Archives of General Psychiatry, 60*, 627–636.

Galbaud du Fort, G., Bland, R.C., Newman, S.C., and Boothroyd, L.J. (1998). Spouse similarity for lifetime psychiatric history in the general population. *Psychological Medicine, 28*, 789–803.

Gaynes, B.N., Magruder, K.M., Burns, B.J., Wagner, H.R., Yarnall, K.S.H., and Broadhead, W.E. (1999). Does a coexisting anxiety disorder predict persistence of depressive illness in primary care patients with major depression? *General Hospital Psychiatry, 21,* 158–167.

Ge, X., Lorenz, F.O., Conger, R.D., Elder, G.H., and Simons, R.L. (1994). Trajectories of stressful life events and depressive symptoms during adolescence. *Developmental Psychology, 30,* 467–483.

Gee, G.C., Spencer, M., Chen, J., Yip, T., and Takeuchi, D.T. (2007). The association between self-reported racial discrimination and 12-month DSM-IV mental disorders among Asian Americans nationwide. *Social Science and Medicine, 64,* 1984–1996.

Gerlsma, C., Emmelkamp, P.M.G., and Arrindell, W.A. (1990). Anxiety, depression, and perception of early parenting: A meta-analysis. *Clinical Psychology Review, 10,* 251–277.

Gibb, B.E., Beevers, C.G., Andover, M.S., and Holleran, K. (2006). The hopelessness theory of depression: A prospective multi-wave test of the vulnerability-stress hypothesis. *Cognitive Therapy and Research, 30,* 763–772.

Gibb, B.E., Butler, A.C., and Beck, J.S. (2003). Childhood abuse, depression, and anxiety in adult psychiatric outpatients. *Depression and Anxiety, 17,* 226–228.

Gladstone, G.L., and Parker, G.B. (2006). Is behavioral inhibition a risk factor for depression? *Journal of Affective Disorders, 95,* 85–94.

Goering, J., Kraft, J., Feins, J., McInnis, D., Holin, M.J., and Elhassan, H. (1999). *Moving to Opportunity for Fair Housing Demonstration Program: Current Status and Initial Findings (accession no. 8771).* Washington, DC: HUD USER.

Gold, P.W., Goodwin, F.K., and Chrousos, G.P. (1988). Clinical and biochemical manifestations of depression: Relation to the neurobiology of stress. *New England Journal of Medicine, 319,* 348–353.

Golding, J.M. (1999). Intimate partner violence as a risk factor for mental disorders: A meta-analysis. *Journal of Family Violence, 14,* 99–132.

Goodman, S.H. (2007). Depression in mothers. *Annual Review of Clinical Psychology, 3,* 107–135.

Goodman, S.H., and Gotlib, I.H. (1999). Risk for psychopathology in the children of depressed mothers: A developmental model for understanding mechanisms of transmission. *Psychological Review, 106,* 458–490.

Grigoriadis, S., and Romans, S. (2006). Postpartum psychiatric disorders: What do we know and where do we go? *Current Psychiatry Reviews, 2,* 151–158.

Gross, D., Fogg, L., Young, M., Ridge, A., Cowell, J., Richardson, R., and Sivan, A. (2006). The equivalence of the Child Behavior Checklist/1½–5 across parent race/ethnicity, income level, and language. *Psychological Assessment, 18,* 313–323.

Gross, J.J. (2001). Emotion regulation in adulthood: Timing is everything. *Current Directions in Psychological Science, 10,* 214–219.

Hammen, C. (1991a). *Depression Runs in Families: The Social Context of Risk and Resilience in Children of Depressed Mothers.* New York: Springer-Verlag.

Hammen, C. (1991b). Generation of stress in the course of unipolar depression. *Journal of Abnormal Psychology, 100,* 555–561.

Hammen, C. (2005). Stress and depression. *Annual Review of Clinical Psychology, 1,* 293–319.

Hammen, C. (2006). Stress generation in depression: Reflections on origins, research, and future directions. *Journal of Clinical Psychology, 62,* 1065–1082.

Hammen, C., and Brennan, P.A. (2002). Interpersonal dysfunction in depressed women: Impairments independent of depressive symptoms. *Journal of Affective Disorders, 72,* 145–156.

Hammen, C., Brennan, P., and Keenan-Miller, D. (2008). Patterns of adolescent depression to age 20: The role of maternal depression and youth interpersonal dysfunction. *Journal of Abnormal Child Psychology, 36*, 1189–1198.

Hammen, C., Henry, R., and Daley, S.E. (2000). Depression and sensitization to stressors among young women as a function of childhood adversity. *Journal of Consulting and Clinical Psychology, 68*, 782–787.

Hankin, B.L., and Abramson, L.Y. (2001). Development of gender differences in depression: An elaborated cognitive vulnerability-transactional stress theory. *Psychological Bulletin, 127*, 773–796.

Hankin, B.L., Abramson, L.Y., Miller, N., and Haeffel, G.J. (2004). Cognitive vulnerability-stress theories of depression: Examining affective specificity in the prediction of depression versus anxiety in three prospective studies. *Cognitive Therapy and Research, 28*, 309–345.

Hariri, A.R., Drabant, E.M., Munoz, K.E., Kolachana, B.S., Mattay, V.S., Egan, M.F., and Weinberger, D.R. (2005). A susceptibility gene for affective disorders and the response of the human amygdala. *Archives of General Psychiatry, 62*, 146–152.

Harkness, K.L., Bruce, A.E., and Lumley, M.N. (2006). The role of childhood abuse and neglect in the sensitization to stressful life events in adolescent depression. *Journal of Abnormal Psychology, 115*, 730–741.

Harrington, R., Fudge, H., Rutter, M., Pickles, A., and Hill, J. (1990). Adult outcomes of childhood and adolescent depression: I. Psychiatric status. *Archives of General Psychiatry, 47*, 465–473.

Hasin, D.S., Goodwin, R.D., Stinson, F.S., and Grant, B.F. (2005). Epidemiology of major depressive disorder: Results from the national epidemiologic survey on alcoholism and related conditions. *Archives of General Psychiatry, 62*, 1097–1106.

Hayes, M., Roberts, S., and Davare, A. (2000). Transactional conflict between psychobiology and culture in the etiology of postpartum depression. *Medical Hypotheses, 54*, 7–17.

Heilemann, M.V., Coffey-Love, M., and Frutos, L. (2004). Perceived reasons for depression among low income women of Mexican descent. *Archives of Psychiatric Nursing, 18*, 185–192.

Heim, C., and Nemeroff, C.B. (2001). The role of childhood trauma in the neurobiology of mood and anxiety disorders: Preclinical and clinical studies. *Biological Psychiatry, 49*, 1023–1039.

Heim, C., Newport, D.J., Heit, S., Graham, Y.P., Wilcox, M., Bonsall, R., Miller, A.H., and Nemeroff, C.B. (2000). Pituitary-adrenal and autonomic responses to stress in women after sexual and physical abuse in childhood. *Journal of the American Medical Association, 284*, 592–597.

Hiott, A., Grzywacz, J., Arcury, T., and Quandt, S. (2006). Gender differences in anxiety and depression among immigrant Latinos. *Families, Systems and Health, 24*, 137–146.

Hollon, S.D., Shelton, R.C., Wisniewski, S., Warden, D., Biggs, M.M., Friedman, E.S., Husain, M., Kupfer, D.J., Nierenberg, A.A., Petersen, T.J., Shores-Wilson, K., and Rush, A.J. (2006). Presenting characteristics of depressed outpatients as a function of recurrence: Preliminary findings from the STAR*D clinical trial. *Journal of Psychiatric Research, 40*, 59–69.

Holmans, P., Weissman, M.M., Zubenko, G.S., Scheftner, W.A., Crowe, R.R., DePaulo, J.R., Jr., Knowles, J.A., Zubenko, W.N., Murphy-Eberenz, K., Marta, D.H., Boutelle, S., McInnis, M.G., Adams, P., Gladis, M., Steele, J., Miller, E.B., Potash, J.B., MacKinnon, D.F., and Levinson, D.F. (2007). Genetics of recurrent early-onset major depression (GenRED): Final genome scan report. *American Journal of Psychiatry, 164*, 248–258.

Holmes, S.J., and Robins, L.N. (1987). The influence of childhood disciplinary experience on the development of alcoholism and depression. *Journal of Child Psychology and Psychiatry, 28*, 399–415.

Holmes, S.J., and Robins, L.N. (1988). The role of parental disciplinary practices in the development of depression and alcoholism. *Psychiatry: Journal for the Study of Interpersonal Processes, 51*, 24–36.

Holsboer, F. (2000). The corticosteroid receptor hypothesis of depression. *Neuropsychopharmacology, 23*, 477–501.

Howren, M., Lamkin, D., and Suls, J. (2009). Associations of depression with C-reactive protein, IL-1, and IL-6: A meta-analysis. *Psychosomatic Medicine, 71*, 171–186.

Huang, C.C., and Warner, L.A. (2005). Relationship characteristics and depression among fathers with newborns. *Social Service Review, 79*, 95–118.

Hughes, M.E., Waite, L., LaPierre, T., and Luo, Y. (2007). All in the family: The impact of caring for grandchildren on grandparents' health. *Journal of Gerontology, 62B*, S108– S119.

Jaser, S.S., Langrock, A.M., Keller, G., Merchant, M.J., Benson, M., Reeslund, K., Champion, J.E., and Compas, B.E. (2005). Coping with the stress of parental depression II: Adolescent and parent reports of coping and adjustment. *Journal of Clinical Child and Adolescent Psychology, 34*, 193–205.

Joorman, J. (2008). Cognitive aspects of depression. In I. Gotlib and C. Hammen (Eds.), *Handbook of Depression* (2nd ed., pp. 298–321). New York: Guilford Press.

Judd, L.L. (1997). The clinical course of unipolar major depressive disorders. *Archives of General Psychiatry, 54*, 989–991.

Judd, L.L., Akiskal, H.S., Maser, J.D., Zeller, P.J., Endicott, J., Coryell, W., Paulus, M.P., Kunovac, J.L., Leon, A.C., Mueller, T.I., Rice, J.A., and Keller, M.B. (1998). A prospective 12-year study of subsyndromal and syndromal depressive symptoms in unipolar major depressive disorders. *Archives of General Psychiatry, 55*, 694–700.

Katon, W. (2003). Clinical and health services relationships between major depression, depressive symptoms, and general medical illness. *Biological Psychiatry, 54*, 216–226.

Kaufman, J., Plotsky, P.M., Nemeroff, C.B., and Charney, D.S. (2000). Effects of early adverse experiences on brain structure and function: Clinical implications. *Biological Psychiatry, 48*, 778–790.

Keller, M.B. (1985). Chronic and recurrent affective disorders: Incidence, course, and influencing factors. In D. Kemali and G. Recagni (Eds.), *Chronic Treatments in Neuropsychiatry* (pp. 111–120). New York: Raven Press.

Kendler, K.S., and Karkowski-Shuman, L. (1997). Stressful life events and genetic liability to major depression: Genetic control of exposure to the environment? *Psychological Medicine, 27*, 539–547.

Kendler, K.S., Bulik, C., Silberg, J., Hettema, J., Myers, J., and Prescott, C. (2000). Childhood sexual abuse and adult psychiatric and substance use disorders in women: An epidemiological and co-twin control analysis. *Archives of General Psychiatry, 57*, 953–959.

Kendler, K.S., Gardner, C.O., and Lichtenstein, P. (2008). A developmental twin study of symptoms of anxiety and depression: Evidence for genetic innovation and attenuation. *Psychological Medicine, 30*, 1–9 [E pub].

Kendler, K.S., Gardner, C.O., and Prescott, C.A. (2002). Toward a comprehensive developmental model for major depression in women. *American Journal of Psychiatry, 159*, 1133–1145.

Kendler, K.S., Gardner, C.O., and Prescott, C.A. (2003). Personality and the experience of environmental adversity. *Psychological Medicine, 33*, 1193–1202.

Kendler, K.S., Gardner, C.O., and Prescott, C.A. (2006). Toward a comprehensive developmental model for major depression in men. *American Journal of Psychiatry, 163*, 115–124.

Kendler, K.S., Gardner, C.O., Gatz, M., and Pedersen, N.L. (2007). The sources of comorbidity between major depression and generalized anxiety disorder in a Swedish national twin sample. *Psychological Medicine, 37*, 453–462.

Kendler, K.S., Gardner, C.O., Neale, M.C., and Prescott, C.A. (2001). Genetic risk factors for major depression in men and women: Similar or different heritabilities and same or partly distinct genes? *Psychological Medicine, 31*, 605–616.

Kendler, K.S., Gatz, M., Gardner, C., and Pedersen, N. (2006). A Swedish National Twin Study of Lifetime Major Depression. *American Journal of Psychiatry, 163*, 109–114.

Kendler, K.S., Karkowski, L.M., and Prescott, C.A. (1998). Stressful life events and major depression: Risk period, long-term contextual threat, and diagnostic specificity. *Journal of Nervous and Mental Disease, 186*, 661–669.

Kendler, K.S., Karkowski, L.M., and Prescott, C.A. (1999). Causal relationship between stressful life events and the onset of major depression. *American Journal of Psychiatry, 156*, 837–841.

Kendler, K.S., Kessler, R.C., Walters, E.E., MacLean, C., Neale, M.C., Heath, A.C., and Eaves, L.J. (1995). Stressful life events, genetic liability, and onset of an episode of major depression in women. *American Journal of Psychiatry, 152*, 833–842.

Kendler, K.S., Kuhn, J., and Prescott, C.A. (2004). The interrelationship of neuroticism, sex, and stressful life events in the prediction of episodes of major depression. *American Journal of Psychiatry, 161*, 631–636.

Kendler, K.S., Kuhn, J.W., Vittum, J., Prescott, C.A., and Riley, B. (2005). The interaction of stressful life events and a serotonin transporter polymorphism in the prediction of episodes of major depression: A replication. *Archives of General Psychiatry, 62*, 529–535.

Kendler, K.S., Thornton, L.M., and Gardner, C.O. (2000). Stressful life events and previous episodes in the etiology of major depression in women: An evaluation of the "kindling" hypothesis. *American Journal of Psychiatry, 157*, 1243–1251.

Kendler, K.S., Thornton, L.M., and Gardner, C.O. (2001). Genetic risk, number of previous depressive episodes, and stressful life events in predicting onset of major depression. *American Journal of Psychiatry, 158*, 582–586.

Kendler, K.S., Thornton, L.M., and Prescott, C.A. (2001). Gender differences in the rates of exposure to stressful life events and sensitivity to their depressogenic effects. *American Journal of Psychiatry, 158*, 587–593.

Kessing, L.V., Hansen, M.G., Andersen, P.K., and Angst, J. (2004). The predictive effect of episodes on the risk of recurrence in depressive and bipolar disorders: A lifelong perspective. *Acta Psychiatrica Scandinavica, 109*, 339–344.

Kessler, R.C. (1997). The effects of stressful life events on depression. *Annual Review of Psychology, 48*, 191–214.

Kessler, R.C., and Magee, W.J. (1993). Childhood adversities and adult depression: Basic patterns of association in a US national survey. *Psychological Medicine, 23*, 679–690.

Kessler, R.C., and Walters, E.E. (1998). Epidemiology of DSM-III-R major depression and minor depression among adolescents and young adults in the National Comorbidity Survey. *Depression and Anxiety, 7*, 3–14.

Kessler, R.C., Berglund, P., Demler, O., Jin, R., Koretz, D., Merikangas, K.R., Rush, A.J., Walters, E.E., and Wang, P.S. (2003). The epidemiology of major depressive disorder: Results from the National Comorbidity Survey Replication (NCS-R). *Journal of the American Medical Association, 289*, 3095–3105.

Kessler, R.C., Berglund, P., Demler, O., Jin, R., Merikangas, K.R., and Walters, E.E. (2005). Lifetime prevalence and age-of-onset distributions of DSM-IV disorders in the National Comorbidity Survey Replication. *Archives of General Psychiatry, 62*, 593–602.

Kessler, R.C., Davis, C.G., and Kendler, K.S. (1997). Childhood adversity and adult psychiatric disorder in the U.S. National Comorbidity Survey. *Psychological Medicine, 27*, 1101–1119.

Kessler, R.C., Nelson, C.B., McGonagle, K.A., Liu, J., Swartz, M., and Blazer, D.G. (1996). Comorbidity of DSM-III-R major depressive disorder in the general population: Results from the U.S. National Comorbidity Survey. *British Journal of Psychiatry, 168*(Suppl.), 17–30.

Kim, P., and Swain, J.E. (2007). Sad dads: Paternal postpartum depression. *Psychiatry, 4,* 36–47.

Klein, D.N. (2003). Patients' versus informants' reports of personality disorders in predicting 7½-year outcome in outpatients with depressive disorders. *Psychological Assessment, 15,* 216–222.

Klein, D.N., and Shih, J.H. (1998). Depressive personality: Associations with DSM-III-R mood and personality disorders and negative and positive affectivity, 30-month stability, and prediction of course of Axis I depressive disorders. *Journal of Abnormal Psychology, 107,* 319–327.

Klein, D.N., Shankman, S.A., and Rose, S. (2006). Ten-year prospective follow-up study of the naturalistic course of dysthymic disorder and double depression. *American Journal of Psychiatry, 163,* 872–880.

Klein, D.N., Shankman, S.A., Lewinsohn, P.M., Rohde, P., and Seeley, J.R. (2004). Family study of chronic depression in a community sample of young adults. *American Journal of Psychiatry, 161,* 646–653.

Kobak, R., Sudler, N., and Gamble, W. (1991). Attachment and depressive symptoms during adolescence: A developmental pathways analysis. *Development and Psychopathology, 3,* 461–474.

Kwak, K. (2003). Adolescents and their parents: A review of intergenerational family relations for immigrant and non-immigrant families. *Human Development, 46,* 115–136.

Lau, J.Y.F., Rijsdijk, F., and Eley, T.C. (2006). I think, therefore I am: A twin study of attributional style in adolescents. *Journal of Child Psychology and Psychiatry, 47,* 696–703.

Lewinsohn, P.M., Rohde, P., and Seeley, J.R. (1998). Major depressive disorder in older adolescents: Prevalence, risk factors, and clinical implications. *Clinical Psychology Review, 18,* 765–794.

Lewinsohn, P.M., Rohde, P., Klein, D.M., and Seeley, J.R. (1999). Natural course of adolescent major depressive disorder: I. Continuity into young adulthood. *Journal of the American Academy of Child and Adolescent Psychiatry, 38,* 56–63.

Lewinsohn, P.M., Rohde, P., Seeley, J.R., Klein, D.N., and Gotlib, I.H. (2000). Natural course of adolescent major depressive disorder in a community sample: Predictors of recurrence in young adults. *American Journal of Psychiatry, 157,* 1584–1591.

Lizardi, H., Klein, D.N., Ouimette, P.C., Riso, L.P., Anderson, R.L., and Donaldson, S.K. (1995). Reports of the childhood home environment in early-onset dysthymia and episodic major depression. *Journal of Abnormal Psychology, 104,* 132–139.

Lovejoy, C.M., Graczyk, P.A., O'Hare, E., and Neuman, G. (2000). Maternal depression and parenting behavior: A meta-analytic review. *Clinical Psychology Review, 20,* 561–592.

Lucki, I. (1998). The spectrum of behaviors influenced by serotonin. *Biological Psychiatry, 44,* 151–162.

Maciejewski, P.K., Prigerson, H.G., and Mazure, C.M. (2001). Sex differences in event-related risk for major depression. *Psychological Medicine, 31,* 593–604.

MacMillan, H.L., Fleming, J.E., Streiner, D.L., Lin, E., Boyle, M.H., Jamieson, E., Duku, E.K., Walsh, C.A., Wong, M.Y.-Y., Beardslee, W.R. (2001). Childhood abuse and lifetime psychopathology in a community sample. *American Journal of Psychiatry, 158,* 1878–1883.

Malik, N., Boris, N., Heller, S., Harden, B., Squires J., Chazan-Cohen, R., Beeber, L.S., Kaczynski, K.J. (2007). Risk for maternal depression and child aggression in Early Head Start families: A test of ecological models. *Infant Mental Health Journal, 28,* 171–191.

Masten, A. (2007). Resilience in developing systems: Progress and promise as the fourth wave rises. *Development and Psychopathology, 19,* 921–930.

Mathews, A., and MacLeod, C. (2005). Cognitive vulnerability to emotional disorders. *Annual Review of Clinical Psychology, 1,* 167–195.

Mathews, C.A., and Reus, V.I. (2001). Assortative mating in the affective disorders: A systematic review and meta-analysis. *Comprehensive Psychiatry, 42,* 257–262.

Mazure, C.M. (1998). Life stressors as risk factors in depression. *Clinical Psychology: Science and Practice, 5,* 291–313.

McGonagle, K.A., and Kessler, R.C. (1990). Chronic stress, acute stress, and depressive symptoms. *American Journal of Community Psychology, 18,* 681–706.

McGuffin, P., Rijsdijk, F., Andrew, M., Sham, P., Katz, R., and Cardno, A. (2003). The heritability of bipolar affective disorder and the genetic relationship to unipolar depression. *Archives of General Psychiatry, 60,* 497–502.

McGuire, S., Manke, B., Saudino, K.J., Reiss, D., Hetherington, E.M., and Plomin, R. (1999). Perceived competence and self-worth during adolescence: A longitudinal behavioral genetic study. *Child Development, 70,* 1283–1296.

Meany, M.J., Szyf, M., and Seckl, J.R. (2007). Epigenetic mechanisms of perinatal programming of hypothalamic-pituitary-adrenal function and health. *Trends in Molecular Medicine, 13,* 269–277.

Melartin, T.K., Rytsala, H.J., Leskela, U.S., Lestela-Mielonen, P.S., Sokero, T.P., and Isometsa, E.T. (2002). Current comorbidity of psychiatric disorders among DSM-IV major depressive disorder patients in psychiatric care in the Vantaa Depression Study. *Journal of Clinical Psychiatry, 63,* 126–134.

Meyer, S.E., Chrousos, G.P., and Gold, P.W. (2001). Major depression and the stress system: A life span perspective. *Development and Psychopathology, 13,* 565–580.

Miller, G.E., and Blackwell, E. (2006). Turning up the heat: Inflammation as a mechanism linking chronic stress, depression, and heart disease. *Current Directions in Psychological Science, 15,* 269–272.

Mineka, S., Watson, D., and Clark, L.A. (1998). Comorbidity of anxiety and unipolar mood disorders. *Annual Review of Psychology, 49,* 377–412.

Moffitt, T.E., Harrington, H., Caspi, A., Kim-Cohen, J., Goldberg, D., Gregory, A.M., and Poulton, R. (2007). Depression and generalized anxiety disorder: Cumulative and sequential comorbidity in a birth cohort followed prospectivity to age 32 years. *Archives of General Psychiatry, 64,* 651–660.

Monroe, S.M., and Harkness, K.L. (2005). Life stress, the "kindling" hypothesis, and the recurrence of depression: Considerations from a life stress perspective. *Psychological Review, 112,* 417–445.

Muntaner, C., Eaton, W.W., Miech, R., and O'Campo, P. (2004). Socioeconomic position and major mental disorders. *Epidemiologic Reviews, 26,* 53–62.

Musselman, D.L., Betan, E., Larsen, H., and Phillips, L.S. (2003). Relationship of depression to diabetes types 1 and 2: Epidemiology, biology, and treatment. *Biological Psychiatry, 54,* 317–329.

Neiderhiser, J.M., and McGuire, S. (1994). Competence during middle childhood. In J.C. DeFries, R. Plomin, and D.W. Fulker (Eds.), *Nature and Nurture During Middle Childhood* (pp. 141–151). Malden, MA: Blackwell.

Neiss, M.B., Sedikides, C., and Stevenson, J. (2006). Genetic influences on level and stability of self-esteem. *Self and Identity, 5,* 247–266.

Neumeister, A., Young, T., and Stastny, J. (2004). Implications of genetic research on the role of the serotonin in depression: Emphasis on the serotonin type 1A receptor and the serotonin transporter. *Psychopharmacology, 174,* 512–524.

Newton-Howes, G., Tyrer, P., and Johnson, T. (2006). Personality disorder and the outcome of depression: Meta-analysis of published studies. *British Journal of Psychiatry, 188,* 13–20.

Nolen-Hoeksema, S. (1991). Responses to depression and their effects on the duration of depressive episodes. *Journal of Abnormal Psychology, 100,* 569–582.

Nolen-Hoeksema, S. (2000). The role of rumination in depressive disorders and mixed anxiety/depressive symptoms. *Journal of Abnormal Psychology, 109,* 504–511.

Nolen-Hoeksema, S., and Girgus, J.S. (1994). The emergence of gender differences in depression during adolescence. *Psychological Bulletin, 115,* 424–443.

Nolen-Hoeksema, S., Morrow, J., and Fredrickson, B.L. (1993). Response styles and the duration of episodes of depressed mood. *Journal of Abnormal Psychology, 102,* 20–28.

O'Campo, P., and Yonas, M. (2005). Health of economically deprived populations in cities. In S. Galea and D. Vlahov (Eds.), *Handbook of Urban Health: Populations, Methods, and Practice* (pp. 43–61). New York: Springer Science and Business Media Publishers.

O'Campo, P., Ahmad, F., and Cyriac, A. (2008). Chapter 12: Role of healthcare professionals in preventing and intervening on IPV. In J. Keeling and T. Mason (Eds.), *Domestic Violence: A Multi-professional Approach for Health Professionals* (pp. 107–115). Maidenhead, UK: Open University Press.

O'Campo, P., Salmon, C., and Burke, C. (2009). Neighbourhoods and mental well-being: What are the pathways? *Health and Place, 1,* 56–68.

Panzarine, S., Slater, E., and Sharps, P. (1995). Coping, social support, and depression symptoms in adolescent mothers. *Journal of Adolescent Health, 17,* 113–119.

Parker, G., and Gladstone, G.L. (1996). Parental characteristics as influences on adjustment in adulthood. In G.R. Pierce, B.R. Sarason, and I.G. Sarason (Eds.), *Handbook of Social Support and the Family* (pp. 195–218). New York: Plenum Press.

Paulson, J., Dauber, S., and Leiferman, J. (2006). Individual and combined effects of postpartum depression in mothers and fathers on parenting behavior. *Pediatrics, 118,* 659–668.

Phinney, J.S., Ong, A., and Madden, T. (2000). Cultural values and intergenerational value discrepancies in immigrant and nonimmigrant families, *Child Development, 71,* 528–539.

Pinderhughes, E.E., Dodge, K.A., Bates, J.E., Pettit, G.S., and Zelli, A. (2000). Discipline responses: Influences of parents' socioeconomic status, ethnicity, beliefs about parenting, stress, and cognitive-emotional processes, *Journal of Family Psychology, 14,* 380–400.

Pine, D.S., Cohen, P., Gurley, D., Brook, J., and Ma, Y. (1998). The risk for early-adulthood anxiety and depressive disorders in adolescents with anxiety and depressive disorders. *Archives of General Psychiatry, 55,* 56–64.

Plotsky, P.M., Owens, M.J., and Nemeroff, C.B. (1998). Psychoneuroendocrinology of depression: Hypothalamic-pituitary-adrenal axis. *Pediatric Clinics of North America, 21,* 293–307.

Post, R.M. (1992). Transduction of psychosocial stress into the neurobiology of recurrent affective disorder. *American Journal of Psychiatry, 149,* 999–1010.

Rajaratnam, J.K., O'Campo, P., Caughy, M.O., and Muntaner C. (2008). The effect of social isolation on depressive symptoms varies by neighborhood characteristics: A study of an urban sample of women with preschool aged children. *International Journal of Mental Health and Addiction, 6,* 464–475.

Rao, U., Hammen, C., and Daley, S.E. (1999). Continuity of depression during the transition to adulthood: A 5-year longitudinal study of young women. *Journal of the American Academy of Child and Adolescent Psychiatry, 38,* 908–915.

Reid, V., and Meadows-Oliver, N. (2007). Postpartum depression in adolescent mothers: An integrative review of the literature. *Journal of Pediatric Health Care, 21,* 289–298.

Ribeiro, S.C.M., Tandon, R., Grunhaus, L., and Greden, J.F. (1993). The DST as a predictor of outcome in depression: A meta-analysis. *American Journal of Psychiatry, 150,* 1618–1629.

Rice, F., Harold, G.T., and Thapar, A. (2005). The link between depression in mothers and offspring: An extended twin analysis. *Behavior Genetics, 35,* 565–577.

Riso, L.P., Miyatake, R.K., and Thase, M.E. (2002). The search for determinants of chronic depression: A review of six factors. *Journal of Affective Disorders, 70,* 103–115.

Robbins, T.W. (2005). Controlling stress: How the brain protects itself from stress. *Nature Neuroscience, 8,* 261–262.

Robertson, E., Grace, S., Wallington, T., and Stewart, D.E. (2004). Antenatal risk factors for postpartum depression: A synthesis of recent literature. *General Hospital Psychiatry, 26,* 289–295.

Rohde, P., Lewinsohn, P.M., and Seeley, J.R. (1991). Comorbidity of unipolar depression: II. Comorbidity with other mental disorders in adolescents and adults. *Journal of Abnormal Psychology, 100,* 214–222.

Rossi, A., Marinangeli, M.G., Butti, G., Scinto, A., Di Cicco, L., Kalyvoka, A., and Petruzzi, C. (2001). Personality disorders in bipolar and depressive disorders. *Journal of Affective Disorders, 65,* 3–8.

Rudolph, K.D. (2002). Gender differences in emotional responses to interpersonal stress during adolescence. *Journal of Adolescent Health, 30*(Suppl. 1), 3–13.

Rudolph, K.D., and Hammen, C. (1999). Age and gender as determinants of stress exposure, generation, and reactions in youngsters: A transactional perspective. *Child Development, 70,* 660–677.

Rugulies, R. (2002). Depression as a predictor for coronary heart disease: A review and meta-analysis. *American Journal of Preventive Medicine, 23,* 51–61.

Rush, A.J., Zimmerman, M., Wisniewski, S.R., Fava, M., Hollon, S.D., Warden, D., Biggs, M.M., Shores-Wilson, K., Shelton, R.C., Luther, J.F., Thomas, B., and Trivedi, M.H. (2005). Comorbid psychiatric disorders in depressed outpatients: Demographic and clinical features. *Journal of Affective Disorders, 87,* 43–55.

Sanderson, W.C., Beck, A.T., and Beck, J.S. (1990). Syndrome comorbidity in patients with major depression or dysthymia: Prevalence and temporal relationships. *American Journal of Psychiatry, 147,* 1025–1028.

Santor, D.A., Bagby, R.M., and Joffe, R.T. (1997). Evaluating stability and change in personality and depression. *Journal of Personality and Social Psychology, 73,* 1354–1362.

Sapolsky, R.M. (1996). Why stress is bad for your brain. *Science, 273,* 749–750.

Scher, C.D., Ingram, R.E., and Segal, Z.V. (2005). Cognitive reactivity and vulnerability: Empirical evaluation of construct activation and cognitive diatheses in unipolar depression. *Clinical Psychology Review, 25,* 487–510.

Schmitz, N., Kugler, J., and Rollnik, J. (2003). On the relation between neuroticism, self-esteem, and depression: Results from the National Comorbidity Survey. *Comprehensive Psychiatry, 44,* 169–176.

Segerstrom, S.C., and Miller, G.E. (2004). Psychological stress and the human immune system: A meta-analytic study of 30 years of inquiry. *Psychological Bulletin, 130,* 601–630.

Segre, L., O'Hara, M., Arndt, S., and Stuart, S. (2007). The prevalence of postpartum depression. *Social Psychiatry and Psychiatric Epidemiology, 42,* 316–321.

Seligman, M.E.P., Reivich, K., Jaycox, L., and Gillham, J. (1995). *The Optimistic Child.* New York: Houghton Mifflin.

Shankman, S.A., and Klein, D.N. (2002). The impact of comorbid anxiety disorders on the course of dysthymic disorder: A 5-year prospective longitudinal study. *Journal of Affective Disorders, 70,* 211–217.

Shattell, M.M., Smith, K.M., Quinlan-Colwell, A., and Villalba, J.A. (2008). Factors contributing to depression in Latinas of Mexican origin residing in the United States: Implications for nurses. *Journal of the American Psychiatric Nurses Association, 14*, 193–204.

Shea, M.T., Pilkonis, P.A., Beckham, E., Collins, J.F., Elkin, I., Sotsky, S.M., and Docherty, J.P. (1990). Personality disorders and treatment outcome in the NIMH treatment of depression collaborative research program. *American Journal of Psychiatry, 147*, 711–718.

Shea, M.T., Widiger, T.A., and Klein, M.H. (1992). Comorbidity of personality disorders and depression: Implications for treatment. *Journal of Consulting and Clinical Psychology, 60*, 857–868.

Sherbourne, C.D., Hays, R.D., and Wells, K.B. (1995). Personal and psychosocial risk factors for physical and mental health outcomes and course of depression among depressed patients. *Journal of Consulting and Clinical Psychology, 63*, 345–355.

Shih, J.H., Eberhard, N.K., Hammen, C., and Brennan, P.A. (2006). Differential exposure and reactivity to interpersonal stress predict sex differences in adolescent depression. *Journal of Clinical Child and Adolescent Psychology, 35*, 103–115.

Silberg, J.L., Rutter, M., and Eaves, L. (2001). Genetic and environmental influences on the temporal association between earlier anxiety and later depression in girls. *Biological Psychiatry, 49*, 1040–1049.

Singer, G.H.S. (2006). Meta-analysis of comparative studies of depression in mothers of children with and without developmental disabilities. *American Journal on Mental Retardation, 111*, 155–169.

Solomon, D.A., Keller, M.B., Leon, A.C., Mueller, T.I., Lavori, P.W., Shea, M.T., Coryell, W., Warshaw, M., Turvey, C., Maser, J.D., and Endicott, J. (2000). Multiple recurrences of major depressive disorder. *American Journal of Psychiatry, 157*, 229–233.

Southwick, S.M., Vythilingham, M., and Charney, D.S. (2005). The psychobiology of depression and resilience to stress: Implications for prevention and treatment. *Annual Review of Clinical Psychology, 1*, 255–291.

Spangler, D.L., Simons, A.D., Monroe, S.M., and Thase, M.E. (1996). Gender differences in cognitive diathesis-stress domain match: Implications for differential pathways to depression. *Journal of Abnormal Psychology, 105*, 653–657.

Stein, M.B., Fuetsch, M., Muller, N., Hofler, M., Lieb, R., and Wittchen, H.-U. (2001). Social anxiety disorder and the risk of depression: A prospective community study of adolescents and young adults. *Archives of General Psychiatry, 58*, 251–256.

Sullivan, P.F., Kendler, K.S., and Neale, M.C. (2003). Schizophrenia as a complex trait: Evidence from a meta-analysis of twin studies. *Archives General Psychiatry, 60*, 1187–1192.

Sullivan, P.F., Neale, M.C., and Kendler, K.S. (2000). Genetic epidemiology of major depression: Review and meta-analysis. *American Journal of Psychiatry, 157*, 1552–1562.

Suls, J., and Bunde, J. (2005). Anger, anxiety, and depression as risk factors for cardiovascular disease: The problems and implications of overlapping affective dispositions. *Psychological Bulletin, 131*, 260–300.

Swendsen, J.D., and Merikangas, K.R. (2000). The comorbidity of depression and substance use disorders. *Clinical Psychology Review, 20*, 173–189.

Targosz, S., Bebbington, P., Lewis, G., Brugha, T., Jenkins, R., Farrell, M., and Meltzer, H. (2003). Lone mothers, social exclusion and depression. *Psychological Medicine, 33*, 715–722.

Tennant, C. (2002). Life events, stress and depression: A review of the findings. *Australian and New Zealand Journal of Psychiatry, 36*, 173–182.

Thase, M. (2008). Neurobiological aspects of depression. In I. Gotlib and C. Hammen (Eds.), *Handbook of Depression* (2nd ed., pp. 187–217). New York: Guilford Press.

Tse, W.S., and Bond, A.J. (2004). The impact of depression on social skills. *Journal of Nervous and Mental Disease, 192*, 260–268.

Uher, R., and McGuffin, P. (2008). The moderation by the serotonin transporter gene of environmental adversity in the aetiology of mental illness: Review and methodological analysis. *Molecular Psychiatry, 13,* 131–146.

Van Os, J., and Jones, P.B. (1999). Early risk factors and adult person-environment relationships in affective disorder. *Psychological Medicine, 29,* 1055–1067.

Van Rossum, E.F.C., Binder, E.B., Majer, M., Koper, J.W., Ising, M., Modell, S., Salyakina, D., Lamberts, S.W., and Holsboer, F. (2006). Polymorphisms of the glucocorticoid receptor gene and major depression. *Biological Psychiatry, 59,* 681–688.

Van Voorhees, B.W., Walters, A.E., Prochaska, M., and Quinn, M.T. (2007). Reducing health disparities in depressive disorders outcomes between non-Hispanic whites and ethnic minorities: A call for pragmatic strategies over the life course. *Medical Care Research and Review, 64,* 157S–194S.

Vesga-Lopez, O., Blanco, C., Keyes, K., Olfson, M., Grant, B.F., and Hasin, D.S. (2008). Psychiatric disorders in pregnant and postpartum women in the United States. *Archives of General Psychiatry, 65,* 805–815.

Wade, T.D., and Kendler, K.S. (2000). Absence of interactions between social support and stressful life events in the prediction of major depression and depressive symptomatology in women. *Psychological Medicine, 30,* 965–974.

Wang, J.L. (2004). The difference between single and married mothers in the 12-month prevalence of major depressive syndrome, associated factors and mental health service utilization. *Social Psychiatry and Psychiatric Epidemiology, 39,* 26–32.

Watson, D., and Clark, L.A. (1984). Negative affectivity: The disposition to experience aversive emotional states. *Psychological Bulletin, 96,* 465–490.

Weedon, M.N., Lango, H., Lindgren, C.M., Wallace, C., Evans, D.M., Mangino, M., Freathy, R.M., Perry, J.R., Stevens, S., Hall, A.S., Samani, N.J., Shields, B., Prokopenko, I., Farrall, M., Dominiczak, A., Johnson, T., Bergmann, S., Beckmann, J.S., Vollenweider, P., Waterworth, D.M., Mooser, V., Palmer, C.N., Morris, A.D., Ouwehand, W.H., Zhao, J.H., Li, S., Loos, R.J., Barroso, I., Deloukas, P., Sandhu, M.S., Wheeler, E., Soranzo, N., Inouye, M., Wareham, N.J., Caulfield, M., Munroe, P.B., Hattersley, A.T., McCarthy, M.I., and Frayling, T.M. (2008). Genome-wide association analysis identifies 20 loci that influence adult height. *Nature Genetics, 40,* 575–583.

Weissman, M.M., Wolk, S., Goldstein, R.B., Moreau, D., Adams, P., Greenwald, S., Klier, C.M., Ryan, N.D., Dahl, R.E., and Wickramaratne, P. (1999a). Depressed adolescents grown up. *Journal of the American Medical Association, 281,* 1707–1713.

Weissman, M.M., Wolk, S., Wickramaratne, P., Goldstein, R.B., Adams, P., Greenwald, S., Ryan, N.D., Dahl, R.E., and Steinberg, D. (1999b). Children with prepubertal-onset major depressive disorder and anxiety grown up. *Archives of General Psychiatry, 56,* 794–801.

Whisman, M.A. (2001). The association between depression and marital dissatisfaction. In S.R.H. Beach (Ed.), *Marital and Family Processes in Depression: A Scientific Foundation for Clinical Practice* (pp. 3–24). Washington, DC: American Psychological Association.

Whisman, M.A., and Bruce, M.L. (1999). Marital dissatisfaction and incidence of major depressive episode in a community sample. *Journal of Abnormal Psychology, 108,* 674–678.

Whisman, M.A., Uebelacker, L.A., and Weinstock, L.M. (2004). Psychopathology and marital satisfaction: The importance of evaluating both partners. *Journal of Consulting and Clinical Psychology, 72,* 830–838.

Yates, W., Mitchell, J., Rush, A.J., Trivedi, M.H., Wisniewski, S.R., Warden, D., Hauger, R.B., Fava, M., Gaynes, B.N., Husain, M.M., and Bryan, C. (2004). Clinical features of depressed outpatients with and without co-occurring general medical conditions in the STAR*D. *General Hospital Psychiatry, 26,* 421–429.

Zammit, S., and Owen M.J. (2006). Stressful life events, 5-HTT genotype and risk of depression. *British Journal of Psychiatry*, *188*, 199–201.

Zimmerman, M., Chelminski, I., and McDermut, W. (2002). Major depressive disorder and axis I diagnostic comorbidity. *Journal of Clinical Psychiatry*, *63*, 187–193.

Zisook, S., Rush, A.J., Albala, A., Alpert, J., Balasubramani, G.K., Fava, M., Husain, M., Sackeim, H., Trivedi, M., and Wisniewski, S. (2004). Factors that differentiate early vs. later onset of major depression disorder. *Psychiatry Research*, *129*, 127–140.

Zlotnick, C., Kohn, R., Keitner, G., and Della Grotta, S.A. (2000). The relationship between quality of interpersonal relationships and major depressive disorder: Findings from the National Comorbidity Survey. *Journal of Affective Disorders*, *59*, 205–215.

Zuckerman, M., and Cloninger, C.R. (1996). Relationships between Cloninger's, Zuckerman's, and Eysenck's dimensions of personality. *Personality and Individual Differences*, *21*, 283–285.

4

Associations Between Depression in Parents and Parenting, Child Health, and Child Psychological Functioning

SUMMARY

Parenting Practices

- Depression is significantly associated with more hostile, negative parenting, and with more disengaged (withdrawn) parenting, both with a moderate effect size. Findings are primarily related to mothers rather than to fathers.
- Depression in mothers is significantly associated with less positive parenting (warmth), with a small effect size. Findings are primarily related to mothers rather than to fathers.
- The poorer parenting qualities may not improve to levels comparable to those of never-depressed parents, despite remission or recovery from episodes of depression.
- These patterns of parenting have been found in depressed mothers of infants and young children as well as in depressed mothers of school-age children and adolescents.
- Less is known about parenting in depressed fathers relative to mothers, but most of the findings from the smaller number of studies are consistent with the findings about mothers.

Child Functioning

- Depression in parents is associated with children's poorer physical health and well-being. Infants and young children of mothers with depression are more likely to use a variety of acute health care services. For older children and adolescents, there is limited evidence to suggest that depression plays a role in visits for stress-related health conditions and increased health care utilization. Adverse health outcomes of accidents, childhood asthma, child maltreatment, and adolescent tobacco and substance use occur more often when a parent is depressed.

- Maternal depression symptoms (and stress) levels are high among caregivers of children with chronic conditions.
- Depression in parents is associated with maladaptive patterns of health care utilization for children. Infants and young children of mothers with depression are more likely to use a variety of acute health care services. For older children and adolescents, there is limited evidence to suggest impact on health care utilization.
- Depression in parents has been consistently found to be associated with children's early signs of (or vulnerabilities to) more "difficult" temperament; more insecure attachment; affective functioning (more negative affect, more dysregulated aggression and heightened emotionality, more dysphoric and less happy affect, particularly for girls; lower cognitive/intellectual/academic performance, cognitive vulnerabilities to depression (more self-blame, more negative attributional style, lower self-worth); poorer interpersonal functioning; and abnormalities in psychobiological systems, including poorer functioning stress response systems (neuroendocrine and autonomic) and cortical activity.
- Depression in parents has been consistently associated with a number of behavior problems and psychopathology in children, including higher rates of depression, earlier age of onset, longer duration, greater functional impairment, higher likelihood of recurrence, higher rates of anxiety, and higher rates and levels of severity of internalizing and externalizing symptoms and disorders in children and adolescents.

Mediators and Moderators

- Depression in parents is more likely to be associated with adverse outcomes in children with the presence of additional risk factors (e.g., poverty, exposure to violence, marital conflict, comorbid psychiatric disorders, absence of father when the mother has depression, and clinical characteristics of the depression, such as severity and duration) than with depression that occurs in the context of more protective factors.

- Parental functioning, prenatal exposure to stress and anxiety, genetic influences, and stressful environments appear to play a role in the development of adverse outcomes in children.

This chapter reviews what is known about the associations among depression in parents and parenting, child health, and child functioning, based on the large number of epidemiological and clinical studies that have documented these associations. Throughout our work, the committee recognized that depression exists in a broader context of comorbidities, correlates, and contexts. In addition, there has been a growing body of research that suggests that parenting styles and processes are not necessarily universal and may differ and have differential impact on children's behavior based on culture and ethnic group variations (Deater-Deckard et al., 1996). Thus, the literature was approached with a caution against interpreting outcomes as owing solely to the depression in the parent as a single risk factor. With this in mind, the committee's task was to review the literature that focused on (1) direct association between depression in parents and parenting, child health, and child functioning; (2) conditions that may make the association stronger or weaker (i.e., moderators); and (3) mechanisms or intermediate steps (i.e., mediators) through which depression in the parent becomes associated with parenting or with outcomes in children. Although a review of the effects of parents' depression on the family (e.g., marital conflict) is not within the study scope, such effects are integrated into the literature summaries when findings bear on moderation (e.g., when maternal depression is more strongly associated with adverse child outcomes in the presence of high marital conflict rather than low marital conflict) or mediation (e.g., when maternal depression is associated with an increase in marital conflict, which is then associated with adverse child outcomes).

PARENTING PRACTICES AND THE DEPRESSED PARENT

Skills in parenting are key to facilitating healthy development in children. Qualities of parenting that have been found to be related to healthy development vary by age of the child. They range from the sensitive, responsive caregiving especially needed by infants to the monitoring that is particularly needed by adolescents. Important aspects of effective parenting across development include providing age-appropriate levels of warmth and structure to help children feel safe and to help regulate their emotions (e.g., Cole, Martin, and Dennis, 2004). Children also are dependent on their parents to facilitate their education and to obtain their medical care.

Parenting practices that do not meet infants' or children's needs to sustain healthy development are one of the primary mechanisms through which parental depression exerts its effects on children (Goodman and Gotlib, 1999). As reviewed by Avenevoli and Merikangas (2006), there is evidence to support broad (e.g., stress), specific (e.g., parenting skills), and structural (e.g., divorce) family factors that explain or modify the association between depression in parents and children's development of depression or other problems. Although more research is needed to determine the effects of specific types of parent behaviors, it is evident that parenting behaviors associated with depression affect children's adjustment.

Indeed, a few studies have tested and found support for a mediation role of parenting in associations between depression and outcomes in children. For example, in a large, longitudinal, population-based study of Canadian youth ages 10 to 15, children's reports of both positive parenting behaviors (i.e., nurturance and monitoring) and negative parenting behaviors (i.e., rejection) mediated the relationship between parental depressive symptoms and children's internalizing (e.g., anxiety, depressive symptoms) and/or externalizing (e.g., aggression, noncompliance) problems (Elgar et al., 2007). Also supporting mediation, Cummings et al. (2008) found that a community sample of 6-year-old children's representations of their attachment to their parents and of interparental conflict partially mediated the relation between parental depressive symptoms and the children's externalizing problems that emerged over the following 3 years. Lim, Wood, and Miller (2008), in a study of mothers with depressive symptoms and their children (n = 242, ages 7–17) with asthma symptoms recruited from pediatric emergency departments, also found evidence consistent with negative parenting as a partial mediator of the relation between maternal depressive symptoms and children's internalizing problems. However, despite the many strengths of this study, the reliance on a cross-sectional design limits conclusions that can be drawn about mediation. In addition to this support for parenting as a mediator, others have found that parenting serves as a moderator of associations between depression in parents and outcomes in children. Among research supportive of moderation is the finding that more positive outcomes in youth with depressed mothers were found among the subset of depressed mothers who used less psychological control, more warmth, and less overinvolvement (Brennan, Le Brocque, and Hammen, 2003).

Researchers have accumulated strong evidence directly linking depression in parents with problematic parenting practices, primarily based on studies using direct observations of parents and children in families of depressed parents. In a meta-analysis of this research, Lovejoy et al. (2000) found significant and moderate effect sizes for the association between both maternal depressive symptoms and disorder and hostile negative parenting (e.g., negative affect, coercive, hostile behavior; mean d = 0.40), disengaged (withdrawn) parenting (e.g., neutral affect, ignoring; mean d = 0.29), and a small but significant adverse association with positive parenting behaviors (engaging a child in a pleasant or affectionate way; mean d = 0.16). These studies reflect the significance of disrupted parenting when a parent suffers from depression and underscore the usefulness of direct observations of parent-child interactions in these families. The authors conclude that depressed mothers who are preoccupied are more likely to become angry when children misbehave or make normal demands on them. Lovejoy et al. (2000) argue that the "findings support the need for intervention with depressed mothers, as their parenting behaviors are a component of the risk associated with living with a depressed mother" (p. 588). Despite the strength of findings linking depression and parenting, the analyses were limited by the literature's focus on younger children. Only 17 percent of the studies in the meta-analysis (n = 8) included children ages 6 or older, and none of the studies focused specifically on the high-risk period of early adolescence, a developmental period associated with increasing rates of depression and increasingly stressful parent-child interactions (Hankin and Abramson, 2001). A few more recent studies, however, have similarly supported links between depression and parenting even among parents of adolescents, as reviewed later in this chapter.

Parenting practices are also of concern because they are associated with depression not only during periods of elevated symptom levels or during episodes that meet diagnostic criteria for depression but also when parents who have experienced depression may be relatively symptom free. Negative parenting has been found to persist even after controlling for the presence of major depressive disorder, suggesting that depressed parents continue to parent poorly following a depressive episode (Seifer et al., 2001).

Depression and Parenting During the Prenatal Period, Infancy, Toddlerhood, and Early Childhood

Although it is not common to consider that one engages in parenting behaviors during pregnancy, in fact there are multiple behaviors associated with depression during pregnancy that are relevant to children's outcomes. These include obtaining prenatal care early and regularly, engaging in healthy patterns of eating (weight gain) and sleeping, and avoiding drugs, alcohol, and cigarettes. Both the symptoms of depression, such as anhedonia (lack of pleasure in everyday experiences) and low energy, and the often correlated stressors may contribute to pregnant women neglecting their physical health and to engaging in behaviors that might provide immediate relief from distress, such as smoking, drinking, or unhealthy eating. Also, pregnant women with depression-related low energy or lethargy may seek less prenatal care or begin their care later in pregnancy than women without depression. Furthermore, depression symptoms, such as appetite or sleep disturbances, suggest that pregnant women with depression may get inadequate nutrition or sleep. All of these behaviors raise concern for fetal development. Among the empirical findings, depression during pregnancy has been associated with more smoking, greater consequences from alcohol use, and poorer overall health (Marcus et al., 2003; Zuckerman et al., 1989). Also, greater total sleep time during the third trimester predicted elevated depression symptoms postpartum (Wolfson et al., 2003). Among adolescent parents with depression, the poorer health behaviors are especially strong (Amaro and Zuckerman, 1991).

A much larger literature has shown depression, especially in mothers, to be associated with qualities of parenting of infants and toddlers. Researchers who observed mothers in face-to-face interaction with their babies or toddlers found higher levels of depressive symptoms to be associated with less maternal responsiveness or sensitivity, less verbal and visual interaction, and more intrusiveness (Campbell et al., 2004; Civic and Holt, 2000; Easterbrooks, Biesecker, and Lyons-Ruth, 2000; Ewell Foster, Garber, and Durlak, 2007; Horwitz et al., 2007; Marchand and Hock, 1998; Murray et al., 1996a; NICHD Early Child Care Research Network, 1999; Oztop and Uslu, 2007). Goodman and Brumley (1990), in a home observation study, found that depressed mothers were emotionally unavailable and withdrawn to the extent that they were less sensitive to their children's behavior, relative to women with no depression. Palaez et al. (2008) found that mothers with elevated depressive symptoms were more likely to be classified as authoritarian or disengaged in their interactions with their toddlers in comparison to mothers with low levels of depressive symptoms. Although mostly limited to small samples and to studies of elevated depression symptom levels rather than diagnoses, and with typically moderate effect sizes, these findings provide consistent support for associations between depression in mothers and patterns of interaction with their infants or young children that are intrusive/harsh or withdrawn/disengaged or both. Each of these parenting styles presents significant risks to the development of infants and toddlers.

Parenting of infants is particularly of concern given its essential role in children's development of secure attachment (Sroufe et al., 2005). Sensitive, responsive caregiving has been found to be the strongest predictor of secure attachment, which raises concerns given findings on depressed parents being less responsive and sensitive. Even beyond infancy, a sense of "felt security" has been found to be essential for healthy development and for preventing the development of psychopathology (Davies, Winter, and Cicchetti, 2006).

Other aspects of parenting of young children that have been found to be associated with depression are behaviors related to the health and well-being of children. For example, a community study of 400 children entering kindergarten in New York (Kavanaugh et al., 2006) reported that mothers with high levels of depressive symptoms were less likely to take their children for dental care (odds ratio = 2.6), read to their children less (odds ratio = 2.6), and were less consistent in their use of discipline (odds ratio = 2.3) than mothers with normal results from depression screening. This theme is also reflected in reports of elevated depressive symptoms in mothers being associated with less use of well-child care by age 12 months, more infant hospitalization, less back positioning for sleeping, and fewer up-to-date vaccinations (Chung et al., 2004; Mandl et al., 1999; Minkovitz et al., 2005).

Radke-Yarrow et al. (1993) conducted a landmark study of unipolar and bipolar depressed mothers and controls and their children, all of whom were under age 8 at study entry. To briefly summarize the findings, they found depression in a mother to be associated with (1) problems in functioning in essential and routine roles, (2) failure to help the child achieve self-regulation, (3) anger and irritability or enmeshing dependency or both, (4) less consistency of mother-child relationship over time, and (5) escalating negative qualities of interaction over time. Radke-Yarrow et al. concluded that psychopathology in a child was especially promoted when the mother's behavior interfered with the child's fundamental tasks, such as self-regulation; long-term dependable security, autonomy, and dependency needs; and positive attitudes about self.

Middle Childhood and Adolescence

Although direct observations of parent-child interactions in samples of depressed parents with older children and adolescents have been less common than with infants and younger children, a few studies have tested and found support for the hypothesis that depression is associated with parenting of adolescents and that the affected parent-child interactions may represent a crucial pathway for parental depression to the development of psychological problems in the adolescents (e.g., Gordon et al., 1989; Simons et al., 1993).

Jaser and colleagues (2008) examined the associations between maternal mood and parenting behaviors through direct observations of mothers with and without a history of depression interacting with their adolescent children during a positive and a negative task. Mothers with a history of depression were significantly more likely to exhibit sad affect and disengaged and antisocial parenting behaviors than mothers with no history of depression across the two interactions, but these differences were largely accounted for by mothers' current depressive symptoms. Mothers' self-reports of their current depressive symptoms were also related to higher levels of observed sadness and antisocial behaviors, as well as both children's and mothers' reports of maternal intrusive and withdrawn parent behaviors. Mothers' prior history of depression and their current depressive symptoms were associated with higher levels of parent and self-reported internalizing problems in adolescents.

Parenting associated with depression is thought to be experienced as stressful by children in middle childhood or adolescence, given that by middle childhood children have the cognitive capacity to perceive, interpret, and draw inferences about their parents' behavior. The stress of living with a depressed parent, relative to living with a parent with no depression, is characterized by more negative and unpredictable parental behaviors (e.g., irritability, inconsistent discipline), less supportive parental behaviors (e.g., less warmth, praise, nurturance, monitoring), and heightened marital conflict (Cummings, Keller, and Davies, 2005). Similar to the situation with younger children, depression leads to disruptions in parenting of older children and adolescents as a result of parental withdrawal (e.g., social withdrawal, avoidance, unresponsiveness to children's needs), parental intrusiveness (e.g., irritability toward children, overinvolvement in their lives), or alternating behaviors between the two (e.g., Field et al., 1996; Forehand, McCombs, and Brody, 1987; Gelfand and Teti, 1990). Depressed mothers exhibit both intrusive and withdrawn behaviors, and the alteration or unpredictability itself may be perceived as stressful by their children (Gelfand and Teti, 1990; Jaser et al., 2005; Palaez et al., 2008).

Exposure to these types of parental behaviors contributes to a chronically stressful environment for children. As noted by Hammen, Shih, and Brennan (2004), "Parenting quality, especially if perceived as being negative by the child, is itself stressful" (p. 512). A series of studies found that, according to parent and adolescent reports in a sample of adolescent children of depressed parents, adolescents were faced with the demands of moderate to high stress related to both parental withdrawal and parental intrusiveness in the past 6 months (Jaser et al., 2005, 2007; Langrock et al., 2002). Parental withdrawal and intrusiveness were moderately positively correlated, indicating that children must cope with parents who exhibit both types of behaviors rather than with parents who are either withdrawn or intrusive. Stressful parent-child interactions characterized by parental withdrawal and parental intrusiveness were significantly correlated with higher levels of children's symptoms of anxiety/depression and aggression.

As with studies of younger children, studies of older children that were designed to test mediation have found that qualities of parenting at least partially mediate associations between depression in parents and the development of behavioral or emotional problems in their children. For example, Jaser et al. (2008) found that regression analyses indicated that the relationship between current maternal depressive symptoms and adolescents' internalizing and externalizing problems were mediated by the observed sadness in mothers' interactions with their children. Similarly, in one of the few studies that included mothers and fathers, Du Rocher Schudlich and Cummings (2007) found that disrupted parenting (e.g., parental rejection, lax control, and psychological control) by mothers and fathers partially mediated the relations between maternal and paternal dysphoric mood and children's internalizing and externalizing problems. As described previously, a large-scale study recently found support for parental behaviors (nurturance, rejection, and monitoring) as mediators in the association between depressive symptoms in both mothers and fathers and 10- to 15-year-olds' emergence of emotional and behavioral problems (Elgar et al., 2007). These findings are strongly supportive of interventions to improve the quality of parenting in order to reduce the effects of parental depression on children.

Maternal Depression Increases Risk for Punitive Parenting and Child Abuse

As much as one needs to be concerned about depression in parents being associated with negative parenting qualities such as rejection, harshness, and intrusiveness, it is of even greater concern that researchers find depression in parents to be associated with maltreatment of children. Much of the latter work has focused on the pathway from maternal history of child maltreatment to depression in the women and, ultimately, maltreatment of the children. Numerous studies demonstrate that a maternal history of childhood maltreatment significantly increases a woman's risk for major depression, substance abuse, and domestic violence (Edwards et al., 2003; Kendler et al., 2000; Lang et al., 2004; MacMillan et al., 2001; Spatz Widom, DuMont, and Czaja, 2007; Springer et al., 2007; Whitfield et al., 2003). These outcomes have, in turn, been clinically implicated as increasing the risk for subsequent maltreatment of the woman's children, either by the woman herself or through her association with a perpetrating partner (Collishaw et al., 2007; Hazen et al., 2006; Koverola et al., 2005; Thompson, Kingree, and Desai, 2004). Several studies have sought to empirically determine the relative contributions of maternal child abuse history and the longer term outcomes of maternal depression, substance abuse, and domestic violence to increased risk for maltreatment of children. Statistical models have focused on a variety of proxy outcome measures, including measures of parenting attitudes, punitive parenting, parental stress, or child abuse potential as quantified by the Child Abuse Potential Inventory (CAP), a 160-item measure of potential for physical abuse.

Using path analysis with a sample of 265 predominately minority women, Mapp (2006) found that the only route from experiencing maternal childhood sexual abuse to increased risk for committing child physical abuse, as quantified by the Parenting Stress Index, was through elevated maternal depression symptom levels as defined by a score of 16 or more on the Center for Epidemiologic Studies Depression Scale (CESD). In a sample of 107 sexually abused and 156 control first-time mothers recruited prenatally and followed up when their children were between 2 and 4 years of age, Schuetze and Eiden (2005) found that maternal depression (CESD ≥ 16) was significantly associated with harsh, punitive parenting when the mother was also experiencing domestic violence. They concluded that the relationship between maternal childhood sexual abuse and adverse parenting was indirect and was mediated by maternal depression and domestic violence.

Comparing CAP scores in physically abused adolescent and adult mothers, de Paúl and Domenech (2000) found a significant interaction between young maternal age, a history of severe physical abuse, and maternal depression that predicted significant risk for child maltreatment measured with the CAP. Using a structured clinical interview, Cohen, Hien, and Batchelder (2008) compared mothers diagnosed as substance abusing (n = 41), depressed (n = 40), and both depressed and substance abusing (n = 47) with control mothers (n = 48) and found that the combination of substance abuse and depression was significantly related to elevated CAP scores as well as to several other measures of aversive parenting. Banyard, Williams, and Siegel (2003), however, found that maternal depression was related only to poor parenting satisfaction but not to other measures of parenting dysfunction or to the actual incidence of child protection intervention in a sample of 174 low-income predominantly African American women, half of whom had documented histories of child sexual abuse. That finding may be explained by their use of a nonstandard measure of depression, a subscale of the Trauma Symptom Checklist, which may account for the lack of effect.

Research thus indicates that maternal depression increases risk for child maltreatment when it occurs in some combination with other factors, such as a maternal history of maltreatment, maternal substance abuse, or domestic violence.

Mediators and Moderators of Associations Between Depression and Parenting

Given the strong and consistent evidence linking depression and parenting, it is important to ask what factors might mediate the relations between parental depressive symptoms and parenting behaviors. For example, as part of a larger study of parents of children with attention deficit hyperactivity disorder (ADHD), Gerdes et al. (2007) found that the association of maternal depressive symptoms and lax parenting was mediated by maternal locus of control and maternal parenting stress, and the relation between maternal depressive symptoms and harsh, overreactive parenting was mediated by maternal parenting stress and maternal self-esteem. That is, beliefs about control over events in one's life, perceived parenting stress, and self-esteem explained at least part of the association between high symptom levels in mothers and their parenting approaches.

Similarly, many factors are likely to moderate the relationship between depressive symptoms and parenting behaviors, although few studies have provided direct tests. General systems and social ecological models (Bronfenbrenner, 1980) suggest that a model to explain associations between depression and parenting must include potential influences beyond the individuals involved. Mothers, including mothers experiencing depression, are embedded in systems that have the capacity to enhance or disrupt their responsiveness to their infants. Theory suggests that social support networks may operate by encouraging and modeling parenting skills (Bronfrenbrenner, 1979) or by serving as a resource for alternate child care, thereby minimizing the negative impact of stress on parenting (Cohen and McKay, 1984). Similarly, stress has been identified as a major determinant of qualities of parenting (Belsky and Jaffee, 2006). In studies of general populations samples of parents (not depressed parents), the effect of stress on parenting has been found to be contingent on social support (Crockenberg, 1981; Cutrona, 1984; Goldstein, Diener, and Mangelsdorf, 1996). Specifically, both stress and social support were found to significantly predict maternal attitudes and interactive behavior. Mothers with high stress were found to be less positive, while mothers with high social support were found to be more positive.

Furthermore, social support has been found to moderate the effects of stress on maternal behavior (Crnic et al., 1983). For example, in a study of low-income African American mothers, although depression levels were not specified, mothers with larger support networks tended to be more responsive during interactions with their child (Burchinal, Follmer, and Bryant, 1996). The study also investigated the influence of structure on the effect of social support, finding that the source (father or grandmother) of social support through co-residence was associated with maternal responsiveness. Among the few studies that considered the role of stress and social support in associations between depression and parenting, the large-scale study by Radke-Yarrow (1998) found that, over time, the effects of mothers' affectively symptomatic behaviors on the quality of the mother-child relationship were moderated by levels of family stress.

Not only are qualities of parenting stressful for children of depressed parents, but also such children are exposed to a greater level of contextual stressors. For example, Adrian and Hammen (1993) found that children of depressed mothers were exposed to stressful events in their families because of increased interpersonal conflict associated with the parent's depression, and that family stress was also (along with depression in the mothers) an important predictor of both internalizing and externalizing problems in children.

Stress clearly needs to be an integral part of a model of associations between depression in parents, parenting, and outcomes in children. As an example of the essential role of stress, Jones, Forehand, and Beach (2000) studied the role of maternal depressive symptoms and family relationship stress in a community sample. Mothers' initial depressive symptoms generated perceived stress in both marital and mother-adolescent relationships a year later. In turn, mother-reported family relationship stress exacerbated her depressive symptoms. Mother-reported stressful family interactions also contributed to higher levels of depressive symptoms in both adolescent girls and boys. Although no evidence of a family stress generation process for fathers was found, father-reported family relationship stress was associated with greater adolescent depressive symptoms.

Beyond social support and stress, other moderators, which may increase or decrease the degree of association between depression and parenting, are the level of depression symptom severity, being in or out of a depressive episode, and level of impairment. There is evidence that problematic parenting behaviors persist, as depressed individuals continue to experience interpersonal impairment when not in a depressive episode (Hammen, 2003). However, more research is needed to determine how parenting qualities change in relation to exacerbation or improvement in depression symptoms.

Depression in women who became mothers as teenagers is also a concern, with teenage parenting considered a moderator of associations between depression in parents and adverse outcomes in children. The subset of children of depressed mothers whose mothers gave birth as teenagers may be worse off than other children of depressed mothers. Being a teenage mother is an independent risk factor for depression and also for adverse outcomes for children, although not all such mothers become depressed and not all of their children develop problems. African American women who become mothers during adolescence are more likely to be depressed than their peers who delay motherhood (Deal and Holt, 1998; Horwitz et al., 1996). Teenagers who become pregnant have been found to engage in more maladaptive parenting behaviors than adult mothers (Garcia-Coll et al., 1986; Hann et al., 1994). They are less likely to be empathic and more likely to value physical punishment than adult mothers (Fox et al., 1987). In our review, we highlight studies that sampled teenage mothers for their potential to help explain associations between depression in parents and child functioning.

Summary

The studies reveal well-replicated findings on the relation between parental depression and impaired parenting for children from infancy (and even fetal development) through adolescence. The findings from studies with extended theoretical models also show that the relation between depression and parenting is complex and needs to be considered in the context of a larger set of moderators and mediators, especially including other parental characteristics and the role of stress and social support. More research is needed to better understand this process.

Next we turn to the literature that has examined associations between depression in parents and children's physical and psychological health. Following that review, we return to parenting as we consider the role of parenting as a mediator of associations between depression in parents and aspects of functioning in children.

DEPRESSION IN PARENTS AND CHILDREN'S FUNCTIONING

Researchers have provided a wealth of data on the psychological and physical health of children whose parents have depression. Understandably, much attention has been focused on risk for the development of depression in the children. These findings are reviewed in this section, highlighting representative work. Researchers also expanded the scope of psychological outcomes studied in children of depressed parents to include other aspects of psychopathology, including other internalizing disorders as well as externalizing disorders. Other aspects of psychological functioning, some of which may themselves be developmental precursors, vulnerabilities, or early signs of disorder, are also included in this review. Similarly, physical health-related constructs include data on health or illness as well as children's receipt of routine health care, safety of the home, and growth. Although a comprehensive review of that literature is beyond the scope of this project, we present representative findings and an overview of the conclusions that can be drawn.

Limitations Stemming from Research Gaps

For each aspect of children's functioning that we examined in association with depression in parents, we reviewed not only the evidence for associations but also any evidence for moderators and mediators of those associations.

As described in Chapter 2, moderators indicate for whom or under what conditions the associations are stronger or weaker. In the literature on children of depressed parents, the most commonly studied moderators include chronicity, severity, and timing of the parent's depression, comorbidities with the parent's depression, and the role of the family and the larger social context, especially stress and social support. Each of these alone and in combination has the potential to exacerbate or protect against the risks to children associated with depression in parents. Empirical support for moderators provides the information for targeting interventions to subgroups of children of depressed parents by revealing those who are at even greater risk for negative outcomes relative to others who also have a parent with depression. Another potential moderator that has generated interest is sex of the child and, when depression in both parents has been studied, the match between the sex of the parent with depression and the sex of the child. However, most studies did not report sex differences, and, as has already been studied, few studies included depression in fathers. Findings from these studies of sex differences are included in this discussion when available. Finally, although theory and related research suggests that a healthy and available second parent might moderate the effect of depression in one parent on child functioning, few studies were found to support such moderation.

Mediators are of particular interest because they reveal the mechanisms through which the depression in the parent becomes associated with the outcomes in the children, with implications for preventive interventions. As shown in Figure 4-1, the Goodman and Gotlib model (1999) identified the most empirically and theory-based mediators for how depression in parents has its effects on children. These are parenting, genetics, prenatal factors (if the mother had been depressed during pregnancy), and stress. Empirical support for mediators, if they precede the outcomes of concern, provides the information needed for designing interventions in that one would have support for targeting the identified mechanisms in an intervention experiment (Kraemer et al., 2001). For example, research showing that depression in parents is associated with declining parenting skills and that the declining parenting skills at least partially explain associations between the depression and adverse outcomes in the children suggests that interventions designed to improve those parenting skills would benefit the children. With regard to genetics, there is a clear genetic risk for depression, as reviewed in Chapter 3. Thus, at least part of the associations found between depression in parents and children's psychological functioning will be explained by genetics. Conclusions about heritability as a mediator, however, are dependent on studies with genetically informed designs such as twin or adoption studies or studies testing the mediating role of molecular genetics, that is, a specific genetic anomaly.

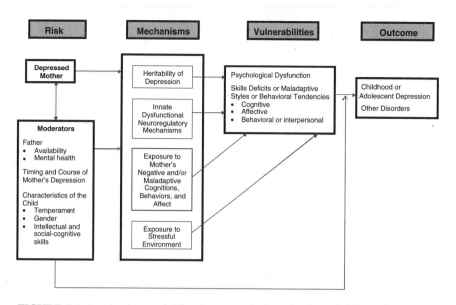

FIGURE 4-1 Integrative model for the transmission of risk to children of depressed mothers.
SOURCE: Reprinted, with permission, from Goodman and Gotlib (1999). Copyright (1999) by the American Psychological Association.

Knowledge of both moderators and mediators thus has clear and direct implications for prevention, as has been described in well-written papers that include a report on the prevention of mental disorders by the Institute of Medicine (1994). Despite these compelling reasons for identifying mediators and moderators, our review revealed that most of the outcome studies did not use research designs that would allow identification of moderators or mediators. Thus we are limited in our ability to draw conclusions on these important questions.

Another important consideration in evaluating this literature is a developmental perspective, as outlined in Chapter 2. That is, it is essential to consider the normative developmental accomplishments expected of children at the ages at which the effects of parental depression are being studied as well as at the time of the child's previous exposures, if any. This is especially important with the risk factor of parental depression given that depression is an episodic disorder. A further aspect of the developmental perspective is that children whose mothers are depressed may have mothers who were depressed during pregnancy and thus they were also exposed during fetal development. Maternal antenatal depression and its often accompanying high levels of stress may be an early life stress that alters developmental processes associated with later hypothalamic-pituitary-adrenal (HPA) axis functioning, potentially resulting in dysregulated stress response systems that have been identified as vulnerabilities to depression (Heim, Plotsky, and Nemeroff, 2004; Kammerer, Taylor, and Glover, 2006).

As with the limitations associated with knowledge of moderators and mediators, the literature is also limited in its ability to draw conclusions from a developmental perspective. Most of the outcomes studied are cross-sectional (both the parent's depression and the child's functioning were studied at the same time) rather than longitudinal (studying the parent's depression and the child's functioning at two or more times to see if changes in depression over time, such as increases in depressive symptom levels, account for changes in child functioning, such as the emergence of psychological problems). Thus most knowledge is about specific outcomes associated with concurrent depression in mothers at specific child ages (e.g., 4-year-old children of mothers who are depressed at that time). We know less about the course of outcomes over time for children exposed at particular times, taking into account the child's age when first exposed to depression in the parent (including potentially prenatally) and the chronicity and patterns of recurrence of the parent's depression. The latter question is complicated by depression being recurrent and the possibility that correlates of depression that matter for children (especially stressors and parenting qualities) may or may not vary with the course of illness (being in episode or in recovery). It is also important to consider the transactional nature of child rearing, in that both parental depression and child functioning continue to influence each other in an ongoing, cyclical manner throughout development (Elgar et al., 2004; Sameroff, 1975). In this review, we present a summary of what is known not only from the cross-sectional studies but also from the longitudinal studies and from studies that include pregnancy measures of depression.

A further limitation of the literature is that the vast majority of studies of parental depression are on depression in mothers rather than fathers. Nonetheless, we reviewed the scant literature on depression in fathers. We also report on the Connell and Goodman (2002) meta-analysis in which we found that, although depression in both mothers and fathers has been shown to affect children's psychological functioning, both internalizing and externalizing problems in children are more strongly associated with depression in mothers than with depression in fathers.

For some children, the primary caregiver is the grandmother. Thus it is relevant to understand the prevalence of depression in grandmothers or grandfathers who care for their grandchildren, the effect of depression in grandparents on their grandchildren, moderators of those associations, and the role of parenting qualities and other mediators in those associations. The committee found very few studies addressing these points. Findings on children raised by grandparents are also complicated by the often stressful circumstances that lead to that caregiving arrangement, such as father absence, maternal drug use or incarceration, high stress and low levels of support, exposure to trauma, and neglect (Gregory, Smith, and Palmieri, 2007). Given these added complications and the scarcity of the literature, we chose to not comprehensively review depression in grandparents who are primary caregivers. However, given the increasing frequency of such family arrangements, this lack of studies represents a critical research gap.

One concern raised about this literature is that often the mother is the reporter on both her own depression and the child outcome (Kraemer et al., 2003). This has particularly raised questions given that one might suspect that depression may negatively bias the mother's perceptions. We took note of Richters's helpful writing on concerns about depression influencing mothers' reports on their children (Richters, 1992). Our review shows that researchers with well-designed studies to address this question continue to find small to moderate support for an association between higher levels of maternal depression and mother's tendency to overreport child behavior problems, relative to a latent criterion variable (Boyle and Pickles, 1997; Fergusson, Lynskey, and Horwood, 1993). There remain important unresolved questions about how to interpret this association. Thus in our review we noted when researchers included additional sources of data, at least for the child outcome, which was more common than not.

Finally, another limitation of the research is that very few studies were designed to test transactional processes. In particular, little is known about the role of having a child with psychological problems on a parent's depression, although there is more literature on the role of children's physical health problems as a causal or exacerbating factor in parents' depression, on which we touch. Children with emotional, behavioral, or physical health problems may contribute to the causes of depression in parents or may exacerbate or help to maintain it once the parent's depression has emerged.

Physical Health and Health Care Utilization Consequences

The health-related outcomes for children when a parent is depressed have been studied in several key areas. First, studies describe the health of the neonate when the mother experiences mental health issues. Second, studies examine how the children of mothers with depressive symptoms have different patterns of physical illness and health care utilization. Third, studies have investigated the role of maternal depression when the child has a chronic health condition. Fourth, investigations explore how the presence of parental depression is linked to a home environment that presents more health risks to the child. Finally, a few studies report on the occurrence of adolescent health risk behaviors when their depressed parents exhibit health risk behaviors. In addition, the patterns of parenting with parental depression often influence how parents supervise, monitor, and model healthy behaviors.

Depression in the parent usually does not exist as a sole factor explaining health-related outcomes in these studies, as in studies of other outcomes. As has been described elsewhere in this report, depression is often accompanied by the circumstances of social disadvantage, marital difficulties, and other coexisting mental health and substance use disorders, and it is acknowledged that any or all of these factors may play a role (independent, additive, mediating, or moderating) in determining health-related and other adverse outcomes for the children of depressed parents. Only a few studies have addressed all of these multiple factors. When the interaction of these factors has been addressed, they are noted. Most studies have investigated depressive symptoms in mothers, not the clinical diagnosis of depression. Except for adolescent reports, data on the impact of depression in fathers or depression in both parents are not available. Given the centrality of developmental issues, we review this literature from that perspective.

Newborns

Antenatal depression, as well as stressful life events and anxiety, which often co-occur with depression, have been linked to complications of pregnancy or delivery (e.g., preeclampsia) and adverse pregnancy outcomes (e.g., low birth weight), at least partially as a function of poor prenatal care and unhealthy habits (smoking, alcohol, drugs) (see the review by Bonari et al., 2004). Among low-income African American women, those with a high level of depressive symptoms were nearly twice as likely to have spontaneous preterm births (Orr, James, and Blackmore Prince, 2002). This was true even after controlling for other health risks related to premature birth. In a more recent, large, prospective cohort study that began early in pregnancy (Li, Liu, and Odouli, 2009), clinically significant levels of depressive symptoms were associated with almost twice the risk of preterm delivery relative to women with no depressive symptoms. Further, the risk for preterm delivery increased with higher levels of severity of depressive symptoms and the results were not associated with the use of antidepressants although they were associated with obesity and stress. Thus depressive symptoms in the mother, although associated with other health risks, played the central role in association with the negative outcomes for infants. The adverse effects of fetal and newborn elevated cortisol that occur with perinatal maternal depression are discussed later in this chapter. In addition, mothers with depressive symptoms are also less likely to continue to breast-feed (Kendall-Tackett, 2005). Another concern about antenatal depression is fetal exposure to the mother's antidepressant medication or substance abuse during pregnancy, although we considered review of that literature outside the scope of this report.

Infants and Young Children

The social-environmental risk factors for child hospitalization in the first two years were examined in a Canadian cohort while controlling for biological risk factors. Elevated maternal depressive symptoms, single parenthood, and income inadequacy each increased the risk of hospitalization 1.5 to 1.8 times, independent of the infant's poor health and prematurity (Guttman, Dick, and To, 2004). In an ambulatory setting, even after controlling for socioeconomic factors, infants or young children of mothers with depressive symptoms were two times more likely to have more acute care visits and three times more likely to have an emergency room visit (Mandl et al., 1999). Among a prospective cohort of infants followed for the first year of life, infants of mothers with the diagnosis of depression were three times more likely to have acute care visits (Chee et al., 2008).

The emergency department is another frequently used acute care venue. In a prospective study, after controlling for disease morbidity and other factors, it was found that 6 months later inner-city mothers with high levels of depressive symptoms were 30 percent more likely to take their school-age children to an inner-city emergency department for asthma care than mothers with low levels of depressive symptoms (Bartlett et al., 2001). In another study, a diverse population of mothers who screened positive for depression were more than three times more likely to have had multiple emergency department visits and to have missed other outpatient visits, relative to mothers without depressive symptoms (Flynn et al., 2004). These increased rates of acute care visits and hospitalization were also found in two studies of socially disadvantaged populations and one community cohort with children up to age 3 years (Casey et al., 2004; Chung et al., 2004; Minkovitz et al., 2005). Maternal depressive symptoms have not been found to influence overall hospitalization rates for older children. However, in a prospective study of urban, economically disadvantaged, 4- to 9-year-olds with asthma, clinically significant maternal mental health symptoms were the strongest psychosocial predictor of hospitalization 9 months later (Weil et al., 1999). Further discussion of the influence of maternal depression on illness management for children with asthma in the inner-city setting is discussed later in this section.

Studies that examined preventive health care utilization found it to be associated with depressive symptoms in mothers (Mandl et al., 1999; Minkowitz et al., 2005). Minkowitz's study determined that higher levels of maternal depressive symptoms at 2 to 4 months postpartum predicted fewer well-child visits up to age 24 months in a prospective primary care sample receiving augmented services to enhance child development. In a study of children starting school, maternal depressive symptom levels were not associated with children's receipt of preventive health care services, but they were associated with children's being less likely to have had preventive dental care (Kavanaugh et al., 2006).

Women with clinically significant levels of depressive symptoms are more likely to report their child's health at age 3 as fair or poor (Kahn et al., 2002). They are also more likely to seek clinical care for childhood somatic disorders, such as syncope (i.e., fainting; Morris et al., 2001), abdominal pain (Levy et al., 2006; Zuckerman and Beardslee, 1987), headaches (Zuckerman and Beardslee, 1987), and injuries (Minkovitz et al., 2005). Increased accident rates have also been shown to occur when mothers are experiencing an episode of depression (Brown and Davidson, 1978).

Among some subgroups of children with specific medical conditions, high levels of maternal depressive symptoms have been found to be more common. This includes conditions with associated psychosocial issues, such as failure to thrive (Stewart, 2007), ADHD (Johnston and Mash, 2001; Lesesne, Visser, and White, 2003), and chronic epilepsy (Shore et al., 2002), and conditions with high daily care demands, such as medical fragility (Meltzer and Mindell, 2006), ventilator technology–dependent (Meltzer and Mindell, 2006), severe burn (El Hamaoui et al., 2006), and major developmental disabilities (Bailey et al., 2007; Manuel et al., 2003; Smith et al., 1993). Many of these studies assess depressive symptoms only on small, cross-sectional cohorts of children with specific diseases and do not determine the severity or chronicity of parental depression or illness course. Stress from caregiving, anxiety, lack of social supports, and disrupted caregiver sleep have all been shown to play a role in how a chronic condition relates to maternal depression (Boman, Lindahl, and Björk, 2003; Manuel et al., 2003; Meltzer and Mindell, 2006; Moore et al., 2006). These descriptive studies overall indicate that parental depression needs to be considered in these populations and that recognizing and treating the depression in parents may be an important adjunct to treatment of the child.

As indicated above (Weil et al., 1999), the influence of maternal depression on illness management has been studied more in depth for children with asthma in inner-city communities than for other illnesses or in other settings. In the prospective study of inner-city children with asthma, mothers with a high level of depressive symptoms, compared with mothers with lower levels of depressive symptoms, were less likely to adhere to medication regimens prescribed for their children, more likely to have poorer understanding of asthma illness management and poorer communication with the health provider, and were less confident in managing their child's illness at home (Bartlett et al., 2004). In addition, the mothers with high levels of depressive symptoms were 2 to 3 times more likely to report recently feeling helpless or frightened and upset by the child's asthma. For families dealing with asthma, the role of maternal depression in disease control has been shown to be mediated by the child's psychological problems as well (Lim, Wood, and Miller, 2008). Findings on depression being associated with parents' greater hostility and lower warmth/nurturance have also been replicated in low-income African American mothers of children with asthma (Celano et al., 2008), with implications for problems in parents' management of these children's persistent health care needs.

Maternal depression and related parenting issues play a role not only in the management but also in the development of asthma. Parenting difficulties early in life, subsequent child psychosocial problems, and immunoglobulin E levels at age 6 were significant predictors of asthma at ages 6–8 years in a longitudinal cohort at high risk for asthma (Klinnert et al., 2001). Maternal depressive symptoms measured at age 6 were strongly correlated with key predictors, parenting, and child psychosocial problems. In a recent large birth cohort study, children with continued exposure over the first 7 years of life to mothers under treatment for depression and anxiety had higher incidence of asthma (odds ratio = 1.25) after controlling for asthma risk factors (Kozyrskyj et al., 2008). These effects were greater in high-income than low-income households.

Only recently have studies been published that examine more closely the interface between maternal mental health, parenting, child behavior, and chronic disease management. These asthma studies illustrate how maternal depression might play a role in adverse outcomes for childhood chronic physical health conditions when psychosocial factors influence the disease process and the diseases require careful parental attention to care management regimes and monitoring.

Other health consequences may occur because of changes in the family environment associated with maternal depression. Mothers of young children with depression are more likely to be smokers (Whitaker, Orzol, and Kahn, 2006), thus exposing children to secondhand smoke that is associated with more respiratory problems (Neuspiel et al., 1989). In a longitudinal study of depressed parents, more respiratory illness was reported in children during middle childhood (Goodwin et al., 2007). Among preschoolers, the children watching the most television were predicted by two factors, maternal depression and maternal overweight status (Burdette et al., 2003). Excessive television viewing in young children has implications for obesity and behavior. Other preventive health parenting practices that may limit optimal health and prevention of disease in children are discussed in the earlier section on parenting practices.

Adolescents

Although rarely studied compared with studies of infants or young children, adolescents' health care utilization also has been found to be associated with depression in parents. In one study at 10-year follow-up, the children of a depressed parent were more likely to have been hospitalized. However, only the subgroup of children who had themselves developed depression had more medical problems reported by their late teens to mid-20s (Kramer et al., 1998). Another report of these offspring after 20 years in middle age also showed an increase in the overall number of medical problems. Substance dependence was also more likely to develop during the adolescent years in this population (Weissman et al., 2006a).

An issue that emerges with adolescence is health risk behaviors, such as the use of tobacco, alcohol, and drugs. It is well known that adolescent health risk-taking behaviors are closely related to parental alcohol and tobacco use patterns. It was particularly informative to note that, in a German longitudinal community study from early adolescence into early adulthood, the odds of illicit drug use doubled if either parent had an affective disorder, even after controlling for parental use (Lieb et al., 2002). Rates did not increase further when both parents were affected—that is, even after accounting for parental use, an affective disorder in either the mother or father increased the likelihood of an adolescent's beginning to use illicit drugs. Similarly, having a parent with depression was associated with a 40 percent increase in adolescents' alcohol and nicotine dependence, even after controlling for parental anxiety and substance use (Lieb et al., 2002).

Overall, there is emerging evidence that depression, at least in mothers if not also in fathers, is related to the use of child health care services and adverse health outcomes in children, from infancy through adolescence. Moreover, the co-occurrence of maternal depression and a chronic health condition in the child places the child at additional risk of poor outcomes. Longitudinal studies that examine more closely the pathways by which depression influences health outcomes are needed to inform effective interventions.

Child Psychological Problems and Well-Being

Particular Aspects of Concern

Researchers have studied a range of aspects of child psychological problems and well-being. Typically, the choice of what to study in the children is justified as being important both in terms of theories and research suggesting (a) why these aspects of functioning are likely to be affected by depression in parents and (b) why these aspects of functioning, if affected, would be of concern regarding the potential for later development of psychopathology.

Not surprisingly, much attention has focused on the likelihood of children of depressed parents becoming depressed themselves. Both theory about the mechanisms whereby maternal depression might contribute to depression in children (Goodman and Gotlib, 1999) and about the developmental pathways to the emergence of depression in children (Cicchetti and Toth, 1998) point to the importance of knowing more about associations between maternal depression and the emergence of depression in children and adolescents. Many of the studies of children of depressed parents have therefore examined associations between depression in parents and depression-related outcomes in their children, including depressive symptom levels and rates of depressive disorder. Some researchers have broadened the construct to internalizing disorders or problems in children, given that anxiety disorders are the most frequent co-occurring disorders in both clinical (Compas et al., 1997) and community samples (Lewinsohn et al., 1991) and that many researchers rely on symptom checklists that yield scores on internalizing problems as a broadband construct.

Among other outcomes associated with depression in parents, researchers have also been interested in externalizing disorders, since elevated rates of conduct problems have been noted since the earliest studies of children of depressed parents (e.g., Welner et al., 1977). From a theoretical perspective, externalizing disorders in children with depressed parents are interesting because they may reflect problems with dysregulated aggression (Radke-Yarrow et al., 1992), a distinct pattern of inherited vulnerability perhaps related to behavior disorders (e.g., alcoholism, substance abuse, antisocial personality disorders) in first-degree relatives (Kovacs et al., 1997; Williamson et al., 1995). Alternatively, externalizing problems in children may reflect particular interactions among genes and cognitive, affective, interpersonal, and other biological systems that lead to the emergence of externalizing rather than (or co-occurring with) internalizing disorders.

Although much of the literature has focused on psychopathology as outcomes for children with depressed mothers, a developmental psychopathology perspective requires an expanded definition of outcomes to also include competence or limits on ability to achieve typical development in the full range of affective/emotional, cognitive, and social/interpersonal functioning.

A separate, important aspect of functioning that is essential to understand in children of depressed parents is temperament or behavioral tendencies. Difficulties in temperament associated with depression in parents could be observed, for example, through infants' behavioral tendencies toward less interest in and active exploration of their environment and novel stimuli, poorer organizational capabilities, and less soothability relative to infants of nondepressed mothers. Mechanisms to explain such associations would primarily be heritability but could also include effects of prenatal exposures to maternal depression and correlated stress. Consistent with both explanations, fetal movement at 36 weeks gestation has been found to account for 21 to 43 percent of the variance in distress to limitations at 1 year and behavioral inhibition at 2 years (negative predictions), both indices of regulatory abilities (DiPietro et al., 2002). Temperament has also been of interest to parental depression researchers because it may be an early sign of vulnerability to the later development of depression (Hayden et al., 2006). Furthermore, temperament is of interest given transactional processes, which suggest that a depressed parent and an infant with a "difficult" temperament may face particular challenges in relation to each other relative to nondepressed parents or children who do not have these temperament qualities.

For several reasons, researchers also have been interested in affective functioning, especially high negative affect and low positive affect in children of depressed parents (Cicchetti, Ackerman, and Izard, 1995; Garber, Braafladt, and Zeman, 1991). First is an understanding that how children manage their emotions may be early signs of some of the underlying personality traits associated with depression in adults (Klein et al., 2002). Second is research showing that high negative affect and low positive affect may be early signs of vulnerability to depression or even early signs of depression. Third, from the transactional perspective, is the understanding that infants and children with these affective tendencies will be especially challenging for parents with depression and may play a critical role in unfolding cycles of mutual negative influences.

Children of depressed mothers may inherit a tendency to experience and express negative emotions (Plomin et al., 1993), may learn such a tendency through modeling, or may have heightened negative emotionality as a function of stress-related HPA axis dysregulation. Even in infancy, problems with negative emotions can be observed by infants showing more distress relative to others (Campbell and Cohn, 1997). Older children may experience more sadness relative to controls.

Positive emotions might be equally important to examine as an outcome for children with depressed mothers, given that depression disorders are uniquely characterized by low positive affect or anhedonia (Clark and Watson, 1991). A dispositional tendency for low positive affect may predispose children to the development of depression. Problems with positive emotions might be noted in infants observed to exhibit less positive affect or enjoyment (Cohn and Campbell, 1992) or in older children experiencing or expressing less positive affect relative to controls. Mechanisms that might help explain the occurrence of low positive affect in children with depressed mothers include heritability, the potential role of temperament and a learned tendency to overcontrol positive affect (or a lower behavioral activation system) (Fowles, 1994), or a frontal lobe pattern of relatively greater left than right frontal cortical activity, which has been associated with lower positive affective responses (Davidson and Fox, 1989). Some aspects of emotional functioning are assessed with such measures as cortisol as an index of stress reactivity, electroencephalogram (EEG) asymmetry as an index of a tendency to experience negative emotions, and infant neurobehavioral functioning as an index of newborns' abilities to control their behavior in response to the physical and social environment. Positive emotionality also has potential for being a partial mediator of associations between depression in parents and the later emergence of depression or other problems in their children. Findings suggestive of this idea include a study that showed that low levels of positive emotionality in 3-year-old children, measured with laboratory tasks and naturalistic observations, predicted higher levels of cognitive vulnerabilities to depression when the children were 7 years old, such as helplessness and depressogenic attributional styles (Hayden et al., 2006).

In addition to emotional functioning, children's competency outcomes in social and cognitive realms are of interest in relation to depression in parents. Interpersonal functioning, ranging from responsiveness of infants to social functioning and competence in older children or adolescents, also is potentially tied to heritability (Goldsmith, Buss, and Lemery, 1997) and learning mechanisms. Deficits in interpersonal functioning are at the core of several theories of depression emerging in childhood (Bemporad, 1994; Cole, 1991; Hammen et al., 2003; Zahn-Waxler, 1993). Behavioral models of depression also suggest the importance of these social skills, traits, or tendencies, in that they could be associated with children's lower likelihood of being reinforced if they lack certain skills or express other behaviors that result in a lack of rewarding relationships (Lewinsohn, 1974; Patterson and Stoolmiller, 1991).

Similarly, cognitive functioning, especially the role of beliefs and attitudes, are central to the etiology of depression in children and adolescents (Garber and Martin, 2002; Hammen, 1992; Seligman et al., 1984), suggesting the importance of examining self-esteem, attributional style, and deficits in cognitive problem-solving skills. Another aspect of cognitive functioning, cognitive/intellectual functioning, is sometimes studied as an outcome in association with depression in parents, although it is sometimes conceptualized as a moderator in models of risk for children with depressed mothers (Goodman and Gotlib, 1999). Trouble concentrating and making decisions, as well as other symptoms, may emerge as early signs of depression in the children and have the strong potential to interfere with intellectual and academic functioning, while associated school failures may independently increase the risk of depression (Lewinsohn et al., 1994).

In the Goodman and Gotlib (1999) model (see Figure 4-1), these domains of child functioning are, for the most part, conceptualized as vulnerability factors. These affective, interpersonal, behavioral, and cognitive variables are conceptualized as early markers of maladaptive processes that may be associated with the later development of psychopathology. We use the term "vulnerability" to refer to individuals' enduring or long-standing life circumstances or conditions that intensify maladaptive processes and thwart the achievement of successful adaptation (Cicchetti, Rogosch, and Toth, 1994; Masten et al., 1999). Risk factors, then, may include the external factors, including depression in a parent as well as other family and broader socioenvironmental factors.

Newborn Neurobehavioral Outcomes

Researchers have reported varying degrees of consistency of support for associations between elevated levels of antenatal depression and poorer newborn neurobehavioral regulation. Studies shows consistent support for antenatal depression being significantly associated with newborns' greater inconsolability (Zuckerman et al., 1990), more crying/fussiness (Diego, Field, and Hernandez-Reif, 2005; Field et al., 2007; Zuckerman et al., 1990), more time in indeterminate sleep (Diego, Field, and Hernandez-Reif, 2005; Field et al., 2001, 2004), and more activity/movement (Field et al., 2004, 2007; Hernandez-Reif et al., 2006). Findings on infant alertness are less consistent, with one study finding a significant association with antenatal depression (Hernandez-Reif et al., 2006), but two others finding no significant association (Field et al., 2007; Zuckerman et al., 1990).

Higher levels of antenatal depression have also been found to be prospectively associated with less optimal scores on several subscales of the Neonatal Behavioral Assessment Scale (NBAS) (Brazelton, 1984). Field and colleagues have been at the forefront of studies revealing higher levels of antenatal depression being associated with less optimal scores on several subscales of the NBAS (Field et al., 2001, 2004; Hernandez-Reif et al., 2006; Jones et al., 1998; Lundy et al., 1999). Across publications, the most replicated finding was for antenatal depression to be associated with lower ability of a newborn to attend to visual and auditory stimuli and the quality of overall alertness. Effect sizes were typically in the range of 0.22 to 0.60. Most studies found that antenatal depression showed minimal to no significant association with newborns' ability to regulate their state in the face of external stimulation or in their having more abnormal reflexes. Other subscales were found to be significantly associated with antenatal depression in some studies and not in others. The inconsistencies in the particular scales that are found to be associated with antenatal depression are likely to be explained by the variability in clinical characteristics of antenatal depression, which would be expected to be a moderator. The inconsistencies are not owing to how antenatal depression was measured, since all but one of the studies relied on symptom scales rather than on diagnoses.

Another plausible explanation for the inconsistencies is comorbid alcohol or substance use during pregnancy. Researchers have found high rates of antenatal depression co-occurring with cigarette smoking, alcohol consumption, and abuse of such substances as cocaine, often in combination with each other (e.g., Amaro and Zuckerman, 1990, 1991; Amaro, Zuckerman, and Cabral, 1989; Zuckerman, Amaro, and Beardslee, 1987; Zuckerman et al., 1989). For example, depression is especially prevalent (35–56 percent) in samples of drug-dependent pregnant women (Burns et al., 1985; Fitzsimons et al., 2007; Regan et al., 1982).

Temperament

Several researchers have found that infants of depressed mothers, relative to controls, have more difficult temperament. Whiffen and Gotlib (1989) found that infants of depressed mothers were perceived as more difficult to care for and more bothersome. A large study in Japan found direct effects of maternal depression on the infant temperament constructs of "frustration tolerance" and "fear of strangers and strange situations" (Sugawara et al., 1999). A meta-analysis found a significant, moderate correlation between postpartum depression and infant temperament, with a 95 percent confidence interval that ranged from 0.26 to 0.37 (Beck, 1996). Although relying on depressed mothers as reporters of their children's temperament has raised concerns (Forman et al., 2003), researchers have found these significant associations even with lab-based measures of temperament (Goldsmith and Rothbart, 1994) and with self-report measures such as those developed by Rothbart (Garstein and Rothbart, 2003), which minimize maternal report bias by asking situation-specific questions and taking advantage of the extent and breadth of experience that mothers have with their infants.

Among the potential moderators or correlated risk factors that have been studied, co-occurring anxiety in mothers has been found to play a role in associations between maternal depression and infant temperament, but the precise role is not clear. It may be that the anxiety, known to be highly correlated with depression, matters more. In one study, maternal trait anxiety predicted difficult infant temperament independent of antenatal and postnatal depression scores (Austin et al., 2005). Another study found that both anxiety and depression in mothers matter. One study, which measured temperament not only with maternal reports but also with observations, found that mild parental dysphoria and mild parental anxiety were associated with two dimensions of child temperament: attention and emotion regulatory difficulties (West and Newman, 2003).

Some of the findings are informative of the developmental perspective, especially of the role of transactional processes. In particular, some researchers have tested the hypothesis that infants' difficult temperament may increase the likelihood of postpartum depression. In one study, infants' difficult temperament was related to maternal depression in mothers of 3-month-olds, and this association was mediated by perceived efficacy in the parenting role (Cutrona and Troutman, 1986). In another study, maternal depression and infant negative emotionality interacted to predict maternal reactivity/sensitivity (Pauli-Pott et al., 2000). Positive infant emotionality was not a predictor. Good marital support was directly associated with maternal reactivity/sensitivity, but not as a moderator.

In a direct test of the role of transactional processes, one group of researchers found that maternal depression and difficult infant temperament, but also fear/shyness, may interact to predict negative outcomes for children as adolescents, but the results vary by temperament factor, the child outcome, and gender. For example, in a longitudinal study that spanned ages 5 through 17, exposure to maternal depression in early childhood predicted increases in boys' externalizing behavior problems over time only among boys whose temperament factor of impulsivity was low (Leve, Kim, and Pears, 2005). Others have found that children with more difficult temperament are more vulnerable to the effects of inadequate parenting, such as that found to be associated with depression in mothers (Goldsmith, Buss, and Lemery, 1997). Mothers of more difficult infants also perceive their parenting to be less efficacious, which in turn is linked to depression in mothers (Cutrona and Troutman, 1986; Porter and Hsu, 2003). Future research not only needs to continue to address the role of child temperament but also needs to include measures of temperament, parenting, and parents' depressive symptoms that are not limited to maternal self-report for all of these variables.

A few researchers have addressed potential mediators of associations between depression in parents and children's temperament, focusing on influences on fetal development. Antidepressant medication treatment during pregnancy, at least in one study, did not predict temperament (Nulman et al., 2002). However, other prenatal or fetal processes may matter. One study found that elevated maternal cortisol at 30–32 weeks of gestation, but not earlier in pregnancy, was significantly associated with greater maternal report of infant negative reactivity, with additive predictions from prenatal maternal anxiety and depression, even after controlling for postnatal maternal psychological state (Davis et al., 2007). In another study, at 2 and 6 months postpartum, mothers who had been depressed in pregnancy and/or postpartum, compared with nondepressed mothers, reported more difficult infants at both times, even after controlling for histories of maternal abuse or prenatal anxiety (McGrath, Records, and Rice, 2008).

Genetics is likely to be another mediator. Temperament itself is highly heritable (Hwang and Rothbart, 2003). Furthermore, genetics may explain associations between maternal depression and infant temperament (and the later development of depression or other disorders) (Gonda et al., 2006; Pezawas et al., 2005). That is, the same set of genes may predict both temperament qualities, such as negative affectivity and depression.

From a methodological perspective, it is important to note that findings on depression's associations with child temperament are not the result of potential biases in depressed parents' perspectives. For example, not all studies relied solely on depressed mothers' perceptions of child temperament. In one study, not only depressed mothers but also their partners perceived their 2-month-olds' temperaments more negatively relative to nondepressed women and their partners (Edhborg et al., 2000). More broadly, current temperament questionnaire measures have been developed to minimize the contribution of reporter bias (Rothbart and Hwang, 2002).

Finally, there is some evidence that difficult temperament is a partial mediator of associations between major depression disorders in parents and children's development of depressive disorders. One longitudinal study, which followed children of depressed parents over a period of 20 years, showed the expected association between depression in one or both parents and having a difficult temperament (Bruder-Costello et al., 2007). Second, they found that difficult temperament in the children increased their likelihood of major depressive disorder. Third, they supported a partial mediational role of temperament in that children's difficult temperament explained an additional 10 percent of the variance in associations between depression in parents and new episodes of major depression in the child.

Attachment

The association between depression in mothers and infants' less secure attachment relationships is well studied, with fairly consistent findings. There is sufficient literature that it has been subject to some meta-analyses. One meta-analysis reviewed effects of maternal mental illness (including both depression and psychosis) on quality of attachment in clinical samples (van Ijzendoorn et al., 1992). They found that maternal mental illness increased the likelihood of insecure attachment relative to norms and relative to samples of children with a range of problems. Another meta-analysis of 16 studies found that maternal depression was not associated with significantly higher rates of disorganized attachment in children relative to middle-class samples or to poverty samples (van IJzendoorn, Schuengel, and Bakersmans-Kranenburg, 1999). This was true even taking into account socioeconomic status, type of depression assessment, and clinical versus community samples. However, severely and chronically depressed parents were not targeted in this particular study population. Another meta-analysis, restricted to studies of clinically diagnosed depression in mothers, found that infants of depressed mothers showed significantly reduced likelihood of secure attachment and marginally raised the likelihood of avoidant and disorganized attachment (Martins and Gaffan, 2000). For example, clinically significant depression in mothers increased the likelihood of disorganized attachment from 17 to 28 percent on average. The reviewed studies predominantly sampled middle-income families with minimal risk factors other than the depression in the mothers. Thus, poverty and other risk factors do not explain this finding.

Affective Functioning

Several studies have found support for associations between depression in mothers and infants' or children's greater negative affect relative to controls. Infants of depressed mothers show more negative affect (crying and fussing) and more self-directed regulatory behaviors (e.g., self-soothing or looking away) (Field, 1992; Tronick and Gianino, 1986). Toddlers show more dysregulated aggression and heightened emotionality (Zahn-Waxler et al., 1984), and adolescents (particularly girls) display more dysphoric and less happy affect (Hops, Sherman, and Biglan, 1990). In one study that examined depressive symptom levels in both mothers and fathers, mothers' but not fathers' depressive symptom levels were associated with preschool-age children's low positive emotionality (Durbin et al., 2005). These studies predominantly, but not exclusively, sampled middle-class populations.

Cognitive/Intellectual/Academic Performance

Various indices of cognitive-intellectual or academic performance have reliably been found to be associated with depression in mothers. Children with depressed mothers, compared with children whose mothers are medically ill or have other psychiatric disorders, have poorer academic performance and other behavioral problems in school (Anderson and Hammen, 1993). Children of depressed mothers or mothers high in depressive symptom levels have been found to score lower on measures of intelligence in several studies (Anderson and Hammen, 1993; Hammen and Brennan, 2001; Hay and Kumar, 1995; Hay et al., 2001; Jaenicke et al., 1987; Kaplan, Beardslee, and Keller, 1987; Murray et al., 1993; Sharp et al., 1995). This literature has been qualitatively reviewed from a developmental perspective, including the role of timing of the depression in the mothers (Sohr-Preston and Scaramella, 2006). For example, a large, federal, early child care study found that chronicity of depressive symptoms over the first 3 years of life was related to maternal sensitivity, and maternal sensitivity moderated associations between maternal depressive symptom levels and 3-year-olds' school readiness and verbal comprehension (NICHD Early Child Care Research Network, 1999).

Among the strongest evidence for moderators of the association between maternal depression and academic functioning is exposure to violence (Silverstein et al., 2006). Essentially, in a large nationally representative sample of kindergarten-aged children, Silverstein et al. found that although depression in mothers was independently strongly associated with children's lower reading, mathematics, and general knowledge, children who had also been exposed to violence scored even lower on those same skills. They also had more behavior problems compared with children who had been exposed to either maternal depression or violence alone. This pattern of findings was stronger for boys than for girls.

School Dropout and Adolescent Sexual Behavior

In a longitudinal study of offspring of depressed and nondepressed mothers followed annually from 6th through 12th grade, higher IQ was found to be protective of dropping out among offspring of never- or moderately depressed mothers but not for adolescents whose mothers had been chronically or severely depressed (Bohon, Garber, and Horomtz, 2007). Similarly, the presence of a male head of household was associated with lower rates of sexual behavior among adolescents of never- or moderately depressed mothers but not among adolescents whose mother's depression was chronic or severe.

Cognitive Vulnerabilities to Depression

One of the strongest predictors of depression in adults and also in children is the presence of cognitive vulnerabilities. Thus, this has been of interest to researchers who study the children of depressed parents. Across multiple studies, depression in mothers and high levels of depressive symptoms in mothers are associated with children, as young as age 5, showing early signs of cognitive vulnerability to depression, including being more likely than controls to blame themselves for negative outcomes, having a more negative attributional style, hopelessness, pessimism, being less likely to recall positive self-descriptive adjectives, and having lower self-worth (Anderson and Hammen, 1993; Garber and Robinson, 1997; Hammen and Brennan, 2001; Hay and Kumar, 1995; Jaenicke et al., 1987; Murray et al., 2001). Adolescents with depressed mothers show early signs of cognitive vulnerability to depression, such as being more likely than other adolescents to blame themselves for negative outcomes and less likely to recall positive self-descriptive adjectives (Hammen and Brennan, 2001; Jaenicke et al., 1987).

Stress and Coping

Of particular concern is a pattern of children of depressed mothers (current or past depression) being more reactive cognitively (e.g., being more likely to think pessimistically) when exposed to failure (Murray et al., 2001; Taylor and Ingram, 1999).

They found, for example, that associations between adolescents' reports of parental stress and parents' reports of adolescents' anxiety/depressive symptoms were related to adolescents' self-reported use of secondary control engagement coping and adolescents' stress reactivity (Jaser et al., 2005, 2008; Langrock et al., 2002). Specifically, increased levels of parent-child stress due to parental withdrawal and parental intrusiveness were associated with higher levels of stress reactivity in children (e.g., heightened emotional and physiological arousal, intrusive thoughts, rumination). Conversely, children's use of coping strategies that involve acceptance of their parents' depression and efforts to reappraise it in more positive ways was related to lower levels of anxiety and depression in children of depressed parents. These findings suggest that teaching children of depressed parents to use more effective coping strategies may be an important target for preventive interventions (Compas et al., 2002).

Beardslee and colleagues have published several papers on this topic, going back several decades, which have informed understanding of the range of functioning in children and adolescents whose parents (mothers and/or fathers) have been depressed. They have found, essentially, that children of depressed mothers vary in their adaptive functioning, and those with more adaptive functioning function better. For example, more flexible approaches to coping and more situationally appropriate strategies are associated with better outcomes (a moderator relationship) (Beardslee, Schultz, and Selman, 1987; Carbonell, Reinherz, and Beardslee, 2005). Results from other studies by Beardslee and colleagues suggest that children may be protected by how they perceive and respond to depression in their parents (Beardslee and Podorefsky, 1988; Solantaus-Simula, Punamaki, and Beardslee, 2002a, 2002b). Specifically, youth who were resilient in the face of parental depression understood that their parents were ill and that they were not to blame for the illness.

Findings from intervention studies in Beardslee's randomized trials are also tests of the role of these constructs in associations between depression in parents and children's well-being (Beardslee et al., 2003, 2008). The concept of understanding on children's part was operationalized to be understanding of the parent's illness at both the fourth and sixth assessment points. Young people whose parents changed the most in response to the intervention had increased the most in understanding their parents' illness. Thus, it was possible to increase understanding through preventive intervention. Others note variability in adolescent children's coping with maternal depression (Klimes-Dougan and Bolger, 1998). For example, children whose mothers' depression is associated with more anger and irritability cope differently than others, boys differ from girls, and, even within families, siblings differ in how they cope with the mother's depression.

Interpersonal Functioning

Beginning with studies of infants, researchers have identified problems in interpersonal functioning associated with depression in mothers. Field (1992) has shown that infants (1) match the negative affective expressions of their mothers when in face-to-face interaction with them, (2) look "depressed," and (3) generalize these styles to the infants' interactions with others. She has also found that infants of depressed mothers whose interaction style is characterized as withdrawn have poorer interactive qualities than those whose style is characterized as intrusive (Jones et al., 1997b). In multiple publications since the early 1980s, Tronick and Cohn have illuminated the nature of infants' responses to face-to-face interaction with mothers who are depressed (Cohn and Tronick, 1983; Cohn et al., 1986). Among their more recent papers, they show that higher symptom levels in mothers and the infants' being male contributed to lower quality mother-infant interactions (Weinberg et al., 2006).

Murray has studied infants, toddlers, and preschool-age children interacting with their depressed mothers. Although some of the studies controlled for other variables, such as conflict in the home, she found that the depression in mothers still accounted for the children's quality of interaction (Murray and Trevarthen, 1986; Murray et al., 1996b, 1999).

Studies of young children interacting with their depressed mothers, best illustrated by the work of Radke-Yarrow and colleagues, revealed that children whose mothers have been depressed engage in excessive compliance, excessive anxiety, and disruptive behavior that, when the children were followed into adolescence, were found to persist over time (Radke-Yarrow, 1998).

Among the few studies of peer interactions, sons but not daughters of depressed mothers were found to display more aggressive behavior during interactions with friends (Hipwell et al., 2005). Kindergarten-age children whose mothers were depressed were more often excluded by peers (Cummings, Keller, and Davies, 2005). The latter effect was mediated by the children's exposure to interparental conflict. Adolescent children of depressed mothers have poorer peer relationships and less adequate social skills than teens of nondepressed control mothers (Beardslee, Schultz, and Selman, 1987; Billings and Moos, 1985; Forehand and McCombs, 1988; Hammen and Brennan, 2003).

Psychobiological Systems: Stress Responses and Cortical Activity

Researchers have found significant associations between maternal depression and two psychobiological systems in children that have been found to play a role in emotion regulation and expression. The first is stress responses measured in either (a) autonomic activity (higher heart rate and lower vagal tone) or (b) stress hormonal levels (higher cortisol as an index of HPA axis activity). Field (1992) found that infants of depressed mothers have higher cortisol levels, especially following interaction with their depressed mothers (Field, 1992). Harsh parenting, which is sometimes associated with maternal depression, has also been linked to higher cortisol levels in children (Hertsgaard et al., 1995). Both findings suggest an association between children's HPA axis functioning and the depressed mothers' failure to provide sensitive, responsive care.

The second significant association with maternal depression is cortical activity in the prefrontal cortex and particularly the pattern of greater relative right frontal EEG asymmetries. This pattern is associated with the experience of withdrawal emotions in children and with depression in adults and adolescents (Davidson et al., 1990; Dawson, 1999; Dawson et al., 1992; Finman et al., 1989). Even 1-week-old infants of depressed mothers, as well as 1-month-old infants, showed greater relative right frontal EEG asymmetry compared with infants of nondepressed mothers, and these early EEGs are correlated with EEGs at 3 months and 3 years (Jones et al., 1997a), suggesting continuity of this effect. Dawson and colleagues saw similar patterns in 18-month-olds (Dawson et al., 1997). These patterns show remarkable stability from as early as age 1 week to age 3 years, suggesting that the early measures are reliably detecting a pattern of individual differences (Dawson et al., 1997, 2003; Jones et al., 1997a). Further, although restricted to a small sample, Dawson found support for both contextual stressors (marital discord and levels of stress) and children's frontal brain activation mediating the association between a history of maternal depression and children's behavior problems when the children were 3 years old.

Among possible moderators of associations between maternal depression and children's frontal brain activation are the extent of exposure to depression in mothers, especially prenatal exposure. For example, the number of prenatal months of exposure to maternal depression marginally predicted left frontal lobe activation from EEG (Ashman and Dawson,

2002; Dawson et al., 1997). However, depression during pregnancy was measured retrospectively when the mothers were 13–15 months postpartum, and depression was defined to include women who were in partial remission or subthreshold. If this finding is replicated, it suggests the need to examine such mechanisms as genetics and intrauterine factors for the association between maternal depression and frontal brain activity in prenatally exposed infants.

Other potential moderators yield mixed findings. For example, abnormalities in neurobiological or neuroendocrine functioning in infants are sometimes specifically found to be associated with face-to-face interaction with their depressed mothers (Field, 1992) and with harsh parenting in particular (Hertsgaard et al., 1995), but others find them to reflect a more general trait (Dawson et al., 2001).

Behavior Problems or Psychopathology

The ultimate outcome of concern among children of depressed parents is the emergence of elevated levels of behavior problems or diagnosable psychopathology. Many studies show that rates of depression are higher in children with depressed mothers, whether the maternal depression is determined by meeting diagnostic criteria or clinically significant levels of depressive symptom scale scores, relative to a variety of controls (Beardslee et al., 1988; Billings and Moos, 1985; Goodman et al., 1994; Lee and Gotlib, 1989; Malcarne et al., 2000; Orvaschel, Walsh-Allis, and Ye, 1988; Weissman et al., 1984; Welner et al., 1977). Studies with adolescents show the same. Adolescents with depressed parents have been found to have higher rates of depression (Beardslee et al., 1988; Beardslee, Schultz, and Selman, 1987; Hammen et al., 1987; Hirsch, Moos, and Reischl, 1985) as well as higher rates of other disorders (Orvaschel, Walsch-Allis, and Ye, 1988; Weissman et al., 1984) relative to controls. Overall, rates of depression in the school-age and adolescent children of depressed mothers have been reported to be between 20 and 41 percent, in contrast to general population rates of about 2 percent in children ages 12 and younger and 15 to 20 percent in adolescents (Lewinsohn et al., 2000). Higher rates among children of depressed parents are associated with greater severity or impairment of the parent's depression and with the addition of other risk factors, such as those associated with poverty.

Not only are rates of depression higher, but depression in children of depressed parents, relative to depression in same-age children of nondepressed parents, has an earlier age of onset and longer duration and is associated with greater functional impairment and a higher likelihood of recurrence (Hammen and Brennan, 2003; Hammen et al., 1990; Keller et al., 1986; Warner et al., 1992).

Beginning in the preschool years, maternal depression is also associated with children's and adolescents' higher levels of internalizing and external- izing behavior problems (attention deficit disorders and disruptive behavior disorders, including violence) and substance abuse (Brennan et al., 2002; Fergusson, Lynskey, and Horwood, 1993; Forehand et al., 1988), anxiety (social phobia, separation anxiety, and other anxiety disorders), and dys- regulated aggression and more externalizing problems, although some re- searchers have found the latter to be specific to daughters (Biederman et al., 2001; Luoma et al., 2001; Orvaschel, Walsch-Allis, and Ye, 1988; Weissman et al., 1984; Zahn-Waxler et al., 1990). The studies from Radke-Yarrow's lab were also seminal in showing that even 5-year-olds of depressed mothers showed more dysregulated aggression and heightened emotionality and had more externalizing problems (Zahn-Waxler et al., 1984, 1990).

Moderators include the sex of the child, clinical characteristics of the parent's depression, and whether the depression is in the mother or the father. For example, maternal depression was associated with higher rates of internalizing problems (e.g., depression, anxiety) in 4-year-old boys and girls, but with externalizing problems (e.g., conduct disorder, attention defi- cit disorder) only in girls (Marchand and Hock, 1998). In middle childhood and adolescence, daughters of depressed mothers may be more likely than sons to show depression (Davies and Windle, 1997; Fergusson, Horwood, and Lynskey, 1995; Hops, 1996), although others have not found sex dif- ferences (Fowler, 2002).

In terms of clinical characteristics, mothers who reported high levels of depressive symptoms reported higher levels of behavior problems in their 5-year-old children, with even stronger associations when those symptoms were severe, chronic, and recent (Brennan et al., 2000). Generally, as ex- pected, longer exposure is associated with worse outcomes for children (NICHD Early Child Care Research Network, 1999; Sohr-Preston and Scaramella, 2006; Trapolini, McMahon, and Ungerer, 2007). Surprisingly, conclusions regarding severity of depression are mixed; some have found that severity is a strong predictor of children's emotional and behavior problems (Hammen and Brennan, 2003), and others have found only small associations (Radke-Yarrow and Klimes-Dougan, 2002).

A few of the studies of psychopathology as an outcome for children or adolescents have tested the bidirectional or transactional role—to what extent do problems in the children contribute to the depression in the par- ents? In two seminal studies on this topic, based on two distinct samples (Gross et al., 2008; Gross, Shaw, and Moilanen, 2008), most associations between maternal and paternal depression and children's internalizing or conduct problems revealed that higher levels of both mothers' and fathers' depressive symptoms predicted later increases in children's internalizing or conduct problems. At the same time, a few findings, specific to particular ages, supported child effects on parental depression. For example, higher levels of aggressive behavior in 5-year-old boys predicted higher levels of maternal depression when the boys were 6 years old (Gross, Shaw, and Moilanen, 2008). These researchers also found that child noncompliance was more strongly associated with depression in mothers than in fathers (Gross et al., 2008).

Across multiple studies, depression in mothers has been found to be more strongly associated with internalizing and externalizing problems in children relative to depression in fathers, as revealed in a meta-analysis (Connell and Goodman, 2002). Nonetheless, depression in fathers is of concern. For example, in a large cohort study, depression in fathers during the postnatal period predicted a greater likelihood of preschool-age boys and girls having emotional and behavioral problems and boys having conduct problems (Ramchandani et al., 2005). These findings were maintained even after accounting for postnatal depression in the mothers and later depression in the fathers. A more recent study found that the problems in the children persist until age 7 (Ramchandani et al., 2008). Another study found different patterns of association with mothers' relative to fathers' depression among young adults (age 24) who had experienced major depressive disorder by age 19 (Rohde et al., 2005). Major depression in fathers was associated with both sons' and daughters' lower psychosocial functioning, whereas for depression in mothers that association was specific to sons. Sons of depressed fathers also had higher levels of suicidal ideation and higher rates of attempts, whereas that association with depression in mothers was not significant. And recurrent depression in fathers but not mothers was associated with depression recurrence in daughters, but not sons. These studies suggest direct and specific associations between depression in fathers and the development of psychological problems in their children.

In order to further examine the relationship of paternal depression to psychopathology in the child, the committee undertook an independent analysis of public use data from the National Comorbidity Survey-Replication (NCS-R)[1] study. The NCS-R offered the opportunity to analyze a data set generalizable to the population in the United States in which the elements of a comprehensive theoretical framework consistent with the goals of our committee could be examined. We conducted our analysis separately among 759 male and 1,035 female respondents, ages 18–35 at the time of the NCS-R interview. The respondents' reported recall indicated that primary independent risk factors for self-reported major depressive disorder diagnosis (defined by *Diagnostic and Statistical Manual of Mental Disorders*, fourth edition) within the past 12 months were recalling

---

[1]Tabulations based on the National Comorbidity Survey-Replication (see http://www.icpsr.umich.edu/CPES/).

(1) each of their parents having sad behavior for 2 or more weeks and (2) their parents' drug and alcohol problems during the respondents' childhood (defined as up to the age of 18). These analyses were conducted incorporating the weighting and design effects from the NCS-R. Control variables in this framework included their parents' immigrant status and ethnicity and the respondent's own age at interview and relationship status. Potential mediating variables in this framework included the respondents' recall of the level of closeness with each of their parents, their recall of each of their parents' social problems, their report of parental neglect during their childhoods, and their report of the experience of trauma during childhood. We statistically tested the mediational effects of these factors and found that an alternate model in which these potential mediating variables were treated as covariates provided a better fit. Hence, we evaluated the independent and potential moderating effects of these variables in multiple logistic regression analyses. In these logistic regression models, we retained independent variables that had p-values less than 0.10 and examined interactions (effect modification) among the variables that met this criterion. Interaction terms with p-values less than 0.05 were retained.

In the models for both sons and daughters, the variables that consistently predicted major depression within the past 12 months were recalling having a *father* who had experienced sadness for 2 or more weeks during the respondent's childhood and having had an experience of trauma before age 18. As shown in Table 4-1, in the multiple logistic regression model, we found that males who recalled their fathers having experienced sadness for 2 or more weeks during their childhoods had rates of major depression in the past 12 months that were modified by their fathers' drug or alcohol problems during their childhoods (effect modification statistically significant, $p = 0.01$). Paradoxically, those whose fathers had experienced sadness and also had drug or alcohol problems during the respondents' childhood had lower rates of major depression in the past 12 months compared to those who fathers had neither risk factor, though this difference was not statistically significant. In contrast, those whose fathers experienced 2 or more weeks of sadness alone and those whose fathers had drug or alcohol problems alone had elevated rates of major depression compared to those with neither risk factor, with odds ratios of 3.65 and 1.73, respectively. In addition, the summary score of paternal closeness during childhood was highly significantly associated with major depression in the past 12 months ($p = 0.01$), with those who perceived less closeness to their fathers more likely to have major depression. Also, males who reported having experienced trauma before the age of 18 were approximately 3.8 times more likely to have had major depression in the past year ($p = 0.02$).

Among females, we again found that having a father who had sadness for 2 or more weeks during the respondent's childhood was a strong (odds

TABLE 4-1 Multiple Logistic Regression Analysis of Major Depression in Past 12 Months Among Males

	Odds ratio (95% C.I.[a])	p-value
Interaction of father sad for 2+ weeks during childhood with father had drug/alcohol problems during childhood (overall p = 0.01)		
Father sad, drug/alcohol problems vs. neither	0.37 (0.07, 1.95)	0.24
Father not sad, drug/alcohol problems vs. neither	1.73 (0.95, 3.15)	0.07
Father sad, no drug/alcohol problems vs. neither	3.65 (1.20, 11.14)	0.02
Mother sad for 2+ weeks during childhood	1.58 (0.79, 3.15)	0.20
Closeness of father: summary score[b]	1.39 (1.08, 1.80)	0.01
Race/ethnicity (overall p = 0.07)		
African-American vs. white	0.75 (0.32, 1.75)	0.51
Hispanic vs. white	0.85 (0.37, 1.94)	0.70
Other vs. white	3.64 (1.23, 10.71)	0.02
Any PTSD before age 18	3.23 (1.36, 7.69)	0.008

NOTES: PTSD = Posttraumatic stress disorder; N = 759, 65 with major depression, 694 without; model p-value = 0.003; generalized R^2 = 0.10; C-statistic = 0.65.

[a]Confidence interval.

[b]For a one standard deviation difference; higher values denote less closeness.

SOURCE: Tabulations based on the National Comorbidity Survey-Replication (see http://www.icpsr.umich.edu/CPES/).

ratio 3.17) and statistically significant (p < 0.0001) predictor of major depression in the past 12 months (Table 4-2), as was experience of trauma before the age of 18 (odds ratio of 3.41, p < 0.0001). Additional statistically significant factors in the model for females predictive of major depression in the past year were lower levels of closeness to the mother during childhood (p = 0.005), greater parental neglect during childhood (p = 0.047), a paradoxical effect of fewer social problems among the respondents' fathers (p = 0.047), increased depression with older age at the time of the interview (p = 0.03) and having never been married compared to having been married or co-habiting (p = 0.02).

These findings underscore the importance of examining the effects of paternal risk factors as well as maternal risk factors for psychopathology in children and that comprehensive models are required to properly quantify the effects of these risk factors, many of which are intercorrelated and may show effect moderation. Further studies of this type are needed, especially those in which more detailed information on personal trauma and neglect

TABLE 4-2 Multiple Logistic Regression Analysis of Major Depression in Past 12 Months Among Females

	Odds ratio (95% C.I.[a])	p-value
Father sad for 2+ weeks during childhood	3.17 (1.80, 5.60)	< 0.0001
Closeness of mother: summary score[b] (higher values denote less closeness)	1.24 (1.07, 1.44)	0.005
Father social problems: summary score[b] (higher values denote more problems)	0.80 (0.65, 0.99)	0.047
Parental neglect: summary score[b] (higher scores denote more neglect)	1.21 (1.01, 1.47)	0.047
Age[b] (years)	1.36 (1.03, 1.80)	0.03
Relationship status (overall p = 0.07)		
Separated, widowed, divorced vs. Married, cohabitating	1.37 (0.72, 2.59)	0.33
Never married vs. married, cohabitating	1.77 (1.09, 2.90)	0.02
Any PTSD before age 18	3.41 (1.98, 5.88)	< 0.0001

NOTES: PTSD = Posttraumatic stress disorder; N = 1,035 (176 with major depression, 859 without); model p-value < 0.0001; generalized R^2 = 0.12; C-statistic = 0.66.

[a]Confidence interval.

[b]For a one standard deviation difference.

SOURCE: Tabulations based on the National Comorbidity Survey-Replication (see http://www.icpsr.umich.edu/CPES/).

history can be included in public use data sets to be further analyzed, e.g., identifying the perpetrator of the trauma or neglect.

Timing of Exposure

The timing of exposure has received quite a bit of attention as a potential moderator, addressing the question: Is there a sensitive period for exposure to maternal depression? Some theories suggest that the first year of life, approximately, may represent a sensitive period given both infants' dependence on their caregivers and the centrality of responsive, sensitive caregiving for children's development of secure attachment and other aspects of emotion regulation (Essex et al., 2001). Two prospective studies conducted in Great Britain came to somewhat different conclusions regarding the role of postpartum depression alone in predicting adverse outcomes for children, regardless of subsequent episodes. Hay and colleagues studied youth from low-income homes. In contrast to cognitive development, for which postnatal depression has been found to be associated with children's later cognitive functioning (at ages 11 and 16) regardless of subsequent exposures to maternal depression, postnatal depression plus at least one subsequent episode of depression in mothers predicted children's behavioral problems at ages 11 and 16 (Hay et al., 2001). In the other British study, which sampled from a more middle-income population, postnatal depression exposure was associated with subsequent behavior problems (at age 5) and symptoms of hyperactivity and conduct disorder (at age 8) (Morrell and Murray, 2003). However, later follow-ups revealed that both postnatal depression and later episodes of depression in mothers predicted depression in the children at age 13, although anxiety was best predicted by postpartum exposure alone (Halligan et al., 2007).

Others concluded that postpartum depression does not predict later functioning in children, but that it is later exposures that matter. For example, in a large study of predominantly low-income Australian mothers and their children, mothers' recent depressive symptoms were associated with their 5-year-old children's socioemotional problems, whereas their postpartum depression levels were not (Brennan et al., 2000).

Other support for the conclusion that postpartum depression combined with later exposures is what matters for children comes from another British study, in which only postpartum depression that continued was associated with children's behavior problems at age 15 months (Cornish et al., 2006) and age 4 years as reported by mothers, fathers, and teachers (Trapolini, McMahon, and Ungerer, 2007).

Persistence of Problems Following Recovery or Remission

Among studies that did not explicitly examine treatment for depression in the parents, the small longitudinal literature reveals that, for the most part, children's problems persist despite the mothers' remission or recovery from depression. Typical of these studies are two that focused on children of preschool age through adolescence. Children of depressed parents continued to be at risk for psychological problems despite reductions in parents' depressive symptoms (Billings and Moos, 1985; Lee and Gotlib, 1991; Timko et al., 2002). Most of the longitudinal studies of infants and toddlers have drawn similar conclusions, that is, children of the recovered mothers showed fewer disturbances than the children of unrecovered mothers but greater disturbances than the children of control mothers who had never been depressed (Cox et al., 1987; Ghodsian, Zayicek, and Wolkind, 1984). Similarly, in a follow-up of low-income children ages 18 months to 4–6 years, Alpern and Lyons-Ruth (1993) showed that both the group of children whose mothers exceeded the clinical cutoff score on a depression rating scale at both times and the group whose mothers were previously but not currently depressed had more behavior problems than the children with never-depressed mothers.

Maternal depression during the first postpartum year predicted lower cognitive ability at age 4 years regardless of the mother's depression status when the child was 4 years old (Cogill et al., 1986). Stein et al. (1991) found that 19-month-olds whose mothers had recovered from depression that had occurred during the first postnatal year showed lower quality interaction with their mothers and with a stranger than did children whose mothers had never been depressed.

There are some exceptions to this finding, and these are intriguing. For example, Field (1992) reported that 75 percent of mothers who had been depressed early in the postpartum period continued to have symptoms at 6 months postpartum. The infants of the remaining 25 percent did not display a depressed style of interaction or have lower Bayley mental and motor scale scores at 1 year of age (Field, 2002).

Another intriguing question that has been addressed by some of the longitudinal studies is: If parenting quality improves with remission of depression, do children benefit? A few studies help to answer that question. Campbell, Cohen, and Meyers (1995), for example, found that mothers who were depressed 2 months postpartum but whose depression remitted by 6 months were significantly more positive and more competent in feeding their infants relative to mothers whose depression was chronic through 6 months postpartum (Campbell, Cohn, and Meyers, 1995). Furthermore, the infants in the depression remission group were significantly more positive in face-to-face interactions with their mothers than were those whose mothers remained depressed, although they did not differ significantly in terms of negative interaction or in the quality of engagement with their mothers in toy play.

Some studies that included an active treatment component for the mothers' depression also included mother-infant assessments, providing an opportunity to more directly test the hypothesis that parenting is one of the mechanisms in the transmission of risk from depressed mothers to their children. Treatment studies are reviewed in Chapter 6, but we focus here on the small subset of treatment studies that allow us to address this issue. A controlled trial of interpersonal psychotherapy in postpartum women with major depression, which was found to be effective in reducing levels of depression, also found significant improvement on self-reported measures of mothers' relationships with their children associated with interpersonal psychotherapy, even though the women did not achieve the levels typical of women with no history of depression (O'Hara et al., 2000). More recent studies continue to show that despite improvement in depression with interpersonal psychotherapy, mother-infant relationships were not improved (Forman et al., 2007).

Similarly, Cooper and Murray (1997), with a community sample screened for depression, found that treated mothers (randomly assigned to either nondirective counseling, cognitive-behavioral therapy, or dynamic psychotherapy), despite significant improvement in mood, were not observed to differ from untreated mothers or early remission mothers either on sensitive-insensitive or intrusive-withdrawn dimensions in face-to-face interactions with their infants (Cooper and Murray, 1997). It should be noted that these studies may have been restricted in their ability to find an impact of treatment on parenting in that the initial level of disturbance in parenting in these community samples may have been relatively minor.

In a third study, Fleming, Klein, and Corter (1992) investigated a community sample of women with self-reported depression who were treated with group therapy. Despite limited changes in ratings of depression, the treated mothers made more noninstrumental approaches to their infants, and the infants decreased in amounts of crying and increased in noncry vocalizations.

In a recent small sample study, in contrast to these three studies of psychotherapy, the intervention for postpartum depression was antidepressant medication treatment (Goodman et al., 2008). Six months after beginning treatment, the postpartum depressed mothers' scores on the Beck Depression Inventory were not significantly different from the well mothers. And although the depressed mothers as a group did not show a significant improvement in parenting over time, reductions in depression, after 12 weeks of treatment, were associated with (1) improvements in the quality of their interaction with their infants and (2) improvement in the infants' quality of interaction, although only for their quality of play. Furthermore, improvements in mothers' quality of interaction after 12 weeks of treatment accounted for changes in infants' positive affect.

Others, such as Weissman et al. (2006b), have examined the effect of parents' treatment for depression on psychopathology in the children, but without examining potential changes in parenting as a possible mechanism. Those studies are reviewed in Chapter 7.

RESEARCH GAPS

Although strong evidence now supports the breadth and extent of associations between depression in parents and adverse outcomes in children, there remain many unanswered questions. In particular, many questions remain regarding mediation and moderation of those associations. In terms of mediation, more studies are needed to test specific aspects of parenting and other potential mediators of associations between depression in parents and child functioning. In this regard, the committee noted the strong potential of studies designed to test the effectiveness of interventions aimed at reducing the level of constructs that have been found to mediate associations between depression in parents and outcomes in children, for example, particular aspects of parenting. Such experimental designs can be strong tests of mediation.

In terms of moderation, more studies are needed to reveal which children of depressed parents are more or less likely to develop problems and which parents with depression are more or less likely to have problems with parenting. Moderators might include parent characteristics, including severity, duration, and impairing qualities of their depression, social context variables, and child characteristics, among others. For example, the moderating roles of the child's sex and the child's ages at times of exposure are still not well understood, with findings suggesting that boys and girls might be affected differently depending on their ages at the times of exposures. More broadly, more studies are needed to quantify percentages of children who are affected (with specific outcomes) and those who are not and what distinguishes them. The committee notes the potential knowledge to be gained by further studies that target interventions to subsets of children with greater or lesser risk (degree of presence of moderators) to determine whether interventions need to be addressed to children at all levels of risk (do they benefit equally?) or might be focused on children at greater risk.

The committee also notes several gaps in the literature related to the physical health of children of depressed parents. More tracking is needed of health care utilization, missed school days, and other aspects of daily functioning in association with depression in parents. In particular, we conclude that more research is needed to understand the role of maternal depression in the health outcomes of children. Furthermore, both psychological and physical health outcomes need to be addressed in longitudinal studies of healthy and chronically ill children in order to know how physical health outcomes relate to psychological outcomes. Finally, tracking of avoidable and desirable health care utilization is needed to understand the impact on health services.

In addition to the research gaps in terms of unanswered questions, the committee also found gaps in relation to study design. First, tests of mediation are most informative when conducted on data from longitudinal designs, with measures of depression, parenting, and child functioning at multiple time points in order to capture the pathways. A second methodological issue concerns the measurement of depression in parents. The committee recognizes the staffing and time constraints that often prohibit the use of diagnostic interviews yet encourages their use whenever possible. Important questions remain about differences in association with parenting and child outcomes when parents' depression meets diagnostic criteria relative to exceeding the clinical cutoff on rating scales. Among groups who exceed clinical cutoffs will be those who would also meet diagnostic criteria and those who do not, despite their high symptom levels. Differences in parenting and child outcomes between those two groups need to be understood.

Third, more studies from a developmental perspective are needed. Such studies need not be longitudinal but require an understanding of child development in their theoretical model, hypotheses, design (especially in terms of the ages of the children studied), and the selection and psychometric properties of the measures. Fourth, the research literature would benefit from improving on the measurement of depression in population-based surveys to enhance their potential value to address these research gaps. Specifically, the committee recognizes the limitations of a single symptom rating scale score, typically reflecting the previous week or two in a parent's life, when the hypotheses typically concern significantly longer term effects on children of exposure to depression in a parent.

Fifth, more research studies are needed to test hypotheses derived from transactional models. As just one example, more studies are needed of child factors that contribute to the development or maintenance of depression in parents, for example, premature birth, chronic or acute health problems, "difficult" temperament, and conduct problems. Finally, as noted throughout this chapter, more studies are needed that examine the differences in parenting styles and children's behavior of the full range of parents who experience depression, including cultural and ethnic groups, those from differing income levels, fathers, and grandparents who are primary caregivers of their grandchildren.

CONCLUSION

Depression interferes with parenting. Depression in mothers of young children is significantly associated with more hostile, negative, and disengaged (withdrawn) parenting. Maternal depression is significantly associated with less positive parenting (warmth). Parenting quality may not improve with recovery from depression. Although depression and parenting of older children are less often studied, findings are clear that depression also interferes with the qualities of parenting needed by children in middle school and in adolescence. Although less is known about parenting in depressed fathers, the accumulating evidence suggests that depression also interferes with healthy parenting in fathers. Families with one or more depressed parents often have additional factors that generally impose risk for children, such as substance use disorders, poverty, exposure to violence, minority status, cultural and linguistic isolation, and marital conflict, which interfere with good parenting qualities and healthy child rearing environments. These additional risk factors are sometimes found to work independently and at other times found to be additive or interactive with the effects of depression in parents.

Depression in parents is also associated with depression in their children as well as with problems in children's daily functioning, physical health and well-being, some childhood chronic conditions, increased utilization of health care, increased likelihood of being abused or neglected, mismanagement of chronic health conditions, and poor school performance. A child with a depressed parent is more likely than other children to evidence other psychological impairment (e.g., temperament, attachment, affective functioning, cognitive/intellectual performance, cognitive vulnerabilities to depression), as well as increased rates of depression and other psychiatric disorders.

REFERENCES

Adrian, C., and Hammen, C. (1993). Stress exposure and stress generation in children of depressed mothers. *Journal of Consulting and Clinical Psychology, 61,* 354–359.

Alpern, L., and Lyons-Ruth, K. (1993). Preschool children at social risk: Chronicity and timing of maternal depressive symptoms and child behavior problems at school and at home. *Development and Psychopathology, 5,* 371–387.

Amaro, H., and Zuckerman, B. (1990). Drug use among adolescent mothers. In A.R. Stiffman and R.A. Feldman (Eds.), *Advances in Adolescent Mental Health, Volume IV: Sexual Activity, Childbearing and Childrearing Pediatrics.* London: Jessica Kingsley Publishers.

Amaro, H., and Zuckerman, B. (1991). Psychoactive substance use and adolescent pregnancy. Compounded risk among inner city adolescent mothers. In M.E. Colten and S. Gore (Eds.), *Adolescent Stress: Causes and Consequences.* Hawthorne, NY: Aldine de Gruyter.

Amaro, H., Zuckerman, B., and Cabral, H. (1989). Patterns and prevalence of drug use among adolescent mothers: A profile of risk. *Pediatrics, 84,* 144–151.

Anderson, C.A., and Hammen, C.L. (1993). Psychosocial outcomes of children of unipolar depressed, bipolar, medically ill, and normal women: A longitudinal study. *Journal of Consulting and Clinical Psychology, 61,* 448–454.

Ashman, S.B., and Dawson, G. (2002). Maternal depression, infant psychobiological development, and risk for depression. In S.H. Goodman and I.H. Gotlib (Eds.), *Children of Depressed Parents: Mechanisms of Risk and Implications for Treatment* (pp. 37–58). Washington, DC: American Psychological Association Books.

Austin, M.-P., Hadzi-Pavlovic, D., Leader, L., Saint, K., and Parker, G. (2005). Maternal trait anxiety, depression and life event stress in pregnancy: Relationships with infant temperament. *Early Human Development, 81,* 183–190.

Avenevoli, S., and Merikangas, K. (2006). Implication of high-risk family studies for prevention of depression. *American Journal of Preventive Medicine, 31,* 126–135.

Bailey, D.B., Jr., Golden, R.N., Roberts, J., and Ford, A. (2007). Maternal depression and developmental disability: Research critique. *Mental Retardation and Developmental Disabilities Research Review, 13,* 321–329.

Banyard, V.L., Williams, L.M., and Siegel, J.A. (2003). The impact of complex trauma and depression on parenting: An exploration of mediating risk and protective factors. *Child Maltreatment, 8,* 334–349.

Bartlett, S.J., Kolodner, K., Butz, A.M., Eggleston, P., Malveaux, F.J., and Rand, C.S. (2001). Maternal depressive symptoms and emergency department use among inner-city children with asthma. *Archives of Pediatric and Adolescent Medicine, 155,* 347–353.

Bartlett, S.J., Krishnan, J.A., Riekert, K.A., Butz, A.M., Malveaux, F.J., and Rand, C.S. (2004). Maternal depressive symptoms and adherence to therapy in inner-city children with asthma. *Pediatrics, 113,* 229–237.

Beardslee, W.R., and Podorefsky, D. (1988). Resilient adolescents whose parents have serious affective and other psychiatric disorders: The importance of self-understanding and relationships. *American Journal of Psychiatry, 145*, 63–69. Reprinted in: S. Chess, A. Thomas, and M.E. Hertzig (Eds.). (1990). *Annual Progress in Child Psychiatry and Child Development.* New York: Bruner-Miesels.

Beardslee, W.R., Gladstone, T.R., Wright, E.J., and Cooper, A.B. (2003). A family-based approach to the prevention of depressive symptoms in children at risk: Evidence of parental and child change. *Pediatrics, 112*, e119–e131.

Beardslee, W.R., Keller, M.B., Lavori, P.W., Klerman, G.K., Dorer, D.J., and Samuelson, H. (1988). Psychiatric disorder in adolescent offspring of parents with affective disorder in a non-referred sample. *Journal of Affective Disorders, 15*, 313–322.

Beardslee, W.R., Schultz, L.H., and Selman, R.L. (1987). Level of social-cognitive development, adaptive functioning, and DSM-III diagnoses in adolescent offspring of parents with affective disorders: Implications for the development of the capacity for mutuality. *Developmental Psychology, 23*, 807–815.

Beardslee, W.R., Wright, E.J., Gladstone, T.R.G., and Forbes, P. (2008). Long-term effects from a randomized trial of two public health preventive interventions for parental depression. *Journal of Family Psychology, 21*, 703–713.

Beck, C.T. (1996). A meta-analysis of the relationship between postpartum depression and infant temperament. *Nursing Research, 45*, 225–230.

Belsky, J., and Jaffee, S.R. (2006). The multiple determinants of parenting. In D. Cicchetti and D.J. Cohen (Eds.), *Developmental Psychopathology: Risk, Disorder, and Adaptation* (pp. 38–85). New York: Wiley.

Bemporad, J.R. (1994). *Dynamic and Interpersonal Theories of Depression.* New York: Plenum Press.

Biederman, J., Rosenbaum, J.F., Faraone, S.V., Hirshfeld-Becker, D.R., Friedman, D., Robin, J.A., and Rosenbaum, J.F. (2001). Patterns of psychopathology and dysfunction in high-risk children of parents with panic disorder and major depression. *American Journal of Psychiatry, 158*, 49–57.

Billings, A.G., and Moos, R.H. (1985). Children of parents with unipolar depression: A controlled 1-year follow-up. *Journal of Abnormal Child Psychology, 14*, 149–166.

Bohon, C., Garber, J., and Horomtz, J.L. (2007). Predicting school dropout and adolescent sexual behavior in offspring of depressed and nondepressed mothers. *Journal of the American Academy of Child and Adolescent Psychiatry, 46*, 15–24.

Boman, K., Lindahl, A., and Björk, O. (2003). Disease-related distress in parents of children with cancer at various stages after the time of diagnosis. *Acta Oncologica, 42*, 137–146.

Bonari, L., Pinto, N., Ahn, E., Einarson, A., Steiner, M., and Koren, G. (2004). Perinatal risks of untreated depression during pregnancy. *Canadian Journal of Psychiatry, 49*, 726–735.

Boyle, M.H., and Pickles, A.R. (1997). Influence of maternal depressive symptoms on ratings of childhood behavior. *Journal of Abnormal Child Psychology, 25*, 399–412.

Brazelton, T.B. (1984). *Neonatal Behavioral Assessment Scale.* Philadelphia: Lippincott.

Brennan, P.A., Hammen, C., Anderson, M.J., Bor, W., Najman, J.M., and Williams, G.M. (2000). Chronicity, severity, and timing of maternal depressive symptoms: Relationships with child outcomes at age five. *Developmental Psychology, 36*, 759–766.

Brennan, P.A., Hammen, C., Katz, A.R., and Le Brocque, R.M. (2002). Maternal depression, paternal psychopathology, and adolescent diagnostic outcomes. *Journal of Consulting and Clinical Psychology, 70*, 1075–1085.

Brennan, P.A., Le Brocque, R., and Hammen, C. (2003). Maternal depression, parent-child relationships, and resilient outcomes in adolescence. *Journal of the American Academy of Child and Adolescent Psychiatry, 42*, 1469–1477.

Bronfenbrenner, U. (1979). Contexts of child rearing: Problems and prospects. *American Psychologist, 34,* 844–850.

Bronfenbrenner, U. (1980). Ecology of childhood. *School Psychology Review, 9,* 294–297.

Brown, G.W., and Davidson, S. (1978). Social class, psychiatric disorder of mother, and accidents to children. *Lancet, 1,* 378–381.

Bruder-Costello, B., Warner, V., Talati, A., Nomura, Y., Bruder, G., and Weissman, M. (2007). Temperament among offspring at high and low risk for depression. *Psychiatry Research, 153,* 145–151.

Burchinal, M.R., Follmer, A., and Bryant, D.M. (1996). The relations of maternal social support and family structure with maternal responsiveness and child outcomes among African American families. *Developmental Psychology, 32,* 1073–1083.

Burdette, H.L., Whitaker, R.C., Kahn, R.S., and Harvey-Berino, J. (2003). Association of maternal obesity and depressive symptoms with television-viewing time in low-income preschool children. *Archives of Pediatrics and Adolescent Medicine, 157,* 894–899.

Burns, K., Melamed J., Burns W., Chasnoff I., and Hatcher R. (1985). Chemical dependence and clinical depression in pregnancy. *Journal of Clinical Psychology, 41,* 851–854.

Campbell, S.B., and Cohn, J.F. (1997). The timing and chronicity of postpartum depression: Implications for infant development. In L. Murray and P. Cooper (Eds.), *Postpartum Depression and Child Development* (pp. 165–197). New York: Guilford Press.

Campbell, S.B., Brownell, C.A., Hungerford, A., Spieker, S.I., Mohan, R., and Blessing, J.S. (2004). The course of maternal depression and maternal sensitivity as predictors of attachment security at 36 months. *Developmental Psychopathology, 16,* 231–252.

Campbell, S.B., Cohn, J.F., and Meyers, T. (1995). Depression in first-time mothers: Mother-infant interaction and depression chronicity. *Developmental Psychology, 31,* 349–357.

Carbonell, D.M., Reinherz, H.Z., and Beardslee, W.R. (2005). Adaptation and coping in childhood and adolescence for those at risk for depression in emerging adulthood. *Child and Adolescent Social Work Journal, 22,* 395–416.

Casey, P., Goolsby, S., Berkowitz, C., Frank, D., Cook, J., Cutts, D., Black, M.M., Zaldivar, N., Levenson, S., Heeren, T., Meyers, A., and the Children's Sentinel Nutritional Assessment Program Study Group. (2004). Maternal depression, changing public assistance, food security, and child health status. *Pediatrics, 113,* 298–304.

Celano, M., Bakeman, R., Gaytan, O., Smith, C.O., Kico, A., and Henderson, S. (2008). Caregiver depressive symptoms and observed family interaction in low-income children with persistent asthma. *Family Process, 47,* 7–20.

Chee, C.Y., Chong, Y.S., Ng, T.P., Lee, D.T., Tan, L.K., and Fones, C.S. (2008). The association between maternal depression and frequent nonroutine visits to the infant's doctor—A cohort study. *Journal of Affective Disorders, 107,* 247–253.

Chung, E.K., McCollum, K.F., Elo, I.T., Lee, H.J., and Culhane, J.F. (2004). Maternal depressive symptoms and infant health practices among low-income women. *Pediatrics, 113,* e523–e529.

Cicchetti, D., and Toth, S. (1998). The development of depression in children and adolescents. *American Psychologist, 53,* 221–241.

Cicchetti, D., Ackerman, B.P., and Izard, C.E. (1995). Emotions and emotion regulation in developmental psychopathology. *Development and Psychopathology, 7,* 1–10.

Cicchetti, D., Rogosch, F.A., and Toth, S.L. (1994). *A Developmental Psychopathology Perspective on Depression in Children and Adolescents.* New York: Plenum Press.

Civic, D., and Holt, V.L. (2000). Maternal depressive symptoms and child behavior problems in a nationally representative normal birthweight sample. *Maternal and Child Health Journal, 4,* 215–221.

Clark, L.A., and Watson, D. (1991). Tripartite model of anxiety and depression: Psychometric evidence and taxonomic implications. *Journal of Abnormal Psychology, 100,* 316–336.

Cogill, S.R., Caplan, H.L., Alexandra, H., Robson, K.M., and Kumar, R. (1986). Impact of maternal postnatal depression on cognitive development of young children. *British Medical Journal*, 292, 1165–1167.

Cohen, L.R., Hien, D.A., and Batchelder, S. (2008). The impact of cumulative maternal trauma and diagnosis on parenting behavior. *Child Maltreatment*, 13, 27–38.

Cohen, S., and McKay, G. (1984). Social support, stress, and the buffering hypothesis: A theoretical analysis. In A. Baum, S.E. Taylor, and J.E. Singer (Eds.), *Handbook of Psychology and Health* (pp. 253–267). Hillsdale, NJ: Lawrence Erlbaum Associates.

Cohn, J.F., and Campbell, S.B. (1992). Influence of maternal depression on infant affect regulation. In D. Cicchetti and S. Toth (Eds.), *Rochester Symposium on Developmental Psychopathology, Vol. 4: A Developmental Approach to Affective Disorders* (pp. 103–130). Rochester, NY: University of Rochester Press.

Cohn, J.F., and Tronick, E.Z. (1983). Three-month-old infants' reaction to simulated maternal depression. *Child Development*, 54, 185–190.

Cohn, J.F., Matias, R., Tronick, E.Z., Lyons-Ruth, K., and Connell, D.B. (1986). Face-to-face interactions, spontaneous and structured, of mothers with depressive symptoms. *New Directions for Child Development*, 34, 31–46.

Cole, D.A. (1991). Preliminary support for a competency-based model of depression in children. *Journal of Abnormal Psychology*, 100, 181–190.

Cole, P.M., Martin, S.E., and Dennis, T.A. (2004). Emotion regulation as a scientific construct: Methodological challenges and directions for child development research. *Child Development*, 75, 317–333.

Collishaw, S., Dunn, J., O'Connor, T.G., and Golding, J., and the Avon Longitudinal Study of Parents and Children Study. (2007). Maternal childhood abuse and offspring adjustment over time. *Development and Psychopathology*, 19, 367–383.

Compas, B.E., Langrock, A.M., Keller, G., Merchant, M.J., and Copeland, M.E. (2002). Children coping with parental depression: Processes of adaptation to family stress. In S.H. Goodman and I.H. Gotlib (Eds.), *Children of Depressed Parents: Mechanisms of Risk and Implications for Treatment* (pp. 227–252). Washington, DC: American Psychological Association.

Compas, B.E., Oppedisano, G., Connor, J.K., Gerhardt, C.A., Hinden, B.R., Achenbach, T.M., and Hammen, C. (1997). Gender differences in depressive symptoms in adolescence: Comparison of national samples of clinically referred and nonreferred youths. *Journal of Consulting and Clinical Psychology*, 65, 617–626.

Connell, A.M., and Goodman, S.H. (2002). The association between psychopathology in fathers versus mothers and children's internalizing and externalizing behavior problems: A meta-analysis. *Psychological Bulletin*, 128, 746–773.

Cooper, P., and Murray, L. (1997). The impact of psychological treatments of post-partum depression on maternal mood and infant development. In L. Murray and P. Cooper (Eds.), *Postpartum Depression and Child Development* (pp. 201–220). New York: Guilford.

Cornish, A.M., McMahon, C.A., Ungerer, J.A., Barnett, B., Kowalenko, N.M., and Tennant, C. (2006). Maternal depression and the experience of parenting in the second postnatal year. *Journal of Reproductive and Infant Psychology*, 24, 121–132.

Cox, A.D., Puckering, C., Pound, A., and Mills, M. (1987). The impact of maternal depression in young children. *Journal of Child Psychology and Psychiatry*, 28, 917–928.

Crnic, K.A., Greenberg, M.T., Ragozin, A.S., Robinson, N.M., and Basham, R.B. (1983). Effects of stress and social support on mothers and premature and full-term infants. *Child Development*, 54, 209–217.

Crockenberg, S.B. (1981). Infant irritability, mother responsiveness, and social support influences on the security of infant-mother attachment. *Child Development*, 52, 857–865.

Cummings, E.M., Keller, P.S., and Davies, P.T. (2005). Towards a family process model of maternal and paternal depressive symptoms: Exploring multiple relations with child and family functioning. *Journal of Child Psychology and Psychiatry*, 46, 479–489.

Cummings, E.M., Schermerhorn, A.C., Keller, P.S., and Davies, P.T. (2008). Parental depressive symptoms, children's representations of family relationships, and child adjustment. *Social Development, 17,* 278–305.

Cutrona, C.E. (1984). Social support and stress in the transition to parenthood. *Journal of Abnormal Psychology, 93,* 378–390.

Cutrona, C.E., and Troutman, B.R. (1986). Social support, infant temperament, and parenting self-efficacy: A mediational model of postpartum depression. *Child Development, 57,* 1507–1518.

Davidson, R.J., and Fox, N.A. (1989). Frontal brain asymmetry predicts infants' response to maternal separation. *Journal of Abnormal Psychology, 98,* 127–131.

Davidson, R.J., Ekman, P., Saron, C., Senulis, R., and Friesen, W.V. (1990). Approach-withdrawal and cerebral asymmetry: Emotional expression and brain physiology I. *Journal of Personality and Social Psychology, 58,* 330–341.

Davies, P.T., and Windle, M. (1997). Gender-specific pathways between maternal depressive symptoms, family discord, and adolescent adjustment. *Developmental Psychology, 33,* 657–668.

Davies, P.T., Winter, M.A., and Cicchetti, D. (2006). The implications of emotional security theory for understanding and treating childhood psychopathology. *Development and Psychopathology, 18,* 707–735.

Davis, E.P., Glynn, L.M., Schetter, C.D., Hobel, C., Chicz-Demet, A., and Sandman, C.A. (2007). Prenatal exposure to maternal depression and cortisol influences infant temperament. *Journal of the American Academy of Child and Adolescent Psychiatry, 46,* 737–746.

Dawson, G. (1999). *The Effects of Maternal Depression on Children's Emotional and Psychobiological Development.* Paper presented at the National Institute of Mental Health Conference on Parenting, October, Bethesda, MD.

Dawson, G., Ashman, S.B., Hessl, D., Spieker, S., Frey, K., Panagiotides, H., and Embry, L. (2001). Autonomic and brain electrical activity in securely- and insecurely-attached infants of depressed mothers. *Infant Behavior and Development, 24,* 135–149.

Dawson, G., Ashman, S.B., Panagiotides, H., Hessl, D., Self, J., Yamada, E., and Embry, L. (2003). Preschool outcomes of children of depressed mothers: Role of maternal behavior, contextual risk, and children's brain activity. *Child Development, 74,* 1158–1175.

Dawson, G., Frey, K., Panagiotides, H., Osterling, J., and Hessl, D. (1997). Infants of depressed mothers exhibit atypical frontal brain activity: A replication and extension of previous findings. *Journal of Child Psychology and Psychiatry, 38,* 179–186.

Dawson, G., Grofer Klinger, L.G., Panagiotides, H., Hill, D., and Spieker, S. (1992). Frontal lobe activity and affective behavior of infants of mothers with depressive symptoms. *Child Development, 63,* 725–737.

de Paúl, J., and Domenech, L. (2000). Childhood history of abuse and child abuse potential in adolescent mothers: A longitudinal study. *Child Abuse and Neglect, 24,* 701–713.

Deal, L.W., and Holt, V.L. (1998). Young maternal age and depressive symptoms: Results from the 1988 National Maternal and Infant Health Survey. *American Journal of Public Health, 88,* 266–270.

Deater-Deckard, K., Bates, J.E., Dodge, K., and Petit, G.S. (1996). Physical discipline among African American and European American mothers: Links to children's externalizing behaviors. *Developmental Psychology, 32,* 1065–1072.

Diego, M., Field, T., and Hernandez-Reif, M. (2005). Prepartum, postpartum and chronic depression effects on neonatal behavior. *Infant Behavior and Development, 28,* 155–164.

DiPietro, J.A., Bornstein, M.H., Costigan, K.A., Pressman, E.K., Hahn, C.S., Painter, K., Smith, B.A., and Yi, L.J. (2002). What does fetal movement predict about behavior during the first two years of life? *Developmental Psychobiology, 40,* 358–371.

Du Rocher Schuldlich, T.D., and Cummings, E.M. (2007). Parental dysphoria and children's adjustment: Marital conflict styles, children's emotional security, and parenting as mediators of risk. *Journal of Abnormal Child Psychology*, 35, 627–639.

Durbin, C., Klein, D.N., Hayden, E.P., Buckley, M.E., and Moerk, K.C. (2005). Temperamental emotionality in preschoolers and parental mood disorders. *Journal of Abnormal Psychology*, 114, 28–37.

Easterbrooks, M.A., Biesecker, G., and Lyons-Ruth, K. (2000). Infancy predictors of emotional availability in middle childhood: The roles of attachment security and maternal depressive symptomatology. *Attachment Human Development*, 2, 170–187.

Edhborg, M., Seimyr, L., Lundh, W., and Widstrom, A.M. (2000). Fussy child—difficult parenthood? Comparisons between families with a "depressed" mother and nondepressed mother 2 months postpartum. *Journal of Reproductive and Infant Psychology*, 18, 225–238.

Edwards, V.J., Holden, G.W., Felitti, V.J., and Anda, R.F. (2003). Relationship between multiple forms of childhood maltreatment and adult mental health in community respondents: Results from the adverse childhood experiences study. *American Journal of Psychiatry*, 160, 1453–1460.

El Hamaoui, Y., Yaalaoui, S., Chihabeddine, K., Boukind, E., Moussaoui, D. (2006). Depression in mothers of burned children. *Archives of Women's Mental Health*, 9, 117–119.

Elgar, F.J., McGrath, P.J., Waschbusch, D.A., Stewart, S.H., and Curtis, L.J. (2004). Mutual influences on maternal depression and child adjustment problems. *Clinical Psychology Review*, 24, 441–459.

Elgar, F.J., Mills, R.S.L., McGrath, P.J., Waschbusch, D.A., and Brownridge, D.A. (2007). Maternal and paternal depressive symptoms and child maladjustment: The mediating role of parental behavior. *Journal of Abnormal Child Psychology*, 35, 943–955.

Essex, M.J., Klein, M.H., Miech, R., and Smider, N.A. (2001). Timing of initial exposure to maternal major depression and children's mental health symptoms in kindergarten. *British Journal of Psychiatry*, 179, 151–156.

Ewell Foster, C.J., Garber, J., and Durlak, J.A. (2007). Current and past maternal depression, maternal interaction behaviors, and children's externalizing and internalizing symptoms. *Journal of Abnormal and Child Psychology*, December 11 [E pub ahead of print].

Fergusson, D.M., Horwood, L.J., and Lynskey, M.T. (1995). Maternal depressive symptoms and depressive symptoms in adolescents. *Journal of Child Psychology and Psychiatry*, 36, 1161–1178.

Fergusson, D.M., Lynskey, M.T., and Horwood, L.J. (1993). The effect of maternal depression on maternal ratings of child behavior. *Journal of Abnormal Child Psychology*, 21, 245–269.

Field, T. (1992). Infants of depressed mothers. *Development and Psychopathology*, 4, 49–66.

Field, T. (2002). Prenatal effects of maternal depression. In S.H. Goodman and I.H. Gotlib (Eds.), *Children of Depressed Parents: Mechanisms of Risk and Implications for Treatment* (pp. 59–88). Washington, DC: American Psychological Association.

Field, T., Diego, M.A., Dieter, J., Hernandez-Reif, M., Schanberg, S., Kuhn, C., Yando, R., and Bendell, D. (2001). Depressed withdrawn and intrusive mothers' effects on their fetuses and neonates. *Infant Behavior and Development*, 24, 27–39.

Field, T., Diego, M., Dieter, J., Hernandez-Reif, M., Schanberg, S., Kuhn, C., Yando, R., and Bendell, D. (2004). Prenatal depression effects on the fetus and the newborn. *Infant Behavior and Development*, 27, 216–229.

Field, T., Diego, M., Hernandez-Reif, M., Figueiredo, B., Schanberg, S., and Kuhn, C. (2007). Sleep disturbances in depressed pregnant women and their newborns. *Infant Behavior and Development*, 30, 127–133.

Field, T., Estroff, D.B., Yando, R., Del Valle, C., Malphurs, J., and Hart, S. (1996). Depressed mothers perceptions of infant vulnerability are related to later development. *Child Psychiatry Human Development, 27*, 43–53.

Finman, R., Davidson, R.J., Colton, M.B., Straus, A.M., and Kagan, J. (1989). Psychophysiological correlates of inhibition to the unfamiliar in children [Abstract]. *Psychophysiology, 26*, S24.

Fitzsimons, H.E., Tuten, M., Vaidya, V., and Jones, H.E. (2007). Mood disorders affect drug treatment success of pregnant drug-dependent women. *Journal of Substance Abuse Treatment, 32*, 19–25.

Fleming, A., Klein, E., and Corter, C. (1992). The effects of a social support group on depression, maternal attitudes and behavior in new mothers. *Journal of Child Psychology and Psychiatry, 33*, 685–698.

Flynn, H.A., Davis, M., Marcus, S.M., Cunningham, R., and Blow, F.C. (2004). Rates of maternal depression in pediatric emergency department and relationship to child service utilization. *General Hospital Psychiatry, 26*, 316–322.

Forehand, R., and McCombs, A. (1988). Unraveling the antecedent-consequence conditions in maternal depression and adolescent functioning. *Behavior Research and Therapy, 26*, 399–405.

Forehand, R., Brody, G., Slotkin, J., Fauber, R., an McCombs, A. (1988). Young adolescent and maternal depression: Assessment, interrelations, and family predictors. *Journal of Consulting and Clinical Psychology, 56*, 422–426.

Forehand, R., McCombs, A., and Brody G.H. (1987). The relationship between parental depressive mood states and child functioning. *Advances in Behaviour Research and Therapy, 9*, 1–20.

Forman, D.R., O'Hara, M.W., Larsen, K., Coy, K.C., Gorman, L.L., and Stuart, S. (2003). Infant emotionality: Observational methods and the validity of maternal reports. *Infancy, 4*, 541–565.

Forman, D.R., O'Hara, M.W., Stuart, S., Gorman, L.L., Larsen, K.E., and Coy, K.C. (2007). Effective treatment for postpartum depression is not sufficient to improve the developing mother-child relationship. *Development and Psychopathology, 19*, 585–602.

Fowler, E.P. (2002). *Longitudinal Reciprocal Relations between Maternal Depressive Symptoms and Adolescent Internalizing and Externalizing Symptoms.* Nashville, TN: Vanderbilt University.

Fowles, D.C. (1994). A motivational theory of psychopathology. *Nebraska Symposium on Motivation, 41*, 181–238. [Review].

Fox, R.A., Baisch, M.J., Goldberg, B.D., and Hochmuth, M.C. (1987). Parenting attitudes of pregnant adolescents. *Psychological Reports, 61*, 403–406.

Garber, J., and Martin, N.C. (2002). Negative cognitions in offspring of depressed parents: Mechanisms of risk. In S.H. Goodman and I.H. Gotlib (Eds.), *Children of Depressed Parents: Mechanisms of Risk and Implications for Treatment* (pp. 121–154). Washington, DC: American Psychological Association.

Garber, J., and Robinson, N.S. (1997). Cognitive vulnerability in children at risk for depression. *Cognition and Emotion, 11*, 619–635.

Garber, J., Braafladt, N., and Zeman, J. (1991). The regulation of sad affect: An information-processing perspective. In J. Garber and K.A. Dodge (Eds.), *The Development of Emotion Regulation and Dysregulation* (pp. 208–242). Cambridge, England: Cambridge University Press.

Garcia-Coll, C.T., Vohr, B., Hoffman, J., and Oh, W. (1986). Maternal and environmental factors affecting developmental outcome of infants of adolescent mothers. *Journal of Behavioral and Developmental Pediatrics, 7*, 230–236.

Gartstein, M.A., and Rothbart, M.K. (2003). Studying infant temperament via the revised infant behavior questionnaire. *Infant Behavior and Development, 26*, 64–86.

Gelfand, D.M., and Teti, D.M. (1990). The effects of maternal depression on children. *Clinical Psychology Review*, 106, 329–353.

Gerdes, A.C., Hoza, B., Arnold, L.E., Pelham, W.E., Swanson, J.M., Wigal, T., and Jensen, P.S. (2007). Maternal depressive symptomatology and parenting behavior: Exploration of possible mediators. *Journal of Abnormal Child Psychology*, 35, 705–714.

Ghodsian, M., Zayicek, E., and Wolkind, S. (1984). A longitudinal study of maternal depression and child behavior problems. *Journal of Child Psychology and Psychiatry*, 25, 91–109.

Goldsmith, H., and Rothbart, M.K. (1994). *Manual for the Laboratory Temperament Assessment Battery*. Version 2.03. Madison: Department of Psychology, University of Wisconsin.

Goldsmith, H.H., Buss, K.A., and Lemery, K.S. (1997). Toddler and childhood temperament: Expanded content, stronger genetic evidence, new evidence for the importance of environment. *Developmental Psychology*, 33, 891–905.

Goldstein, L.H., Diener, M.L., and Mangelsdorf, S.C. (1996). Maternal characteristics and social support across the transition to mother hood: Associations with maternal behavior. *Journal of Family Psychology*, 10, 60–71.

Gonda, X., Rihmer, Z., Zsombok, T., Bagdy, G., Akiskal, K.K., and Akiskal, H.S. (2006). The 5HTTLPR polymorphism of the serotonin transporter gene is associated with affective temperaments as measured by TEMPS-A. *Journal of Affective Disorders*, 91, 125–131.

Goodman, S.H., and Brumley, H.E. (1990). Schizophrenic and depressed mothers: Relational deficits in parenting. *Developmental Psychology*, 26, 31–39.

Goodman, S.H., and Gotlib, I.H. (1999). Risk for psychopathology in the children of depressed mothers: A developmental model for understanding mechanisms of transmission. *Psychological Review*, 106, 458–490.

Goodman, S.H., Adamson, L.B., Riniti, J., and Cole, S. (1994). Mothers' expressed attitudes: Associations with maternal depression and children's self-esteem and psychopathology. *Journal of the American Academy of Child and Adolescent Psychiatry*, 33, 1265–1274.

Goodman, S.H., Broth, M.R., Hall, C.M., and Stowe, Z.N. (2008). Treatment of postpartum depression in mothers: Secondary benefits to the infants. *Infant Mental Health Journal*, 29, 492–513.

Goodwin, R.D., Wickramaratne, P., Nomura, Y., and Weissman, M.M. (2007). Familial depression and respiratory illness in children. *Archives of Pediatrics and Adolescent Medicine*, 161, 487–494.

Gordon, D., Burge, D., Hammen, C., Adrian, C., Jaenicke, C., and Hiroto, D. (1989). Observations of interactions of depressed women with their children. *American Journal of Psychiatry*, 146, 50–55.

Gregory, C., Smith, G.C., and Palmieri, P.A. (2007). Risk of psychological difficulties among children raised by custodial grandparents. *Psychiatric Services*, 58, 1303–1310.

Gross, H.E., Shaw, D.S., and Moilanen, K.L. (2008). Reciprocal associations between boys' externalizing problems and mothers' depressive symptoms. *Journal of Abnormal Child Psychology*, 36, 693–709.

Gross, H.E., Shaw, D.S., Moilanen, K.L., Dishion, T.J., and Wilson, M.N. (2008). Reciprocal models of child behavior and depressive symptoms in mothers and fathers in a sample of children at risk for early conduct problems. *Journal of Family Psychology*, 22(5), 742–751.

Guttmann, A., Dick, P., and To, T. (2004). Infant hospitalization and maternal depression, poverty and single parenthood—a population-based study. *Child: Care, Health, and Development*, 30, 67–75.

Halligan, S.L., Murray, L., Martins, C., and Cooper, P.J. (2007). Maternal depression and psychiatric outcomes in adolescent offspring: A 13-year longitudinal study. *Journal of Affective Disorders, 97,* 145–154.

Hammen, C. (1992). Cognitive, life stress, and interpersonal approaches to a developmental psychopathology model of depression. *Development and Psychopathology, 4,* 189–206.

Hammen, C. (2003). Interpersonal stress and depression in women. *Journal of Affective Disorders, 74,* 49–57.

Hammen, C., and Brennan, P.A. (2001). Depressed adolescents of depressed and nondepressed mothers: Tests of an interpersonal impairment hypothesis. *Journal of Consulting and Clinical Psychology, 69,* 284–294.

Hammen, C., and Brennan, P.A. (2003). Severity, chronicity, and timing of maternal depression and risk for adolescent offspring diagnoses in a community sample. *Archives of General Psychiatry, 60,* 253–258.

Hammen, C., Burge, D., Burney, E., and Adrian, C. (1990). Longitudinal study of diagnoses in children of women with unipolar and bipolar affective disorder. *Archives of General Psychiatry, 47,* 1112–1117.

Hammen, C., Gordon, D., Burge, D., Adrian, C., Jaenicke, C., and Hiroto, D. (1987). Maternal affective disorders, illness, and stress: Risk for children's psychopathology. *American Journal of Psychiatry, 144,* 736–741.

Hammen, C., Shih, J., Altman, T., and Brennan, P.A. (2003). Interpersonal impairment and the prediction of depressive symptoms in adolescent children of depressed and nondepressed mothers. *Journal of the American Academy of Child and Adolescent Psychiatry, 42,* 571–577.

Hammen, C., Shih, J.H., and Brennan, P.A. (2004). Intergenerational transmission of depression: Test of an interpersonal stress model in a community sample. *Journal of Consulting and Clinical Psychology, 72,* 511–522.

Hankin, B.L. and Abramson, L.Y. (2001). Development of gender differences in depression: An elaborated cognitive vulnerability-transactional stress theory. *Psychological Bulletin, 127,* 773–796.

Hann, D.L., Osofsky, J., Barnard, N., and Leonard, D. (1994). Dyadic affect regulation in three caregiving environments. *American Journal of Orthopsychiatry, 64,* 263–269.

Hay, D.F., and Kumar, R. (1995). Interpreting the effects of mothers' postnatal depression on children's intelligence: A critique and re-analysis. *Child Psychiatry and Human Development, 25,* 165–181.

Hay, D.F., Pawlby, S., Sharp, D., Asten, P., Mills, A., and Kumar, R. (2001). Intellectual problems shown by 11-year-old children whose mothers had postnatal depression. *Journal of Child Psychology and Psychiatry and Allied Disciplines, 42,* 871–889.

Hayden, E.P., Klein, D.N., Durbin, E., and Olino, T.M. (2006). Positive emotionality at age 3 predicts cognitive styles in 7-year-old children. *Development and Psychopathology, 18,* 409–423.

Hazen, A.L., Connelly, C.D., Kelleher, K.J., Barth, R.P., and Landsverk, J.A. (2006). Female caregivers' experiences with intimate partner violence and behavior problems in children investigated as victims of maltreatment. *Pediatrics, 117,* 99–109.

Heim, C., Plotsky, P.M., and Nemeroff, C.B. (2004). Importance of studying the contributions of early adverse experience to neurobiological findings in depression. *Neuropsychopharmacology, 29,* 641–648.

Hernandez-Reif, M., Field, T., Diego, M., and Ruddock, M. (2006). Greater arousal and less attentiveness to face/voice stimuli by neonates of depressed mothers on the Brazelton Neonatal Behavioral Assessment Scale. *Infant Behavior and Development, 29,* 594–598. [E pub 2006].

Hertsgaard, L., Gunnar, M., Erickson, M., and Nachmias, M. (1995). Adrenocortical response to the strange situation in infants with disorganized/disoriented attachment relationships. *Child Development, 66*, 1100–1106.

Hipwell, A.E., Murray, L., Ducournau, P., and Stein, A. (2005). The effects of maternal depression and parental conflict on children's peer play. *Child: Care, Health and Development, 31*, 11–23.

Hirsch, B.J., Moos, R.H., and Reischl, T.M. (1985). Psychosocial adjustment of adolescent children of a depressed, arthritic, or normal parent. *Journal of Abnormal Psychology, 94*, 154–164.

Hops, H. (1996). Intergenerational transmission of depressive symptoms: Gender and developmental considerations. In C. Mundt, M.J. Goldstein, K. Hahlweg, and P. Fiedler (Eds.), *Interpersonal Factors in the Origin and Course of Affective Disorders* (pp. 113–128). London: Gaskell/Royal College of Psychiatrists.

Hops, H., Sherman, L., and Biglan, A. (1990). Maternal depression, marital discord, and children's behavior: A developmental perspective. In G.R. Patterson (Ed.), *Depression and Aggression in Family Interaction* (pp. 185–208). Hillsdale, NJ: Erlbaum.

Horwitz, S.M., Briggs-Gowan, M.J., Storger-Isser, A., and Carter, A.S. (2007). Prevalence, correlates and persistence of maternal depression. *Journal of Women's Health, 16*, 678–691.

Horwitz, S.M., Bruce, M.L., Hoff, R.A., Harley, I., and Jekel, J.F. (1996). Depression in former school-age mothers and community comparison subjects. *Journal of Affective Disorders, 40*, 95–103.

Hwang, J., and Rothbart, M.K. (2003). Behavior genetics studies of infant temperament: Findings vary across parent-report instruments. *Infant Behavior and Development, 26*, 112–114.

Institute of Medicine. (1994). *Reducing Risks for Mental Disorders: Frontiers for Preventive Intervention Research.* Washington, DC: National Academy Press.

Jaenicke, C., Hammen, C.L., Zupan, B., Hiroto, D., Gordon, D., Adrian, C., and Burge, D. (1987). Cognitive vulnerability in children at risk for depression. *Journal of Abnormal Child Psychology, 15*, 559–572.

Jaser, S.S., Champion, J.E., Reeslund, K.L., Keller, G., Merchant, M.J., Benson, M., and Compas, B.E. (2007). Cross-situational coping with peer and family stressors in adolescent offspring of depressed parents. *Journal of Adolescence, 30*, 917–932. [E pub 2007].

Jaser, S.S., Fear, J.M., Reeslund, K.L., Champion, J.E., Reising, M.M., and Compas, B.E. (2008). Maternal sadness and adolescents' responses to stress in offspring of mothers with and without a history of depression. *Journal of Clinical Child and Adolescent Psychology, 37*, 736–746.

Jaser, S.S., Langrock, A.M., Keller, G., Merchant, M.J., Benson, M.A., Reeslund, K., Champion, J.E., and Compas, B.E. (2005). Coping with the stress of parental depression II: Adolescent and parent reports of coping and adjustment. *Journal of Clinical Child and Adolescent Psychology, 34*, 193–205.

Johnston, C., and Mash, E.J. (2001). Families of children with attention-deficit/hyperactivity disorder: Review and recommendations for future research. *Clinical Child and Family Psychology Review, 4*, 183–207.

Jones, D.J., Forehand, R., and Beach, S.R. (2000). Maternal and paternal parenting during adolescence: Forecasting early adult psychosocial adjustment. *Adolescence, 35*, 513–530.

Jones, N.A., Field, T., Davalos, M., and Pickens, J. (1997a). EEG stability in infants/children of depressed mothers. *Child Psychiatry and Human Development, 28*, 59–70.

Jones, N.A., Field, T., Fox, N.A., Davalos, M., Malphurs, J., Carraway, K., Schanberg, S., and Kuhn, C. (1997b). Infants of intrusive and withdrawn mothers. *Infant Behavior and Development, 20*, 175–186.

Jones, N.A., Field, T., Fox, N.A., Davalos, M., Lundy, B., and Hart, S. (1998). Newborns of mothers with depressive symptoms are physiologically less developed. *Infant Behavior and Development, 21,* 537–541.

Kahn, R.S., Zuckerman, B., Bauchner, H., Homer, C.J., and Wise, P.H. (2002). Women's health after pregnancy and child outcomes at age 3 years: A prospective cohort study. *American Journal of Public Health, 92,* 1312–1318.

Kammerer, M., Taylor, A., and Glover, V. (2006). The HPA axis and perinatal depression: A hypothesis. *Archives of Women's Mental Health, 9,* 187–196.

Kaplan, B.J., Beardslee, W.R., and Keller, M.B. (1987). Intellectual competence in children of depressed parents. *Journal of Clinical Child Psychology, 16,* 158–163.

Kavanaugh, M., Halterman, J.S., Montes, G., Epstein, M., Hightower, A.D., and Weitzman, M. (2006). Maternal depressive symptoms are adversely associated with prevention practices and parenting behaviors for preschool children. *Ambulatory Pediatrics, 6,* 32–37.

Keller, M.B., Beardslee, W.R., Dorer, D.J., Lavori, P.W., Samuelson, H., and Klerman, G.R. (1986). Impact of severity and chronicity of parental affective illness on adaptive functioning and psychopathology in children. *Archives of General Psychiatry, 43,* 930–937.

Kendall-Tackett, K.A. (2005). *Depression in New Mothers.* Binghamton, NY: Haworth.

Kendler, K.S., Bulik, C.M., Silberg, J., Hettema, J.M., Myers, J., and Prescott, C.A. (2000). Childhood sexual abuse and adult psychiatric and substance use disorders in women: An epidemiological and cotwin control analysis. *Archives of General Psychiatry, 57,* 953–959.

Klein, D.N., Durbin, C.E., Shankman, S.A., and Santiago, N.J. (2002). Depression and personality. In I.H. Gotlib and C.L. Hammen (Eds.), *Handbook of Depression* (pp. 115–140). New York: Guilford.

Klimes-Dougan, B., and Bolger, A.K. (1998). Coping with maternal depressed affect and depression: Adolescent children of depressed and well mothers. *Journal of Youth and Adolescence, 27,* 1–15.

Klinnert, M.D., Nelson, H.S., Price, M.R., Adinoff, A.D., Leung, D.Y.M., and Mrazek, K.A. (2001). Onset and persistence of childhood asthma: Predictors from infancy. *Pediatrics, 108,* e69.

Kovacs, M., Devlin, B., Pollock, M., Richards, C., and Mukerji, P. (1997). A controlled family history study of childhood-onset depressive disorder. *Archives of General Psychiatry, 54,* 613–623.

Koverola, C., Papas, M.A., Pitts, S., Murtaugh, C., Black, M.M., and Dubowitz, H. (2005). Longitudinal investigation of the relationship among maternal victimization, depressive symptoms, social support, and children's behavior and development. *Journal of Interpersonal Violence, 20,* 1523–1546.

Kozyrskyj, A.L., Mai, X.M., McGrath, P., HayGlass, K.T., Becker, A.B., and MacNeil, B. (2008). Continued exposure to maternal distress in early life is associated with an increased risk of childhood asthma. *American Journal of Respiratory and Critical Care Medicine, 177,* 142–147.

Kraemer, H.C., Measelle, J.R., Ablow, J.C., Essex, M.J., Boyce, W., and Kupfer, D.J. (2003). A new approach to integrating data from multiple informants in psychiatric assessment and research: Mixing and matching contexts and perspectives. *American Journal of Psychiatry, 160,* 1566–1577.

Kraemer, H.C., Stice, E., Kazdin, A., Offord, D., and Kupfer, D.J. (2001). How do risk factors work together? Mediators, moderators, and independent, overlapping, and proxy risk factors. *American Journal of Psychiatry, 158,* 848–856.

Kramer, R.A., Warner, V., Olfson, M., Ebanks, C.M., Weissman, M.M., and Chaput, F. (1998). General medical problems among the offspring of depressed parents: A 10-year follow-up. *Journal of the American Academy of Child and Adolescent Psychiatry, 37,* 602–611.

Lang, A.J., Stein, M.B., Kennedy, C.M., and Foy, D.W. (2004). Adult psychopathology and intimate partner violence among survivors of childhood maltreatment. *Journal of Interpersonal Violence, 19*, 1102–1118.

Langrock, A.M., Compas, B.E., Keller, G., Merchant, M.J., and Copeland, M.E. (2002). Coping with the stress of parental depression: Parents' reports of children's coping, emotional, and behavioral problems. *Journal of Clinical Child and Adolescent Psychology, 31*, 312–324.

Lee, C.M., and Gotlib, I.H. (1989). Clinical status and emotional adjustment of children of depressed mothers. *American Journal of Psychiatry, 146*, 478–483.

Lee, C.M., and Gotlib, I.H. (1991). Adjustment of children of depressed mothers: A ten-month follow-up. *Journal of Abnormal Psychology, 100*, 473–477.

Lesesne, C.A., Visser, S.N., and White, C.P. (2003). Attention-deficit/hyperactivity disorder in school-aged children: Association with maternal mental health and use of health care resources. *Pediatrics, 111*, 1232–1237.

Leve, L.D., Kim, H.K., and Pears, K.C. (2005). Childhood temperament and family environment as predictors of internalizing and externalizing trajectories from ages 5 to 17. *Journal of Abnormal Child Psychology, 33*, 505–520.

Levy, R.L., Langer, S.L., Walker, L.S., Feld, L.D., and Whitehead, W.E. (2006). Relationship between the decision to take a child to the clinic for abdominal pain and maternal psychological distress. *Archives of Pediatrics and Adolescent Medicine, 160*, 961–965.

Lewinsohn, P.M. (1974). *A Behavioral Approach to Depression*. Oxford, England: John Wiley and Sons.

Lewinsohn, P.M., Roberts, R.E., Seeley, J.R., Rohde, P., Gotlib, I.H., and Hops, H. (1994). Adolescent psychopathology: II. Psychosocial risk factors for depression. *Journal of Abnormal Psychology, 103*, 302–315.

Lewinsohn, P.M., Rohde, P., Seeley, J.R., and Hops, H. (1991). Comorbidity of unipolar depression: I. Major depression with dysthymia. *Journal of Abnormal Psychology, 100*, 205–213.

Lewinsohn, P.M., Rohde, P., Seeley, J.R., Klein, D.N., and Gotlib, I.H. (2000). Natural course of adolescent major depressive disorder in a community sample: Predictors of recurrence in young adults. *American Journal of Psychiatry, 157*, 1584–1591.

Li, D., Liu, L., and Odouli, R. (2009). Presence of depressive symptoms during pregnancy and the risk of preterm delivery: A prospective cohort study. *Human Reproduction, 24*, 146–153. [Epub 2008].

Lieb, R., Isensee, B., Hofler, M., Pfister, H., and Wittchen, H.-U. (2002). Parental major depression and the risk of depression and other mental disorders in offspring. *Archives of General Psychiatry, 59*, 365–374.

Lim, J., Wood, B.L., and Miller, B.D. (2008). Maternal depression and parenting in relation to child internalizing symptoms and asthma disease activity. *Journal of Family Psychology, 22*, 264–273.

Lovejoy, M.C., Graczyk, P.A., O'Hare, E., and Neuman, G. (2000). Maternal depression and parenting behavior: A meta-analytic review. *Clinical Psychology Review, 20*, 561–592.

Lundy, B., Jones, N.A., Field, T., Nearing, G., Davalos, M., Pietro, P.A., Schanberg, S., and Kuhn, C. (1999). Prenatal depression effects on neonates. *Infant Behavior and Development, 22*, 119–129.

Luoma, I., Tamminen, T., Kaukonen, P., Laippala, P., Puura, K., Salmelin, R., and Almqvist, F. (2001). Longitudinal study of maternal depressive symptoms and child well-being. *Journal of the American Academy of Child and Adolescent Psychiatry, 40*, 1367–1374.

MacMillan, H.L., Fleming, J.E., Streiner, D.L., Lin, E., Boyle, M.H., Jamieson, E., Duku, E.K., Walsh, C.A., Wong, M.Y., and Beardslee, W.R. (2001). Childhood abuse and lifetime psychopathology in a community sample. *American Journal of Psychiatry, 158,* 1878–1883.

Malcarne, V.L., Hamilton, N.A., Ingram, R.E., and Taylor, L. (2000). Correlates of distress in children at risk for affective disorder: Exploring predictors in the offspring of depressed and nondepressed mothers. *Journal of Affective Disorders, 59,* 243–251.

Mandl, K.D., Tronick, E.Z., Brennan, T.A., Alpert, H.R., and Homer, C.J. (1999). Infant health care use and maternal depression. *Archives of Pediatric and Adolescent Medicine, 153,* 808–813.

Manuel, J., Naughton, M.J., Balkrishnan, R., Paterson Smith, B.P., and Koman, L.A. (2003). Stress and adaptation in mothers of children with cerebral palsy. *Journal of Pediatric Psychology, 28,* 197–201.

Mapp, S.C. (2006). The effects of sexual abuse as a child on the risk of mothers physically abusing their children: A path analysis using systems theory. *Child Abuse and Neglect, 30,* 1293–1310.

Marchand, J.F., and Hock, E. (1998). The relation of problem behaviors in preschool children to depressive symptoms in mothers and fathers. *Journal of Genetic Psychology, 159,* 353–366.

Marcus, S.M., Flynn, H.A., Blow, F.C., and Barry, K.L. (2003). Depressive symptoms among pregnant women screened in obstetrics settings. *Journal of Women's Health, 12,* 373–380.

Martins, C., and Gaffan, E. (2000). Effects of early maternal depression on patterns of infant-mother attachment: A meta-analytic investigation. *Journal of Child Psychology and Psychiatry, 41,* 737–746.

Masten, A.S., Hubbard, J.J., Gest, S.D., Tellegen, A., Garmezy, N., and Ramirez, M. (1999). Competence in the context of adversity: Pathways to resilience and maladaptation from childhood to late adolescence. *Development and Psychopathology, 11,* 143–169.

McGrath, J.M., Records, K., and Rice, M. (2008). Maternal depression and infant temperament characteristics. *Infant Behavior and Development, 31,* 71–80.

Meltzer, L.J., and Mindell, J.A. (2006). Impact of a child's chronic illness on maternal sleep and daytime functioning. *Archives of Internal Medicine, 166,* 1749–1755.

Minkovitz, C.S., Strobino, D., Scharfstein, D., Hou, W., Miller, T., Mistry, K.B., and Swartz, K. (2005). Maternal depressive symptoms and children's receipt of health care in the first 3 years of life. *Pediatrics, 115,* 306–314.

Moore, K., David, T.J., Murray, C.S., Child, F., and Arkwright, P.D. (2006). Effect of childhood eczema and asthma on parental sleep and well-being: A prospective comparative study. *British Journal of Dermatology, 154,* 514–518.

Morrell, J., and Murray, L. (2003). Parenting and the development of conduct disorder and hyperactive symptoms in childhood: A prospective longitudinal study from 2 months to 8 years. *Journal of Child Psychology and Psychiatry, 44,* 489–508.

Morris, J.A., Blount, R.L, Brown, R.T., and Campbell, R.M. (2001). Association of parental psychological and behavioral factors and children's syncope. *Journal of Consulting and Clinical Psychology, 69,* 851–857.

Murray, L., and Trevarthen, C. (1986). The infant's role in mother-infant communications. *Journal of Child Language, 13,* 15–29.

Murray, L., Fiori-Cowley, A., Hooper, R., and Cooper, P. (1996a). The impact of postnatal depression and associated adversity on early mother-infant interactions and later infant outcomes. *Child Development, 67,* 2512–2526.

Murray, L., Hipwell, A., Hooper, R., Stein, A., and Cooper, P. (1996b). The cognitive development of 5-year-old children of postnatally depressed mothers. *Journal of Child Psychology and Psychiatry, 37,* 927–935.

Murray, L., Kempton, C., Woolgar, M., and Hooper, R. (1993). Depressed mothers' speech to their infants and its relation to infant gender and cognitive development. *Journal of Child Psychology and Psychiatry*, 34, 1083–1101.

Murray, L., Sinclair, D., Cooper, P., Ducournau, P., Turner, P., and Stein, A. (1999). The socio-emotional development of 5-year-old children of postnatally depressed mothers. *Journal of Child Psychology and Psychiatry*, 40, 1259–1271.

Murray, L., Woolgar, M., Cooper, P., and Hipwell, A. (2001). Cognitive vulnerability to depression in 5-year-old children of depressed mothers. *Journal of Child Psychology and Psychiatry*, 42, 891–899.

Neuspiel, D.R., Rush, D., Butler, N.R., Golding, J., Bijur, P.E., and Kurzon, M. (1989). Parental smoking and post-infancy wheezing in children: A prospective cohort study. *American Journal of Public Health*, 79, 168–171.

NICHD Early Child Care Research Network. (1999). Chronicity of maternal depressive symptoms, maternal sensitivity, and child functioning at 36 months. *Developmental Psychology*, 35, 1297–1310.

Nulman, I., Rovet, J., Stewart, D.E., Wolpin, J., Pace-Asciak, P., Shuhaiber, S., and Koren, G. (2002). Child development following exposure to tricyclic antidepressants or fluoxetine throughout fetal life: A prospective, controlled study. *American Journal of Psychiatry*, 159, 1889–1895.

O'Hara, M.W., Stuart, S., Gorman, L., and Wenzel, A. (2000). Efficacy of interpersonal psychotherapy for postpartum depression. *Archives of General Psychiatry*, 57, 1039–1045.

Orr, S.T., James, S.A., and Blackmore Prince, C. (2002). Maternal prenatal depressive symptoms and spontaneous preterm births among African-American women in Baltimore, Maryland. *American Journal of Epidemiology*, 156, 797–802.

Orvaschel, H., Walsh-Allis, G., and Ye, W. (1988). Psychopathology in children of parents with recurrent depression. *Journal of Abnormal Child Psychology*, 16, 17–28.

Oztop, D., and Uslu, R. (2007). Behavioral, interactional and developmental symptomatology in toddlers of depressed mothers: A preliminary clinical study within the DC:0-3 framework. *Turkish Journal of Pediatrics*, 49, 171–178.

Palaez, M., Field, T., Pickens, J.N., and Hart, S. (2008). Disengaged and authoritarian parenting behavior of depressed mothers with their toddlers. *Infant Behavior and Development*, 31, 145–148. [E pub].

Patterson, G.R., and Stoolmiller, M. (1991). Replication of a dual failure model for boys' depressed mood. *Journal of Consulting and Clinical Psychology*, 59, 491–498.

Pauli-Pott, U., Mertesacker, B., Bade, U., Bauer, C., and Beckmann, D. (2000). Contexts of relations of infant negative emotionality to caregiver's reactivity/sensitivity. *Infant Behavior and Development*, 23, 23–29.

Pezawas, L., Meyer-Lindenberg, A., Drabant, E.M., Verchinski, B.A., Munoz, K.E., Kolachana, B.S., Egan, M.F., Mattay, V.S., Hariri, A.R., and Weinberger, D.R. (2005). 5-HTTLPR polymorphism impacts human cingulate-amygdala interactions: A genetic susceptibility mechanism for depression. *Nature Neuroscience*, 8, 828–834.

Plomin, R., Emde, R.N., Braungart, J.M., Campos, J., Corley, R.P., Fulker, D.W., Kagan, J., Reznick, J.S., Robinson, J., Zahn-Waxler, C., and Defries, J.C. (1993). Genetic change and continuity from fourteen to twenty months: The MacArthur Longitudinal Twin Study. *Child Development*, 64, 1354–1376.

Porter, C.L., and Hsu, H.-C. (2003). First-time mothers' perceptions of efficacy during the transition to motherhood: Links to infant temperament. *Journal of Family Psychology*, 17, 54–64.

Radke-Yarrow, M. (1998). *Children of Depressed Mothers: From Early Childhood to Maturity*. New York: Cambridge University Press.

Radke-Yarrow, M., and Klimes-Dougan, B. (2002). Parental depression and offspring disorders: A developmental perspective. In S.H. Goodman and I.H. Gotlib (Eds.), *Children of Depressed Parents: Mechanisms of Risk and Implications for Treatment* (pp. 155–174). Washington, DC: American Psychological Association.

Radke-Yarrow, M., E., Nottelmann, E., Belmont, B., and Welsh, J.D. (1993). Affective interactions of depressed and nondepressed mothers and their children. *Journal of Abnormal Child Psychology, 21,* 683–695.

Radke-Yarrow, M., Nottelmann, E., Martinez, P., Fox, M.B., and Belmont, B. (1992). Young children of affectively ill parents: A longitudinal study of psychosocial development. *Journal of the American Academy of Child and Adolescent Psychiatry, 31,* 68–77.

Ramchandani, P.G., Stein, A., Evans, J., O'Connor, T.G. and the ALSPAC Study Team. (2005). Paternal depression in the postnatal period and child development: A prospective population study. *Lancet, 365,* 2201–2205.

Ramchandani, P.G., Stein, A., O'Connor, T.G., Heron, J., Murray, L., and Evans, J. (2008). Depression in men in the postnatal period and later child psychopathology: A population cohort study. *Journal of the American Academy of Child and Adolescent Psychiatry, 47,* 390–398.

Regan, D., Leifer, B., Matteucci, T., and Finnegan, L. (1982). Depression in pregnant drug-dependent women. *National Institute on Drug Abuse Research Monograph, 41,* 466–472.

Richters, J.E. (1992). Depressed mothers as informants about their children: A critical review of the evidence for distortion. *Psychological Bulletin, 112,* 485–499.

Rohde, P., Lewinsohn, P.M., Klein, D.N., and Seeley, J.R. (2005). Association of parental depression with psychiatric course from adolescence to young adulthood among formerly depressed individuals. *Journal of Abnormal Psychology, 114,* 409–420.

Rothbart, M.K., and Hwang, J. (2002). Measuring infant temperament. *Infant Behavior and Development, 25,* 113–116.

Sameroff, A.J. (1975). Transactional models in early social relations. *Human Development, 18,* 65–79.

Schuetze, P., and Eiden, R.D. (2005). The relationship between sexual abuse during childhood and parenting outcomes: Modeling direct and indirect pathways. *Child Abuse and Neglect, 29,* 645–659.

Seifer, R., Dickstein, S., Sameroff, A.J., Magee, K.D., and Hayden, L.C. (2001). Infant mental health and variability of parental depression symptoms. *Journal of the American Academy of Child and Adolescent Psychiatry, 40,* 1375–1382.

Seligman, M.E., Peterson, C., Kaslow, N.J., Tanenbaum, R.L., Alloy, L.B., and Abramson, L.Y. (1984). Attributional style and depressive symptoms among children. *Journal of Abnormal Psychology, 93,* 235–238.

Sharp, D., Hale, D.F., Pawlby, S., Schmucker, G., Allen, H., and Kumar, R. (1995). The impact of postnatal depression on boys' intellectual development. *Journal of Child Psychology and Psychiatry, 36,* 1315–1336.

Shore, C.P., Austin, J.K., Huster, G.A., and Dunn, D.W. (2002). Identifying risk factors for maternal depression in families of adolescents with epilepsy. *Journal for Specialists in Pediatric Nursing, 7,* 71–80.

Silverstein, M., Augustyn, M., Cabral, H., and Zuckerman, B. (2006). Maternal depression and violence exposure: Double jeopardy for child school functioning. *Pediatrics, 118,* e792–e800.

Simons, R.L., Lorenz, F.O., Wu, C.-I., and Conger, R.D. (1993). Social network and marital support as mediators and moderators of impact of stress and depression on parental behavior. *Developmental Psychology, 29,* 368–381.

Smith, T.B., Innocenti, M.S., Boyce, G.C., and Smith, C.S. (1993). Depressive symptomatology and interaction behaviors of mothers having a child with disabilities. *Psychological Reports*, 73, 1184–1186.

Sohr-Preston, S.L., and Scaramella, L.V. (2006). Implications of timing of maternal depressive symptoms for early cognitive and language development. *Clinical Child and Family Psychology Review*, 9, 65–83.

Solantaus-Simula, T., Punamaki, R.-L., and Beardslee, WR. (2002a). Children's responses to low parental mood. I: Balancing between active empathy, overinvolvement, indifference and avoidance. *Journal of the American Academy of Child and Adolescent Psychiatry*, 41, 278–286.

Solantaus-Simula, T., Punamaki, R.-L., and Beardslee, W.R. (2002b). Children's responses to low parental mood. II: Associations with family perceptions of parenting styles and child distress. *Journal of the American Academy of Child and Adolescent Psychiatry*, 41, 287–295.

Spatz Widom, C., DuMont, K., and Czaja, S.J. (2007). A prospective investigation of major depressive disorder and comorbidity in abused and neglected children grown up. *Archives of General Psychiatry*, 64, 49–56.

Springer, K.W., Sheridan, J., Kuo, D., and Carnes, M. (2007). Long-term physical and mental health consequences of childhood physical abuse: Results from a large population-based sample of men and women. *Child Abuse and Neglect*, 31, 517–530.

Sroufe, L.A., Egeland, B., Carlson, E.A., and Collins, W.A. (2005). *The Development of the Person: The Minnesota Study of Risk and Adaptation from Birth to Adulthood*. New York: Guilford.

Stein, A., Gath, D.H., Buchere, J., Bond, A., Day, A., and Cooper, P.J. (1991). The relationship between post-natal depression and mother-child interaction. *British Journal of Psychiatry*, 158, 46–52.

Stewart, R.C. (2007). Maternal depression and infant growth: A review of recent evidence. *Maternal and Child Nutrition*, 3, 94–107.

Sugawara, M., Kitamura, T., Toda, M.A., and Shima, S. (1999). Longitudinal relationship between maternal depression and infant temperament in a Japanese population. *Journal of Clinical Psychology*, 55, 869–880.

Taylor, L., and Ingram, R.E. (1999). Cognitive reactivity and depressotypic information processing in children of depressed mothers. *Journal of Abnormal Psychology*, 108, 202–210.

Thompson, M.P., Kingree, J.B., and Desai, S. (2004). Gender differences in long-term health consequences of physical abuse of children: Data from a nationally representative survey. *American Journal of Public Health*, 94, 599–604.

Timko, C., Cronkite, R.C., Berg, E.A., and Moos, R.H. (2002). Children of parents with unipolar depression: A comparison of stably remitted, partially remitted, and nonremitted parents and nondepressed controls. *Child Psychiatry and Human Development*, 32, 165–185.

Trapolini, T., McMahon, C.A., and Ungerer, J.A. (2007). The effect of maternal depression and marital adjustment on young children's internalizing and externalizing behaviour problems. *Child: Care, Health and Development*, 33, 794–803.

Tronick, E.Z., and Gianino, A.F., Jr. (1986). The transmission of maternal disturbance to the infant. In E.Z. Tronick and T. Field (Eds.), *Maternal Depression and Infant Disturbance* (pp. 5–11). San Francisco: Jossey-Bass.

van IJzendoorn, M.H., Goldberg, S., Kroonenberg, P.M., and Frenkel, O.J. (1992). The relative effects of maternal and child problems on the quality of attachment: A meta-analysis of attachment in clinical samples. *Child Development*, 63, 840–858.

van IJzendoorn, M.H., Schuengel, C., and Bakersmans-Kranenburg, M.K. (1999). Disorganized attachment in early childhood: Meta-analysis of precursors, concomitants and sequelae. *Development and Psychopathology, 11*, 225–249.

Warner, V., Weissman, M.M., Fendrich, M., Wickramaratne, P., and Moreau, D. (1992). The course of major depression in the offspring of depressed parents: Incidence, recurrence, and recovery. *Archives of General Psychiatry, 49*, 795–801.

Weil, C.M., Wade, S.L., Bauman, L.J., Lynn, H., Mitchell, H., and Lavigne, J. (1999). The relationship between psychosocial factors and asthma morbidity in inner-city children with asthma. *Pediatrics, 104*, 1274–1280.

Weinberg, K.M., Olson, K.L., Beeghly, M., and Tronick, E.Z. (2006). Making up is hard to do, especially for mothers with high levels of depressive symptoms and their infant sons. *Journal of Child Psychology and Psychiatry, 47*, 670–683.

Weissman, M.M., Pilowsky, D.J., Wickramaratne, P.J., Talati, A., Wisniewski, S.R., Fava, M., Hughes, C.W., Garber, J., Malloy, E., King, C.A., Cerda, G., Sood, A.B., Alpert, J.E., Trivedi, M.H., and Rush, A.J. (2006b). Remissions in maternal depression and child psychopathology: A STAR*D-child report. *Journal of the American Medical Association, 295*, 1389–1398.

Weissman, M.M., Prusoff, B., Gammon, G.D., Merikangagas, K.R., Leckman, J.F., and Kidd, K.K. (1984). Psychopathology in the children (ages 6–18) of depressed and normal parents. *Journal of the American Academy of Child and Adolescent Psychiatry, 23*, 78–84.

Weissman, M.M., Wickramaratne, P., Nomura, Y., Warner, V., Pilowsky, D., and Verdeli, H. (2006a). Offspring of depressed parents: 20 years later. *American Journal of Psychiatry, 163*, 1001–1008.

Welner, Z., Welner, A., McCrary, M.D., and Leonard, M.A. (1977). Psychopathology in children of inpatients with depression: A controlled study. *Journal of Nervous and Mental Disease, 164*, 408–413.

West, A.E., and Newman, D.L. (2003). Worried and blue: Mild parental anxiety and depression in relation to the development of young children's temperament and behavior problems. *Parenting: Science and Practice, 3*, 133–154.

Whiffen, V.E., and Gotlib, I.H. (1989). Infants of postpartum depressed mothers: Temperament and cognitive status. *Journal of Abnormal Psychology, 98*, 274–279.

Whitaker, R.C., Orzol, S.M., and Kahn, R.S. (2006). Maternal mental health, substance use, and domestic violence in the year after delivery and subsequent behavior problems in children at age 3 years. *Archives of General Psychiatry, 63*, 551–560.

Whitfield, C.L., Anda, R.F., Dube, S.R., and Felitti, V.J. (2003). Violent childhood experiences and the risk of intimate partner violence in adults: Assessment in a large health maintenance organization. *Journal of Interpersonal Violence, 18*, 166–185.

Williamson, D.E., Ryan, N.D., Birmaher, B., Dahl, R., Kaufman, J., Rao, U., and Puig-Antich, J. (1995). A case-control family history study of depression in adolescents. *Journal of the American Academy of Child and Adolescent Psychiatry, 34*, 1596–1607.

Wolfson, A.R., Crowley, S.J., Anwer, U., and Bassett, J.L. (2003). Changes in sleep patterns and depressive symptoms in first-time mothers: Late trimester to 1-year postpartum. *Behavioral Sleep Medicine, 1*, 54–68.

Zahn-Waxler, C. (1993). Warriors and worriers: Gender and psychopathology. Special issue: Toward a developmental perspective on conduct disorder. *Development and Psychopathology, 5*, 79–89.

Zahn-Waxler, C., Cummings, E.M., Iannotti, R.J., and Radke-Yarrow, M. (1984). Young offspring of depressed parents: A population at risk for affective problems. *New Directions for Child and Adolescent Development, 26*, 81–105.

Zahn-Waxler, C., Iannotti, R.J., Cummings, E.M., and Denham, S. (1990). Antecedents of problem behaviors in children of depressed mothers. *Development and Psychopathology, 2,* 271–291.

Zuckerman, B.S., and Beardslee, W.R. (1987). Maternal depression: A concern for pediatricians. *Pediatrics, 79,* 110–117.

Zuckerman, B.S., Amaro, H., and Beardslee, B. (1987). Mental health of adolescent mothers: The implications of depression and drug use. *Journal of Developmental and Behavioral Pediatrics, 8,* 111–116.

Zuckerman, B., Amaro, H., Bauchner, H., and Cabral, H. (1989). Depressive symptoms during pregnancy: Relationship to poor health behaviors. *American Journal of Obstetrics and Gynecology, 160,* 107–111.

Zuckerman, B., Bauchner, H., Parker, S., and Cabral, H. (1990). Maternal depressive symptoms during pregnancy, and newborn irritability. *Journal of Developmental and Behavioral Pediatrics, 11,* 190–194.

5

Screening for Depression in Parents

SUMMARY

Primary Care Settings

- Studies show that primary care screening of adults increases the recognition of depressed individuals (two- to three-fold) and has a small effect on the persistence of depression; however, depressive symptoms in adults are more likely to improve when screening is accompanied by a systematic approach that provides further evaluation and treatment than with screening alone.
- Studies that have examined the mental health outcomes of adult depression screening in primary care settings rarely identify if the adult is a parent; have not addressed its impact on parental function; do not inquire about comorbid conditions (e.g., anxiety disorders, substance use); rarely assess adult treatment preferences; and rarely consider barriers to utilization of services or the two-generation impact of depression.
- Evidence shows that effective brief depression screening tools are available for adults. Professional organizations and experts recommend routine use of these screening tools for adults in primary care and obstetric settings if systematic follow-up is in place. However, parents are not routinely screened in clinical practice and screened adults are generally only identified as parents during the perinatal period.
- A variety of programs have focused on screening mothers during

183

routine pregnancy and postpartum clinical visits and other child health visits. These approaches provide opportunities to identify individuals who are at a higher risk for depression, provide education and support, assess parental function, and link child development screening with maternal depression screening.

Other Settings

- Studies have examined screening for depression in parents—particularly mothers—in existing community programs (e.g., early Head Start, those serving homeless women, substance use disorder treatment, home visitation), where individuals who are at higher risk of depression are seen. Although these settings and programs offer opportunities to reach parents and their children at greater risk for depression, screening is not routine.

Implementation

- Little information is available in either public or private settings about the complex process of implementing a systematic approach to maternal or paternal depression screening and follow-up, including time, resources needed, workforce and training competency and capacity, and the impact of engagement and education of depressed parents on the parents as well as their children.

This chapter addresses screening parents for depression in primary care and other health and community programs. First, the evidence basis for screening adults for depression and the use of brief clinical screening tools is discussed. Next, this chapter discusses the current research on parental depression screening at both maternal postpartum and well-child visits. When available, the discussion includes comparison to other informal and diagnostic approaches to the assessment of depression in these settings. Because successful screening and intervention involve a systematic approach, rather than only a questionnaire, the chapter discusses the challenges in implementation of screening with attention to parental, health provider, and health care system issues. Screening is the initial step in a systematic approach to detection and treating parents with depression. Finally, we consider promising approaches to parental depression screening and assessment in public health settings and with high-risk populations served by homeless, home visitation and substance use programs.

In addressing the impact that depression has on children, the committee considered screening for other factors, such as poor developmental outcomes or parenting impairment. Linking developmental screening of the young child to parental depression screening is one option that is discussed. However, screening for parental skills is conducted in research settings with longer instruments (i.e., Parenting Stress Index, Abidin, 1995) with young children. Clinical studies are not available that use screening tools to address the issue of parental skills for children of multiple ages in the context of depression.

PRIMARY CARE SETTINGS

The substantial numbers of adults with depression who are untreated, along with the underrecognition of depression by primary care providers, has led to examination of the use of brief screening procedures for depressive symptoms to address this problem. Review of the research evidence by the U.S. Preventive Services Task Force has shown that, with screening of patients in the primary care setting and provision of this information to the clinician, the number of patients recognized as depressed increases 2–3 times (Pignone et al., 2002). Meta-analysis of studies with screening and feedback showed that this strategy significantly decreased the risk for persistent depression 6 months later by 9 percent (relative risk, RR = 0.9; confidence interval, CI = 0.82–0.98) (Pignone et al., 2002). Many of the screening studies assessed later depression status but did not consider patient factors (e.g., acceptance of diagnosis, treatment preferences). Clinical outcomes were most likely to improve in studies in which screening was accompanied by a systematic approach, beyond the actual screening measures, to improve the quality of depression care, including patient education and follow-up. Thus, although screening alone will increase recognition, the best outcomes occurred when primary care settings implemented quality improvement programs that supported patient education and initiation of therapy.

As a result of its evidence-based review, the U.S. Preventive Services Task Force (USPSTF) in 2002 recommended primary care screening for depression, with a brief measure or two verbal questions, combined with a systematic approach, to assist those who screen positive with further evaluation and assistance (U.S. Preventive Services Task Force, 2002). When applying these recommendations to the specific issue of parental depression, however, there are limitations. None of the studies reviewed by the USPSTF identified status as a parent during screening, and women in the postpartum period were excluded from the studies reviewed. The potential two-generation benefit to the parent, usually the mother, and her children from identification of depressive symptoms and assistance to reduce their impact has not been considered in the reviews of the benefits of screening.

Currently, the American College of Obstetrics and Gynecology and the American Academy of Family Practice follow the recommendations of the task force for adult depression screening. National guidelines by the American Academy of Pediatrics and other national groups address screening for maternal depression and its impact on child development only in infancy, with a focus on the postpartum period (Hagen, Shaw, and Duncan, 2008; Jellinek, Patel, and Froehle, 2002). The main thrust of screening activities at pediatric well-child visits has been directed to detection of developmental delays in young children. The use of formal screening measures for developmental delays at three time periods in infancy and early childhood, with particular attention to language and social delays, is now recommended by the American Academy of Pediatrics (American Academy of Pediatrics and Council on Children with Disabilities, 2006). Although maternal depression is associated with child developmental and behavioral outcomes, as discussed in Chapter 4, these recommendations do not mention either screening for maternal depressive symptoms with developmental screening or screening mothers when developmental delays are found.

Depression is prevalent among women in the childbearing years, but, for many healthy women, their most frequent contact with health care professionals may be through their perinatal care or the care of their children. Thus, screening for depression, in addition to being provided during adult primary care, may need to access parents during obstetrical and pediatric care encounters. The available evidence about screening of parents in these settings needs to be examined. Community services that serve parents at higher risk for depression also offer the opportunity for screening and are discussed in this chapter.

The Screening Process

It has been shown that clinicians do not detect depressive symptoms in nearly half of mothers when they use informal inquiry to screen (Evins, Theofrastous, and Galvin, 2000; Heneghan et al., 2000; Olson et al., 2005). Inconsistent inquiry, the use of less specific questions, and the use of global impression rather than diagnostic criteria are some of the reasons (Olson et al., 2002). To enhance clinician detection of depressive symptoms, various measures have been used for depression screening, ranging from two-item questionnaires to structured clinical interviews. Generally, the tools that are most useful in busy clinical settings are brief, directly address symptoms found in the criteria listed in the *Diagnostic and Statistical Manual of Mental Disorders*, 4th edition, text revision (DSM-IV), are adaptable to specific patient populations (based on age, education, and ethnicity), and are capable of measuring the change in severity over time.

Specific maternal measures for the postpartum period have been developed. The performance characteristics of tools for postpartum depression screening are summarized in a recent review (Boyd, Le, and Somberg, 2005). The Edinburgh Postpartum Depression Scale (EPDS) is the most widely used and has moderate to good reliability. It assesses symptoms of depression and anxiety rather than depression alone, as in other screening measures. The different cutoff scores used in studies limit comparisons of the EPDS with other measures (Gaynes et al., 2005). Screening adults with two questions[1] about mood and anhedonia (low positive affect) has been found to perform as well as longer measures (Whooley et al., 1997). A three-question screen[2] derived from an eight-item depression screen (Burnam et al., 1988) has been used clinically with mothers (Kemper and Babonis, 1992); however, the three-question screen has been validated against the eight-item instrument rather than a psychiatric interview. Small studies in high-risk populations have compared the EPDS with the Patient Health Questionnaire-2 (PHQ-2), but they have not used diagnostic interviews as the gold standard (Cutler et al., 2007; Kabir, Sheeder, and Kelly, 2008). Table 5-1 lists four screening tools that are commonly used in clinical settings and available without cost. It is important to remember that, although a positive screen reveals depressive symptoms that might influence parenting, the positive predictive value for major depression is 35 to 50 percent with these screeners when validated by psychiatric interview (Boyd, Le, and Somberg, 2005; Kroenke, Spitzer, and Williams, 2003). Thus, positive results on a screener indicate depressive symptoms and higher rates of minor (subthreshold) depression; individual patients need to be evaluated to determine if major depression is present.

The screening process has been shown to be efficient, but it is more effective in clinical settings by using a two-step process. If a limited two-question screen is positive, then a nine-item diagnostic measure has then been administered. Both the PHQ-2 and the PHQ-9 have been evaluated by comparing the score with a clinical interview using DSM-IV criteria as well as scoring criteria developed to identify the presence and severity of depression (Kroenke, Spitzer, and Williams, 2003; Spitzer et al., 2000). Better case finding in primary care practice also occurred when follow-up questions asked whether the patient wanted help with the problem (Arroll et al., 2005). The use of a brief measure with simple scoring has the advantage of ease of implementation and less scoring error. Confirmation with a

---

[1]The two questions asked were (1) "During the past month, have you often been bothered by feeling down, depressed, or hopeless?" and (2) "During the past month, have you often been bothered by little interest or pleasure in doing things?" (Whooley et al., 1997).

[2]The three questions selected were: (1) "How much of the time in the past week has this statement been true for you? I feel depressed"; (2) "Have you had 2 or more years in your life when you felt depressed or sad on most days even if you felt 'okay' sometimes?"; and (3) unclear from the article (Kemper and Babonis, 1992).

TABLE 5-1 Summary of Brief Paper-Based Depression Screening Tools

Tool	Validation	Time	Description
Edinburgh Postpartum Depression Screen (EPDS)	Sensitivity = 0.86 Specificity = 0.78 For positive screen ≥ 10	5–10 minutes Self-administered, could be self-scored if scoring instructions are provided to patient	Has been the subject of a number of psychometric studies that provide support for its accuracy, validity, and standardization in Britain, Canada, and the United States. The EPDS consists of 10 multiple-choice items that produce a "possible depression" score and a single question focusing on potential suicidal ideation. Downloadable from http://www.dbpeds.org/articles/detail.cfm?TextID=485.
Patient Health Questionnaire (PHQ-9)	Sensitivity = 0.88 Specificity = 0.88 For positive screen ≥ 10	5–10 minutes Self-administered and self-scored, patient can access this online through http://www.pfizer.com or can obtain it from physician	The nine-item questionnaire is a diagnostic measure that assesses DSM-IV symptoms present in the past 2 weeks. It can be used both for diagnosis and monitoring symptom severity during treatment. Can be downloaded from http://www.depression-primarycare.org/. or http://www.pfizer.com/pfizer/download/do/phq-9.pdf. Laminated copies can be obtained from Pfizer, Inc. (the company holding the copyright on all versions).
PHQ-2 2-question screen	Sensitivity = 0.83 Specificity = 0.92 For positive screen ≥ 3	< 1 minute Self-administered or can be asked	See above. The two questions from the PHQ-9 for mood and anhedonia are used. Scored 1–3 for each question and summed. Recommended that the physician follow up with a more comprehensive screening tool.
RAND 3-question screen	Sensitivity = 1.00 Specificity = 0.88 For positive screen—see footnote 2 in chapter	< 1 minute Self-administered	This is a three-item adaptation (Kemper and Babonis, 1992) of the eight-item depression screener developed by RAND (Burnam et al., 1988) from longer screening instruments. The eight-item measure has been validated by psychiatric interview (sensitivity 0.70–0.71, specificity 0.91–0.96). The reported sensitivity and specificity for the three-item screen are not against the psychiatric interview but a comparison between the three- and eight-item instruments.

second step reduces the false positive rate and leads to appropriate referrals when mental health resources are limited.

Clinicians can also be assisted in understanding severity and making treatment plans when follow-up questions ask about the functional impact on daily life. Although impact on activities of daily living at work or at home is one of the criteria for clinical depressive disorder, the adult studies of screening measures have not considered functional status as a parent in their assessment. One study of parents found over three-quarters of parents screening positive with the PHQ-9 felt their function as a parent was affected (Grupp-Phelan, Whitaker, and Naish, 2003). We could find no studies of depression screening in the adult care setting that addressed the two-generation impact of parental depression.

Screening Selected Parental Populations in Health Settings

When addressing depression in parents, mothers, as the primary caregiver of young children, have been the prime focus of screening in the perinatal period and beyond. Targeted screening of mothers at higher risk for depression or adverse outcomes is one approach to depression screening that has been taken. The postpartum period for mothers has received attention as a specific time to screen. The unique triggers and social issues of this time period have led to recommendations for pediatricians, obstetricians, and family physicians to screen postpartum women. It is particularly during this period of parenting that depression has been widely recognized as impacting the parenting and nurturance of the child. Publicity about severe cases of postpartum depression has led to increased awareness and promotion of screening and education.

Most of the data on women who screen positive for depressive symptoms has come from population surveys, not clinical populations. A meta-analysis of studies (O'Hara and Swain, 1996) reported an average rate of postpartum depression of 13 percent. It found the rate differed by client history. For women with a history of depression, the rate was estimated to be 25 percent. For women with depression during pregnancy, the postpartum rate was about 50 percent. Women who were unmarried, had an unplanned pregnancy, had little social support or inadequate financial resources were more likely to be depressed. Among these stressors, low-income status has been shown to be one of the strongest predictors of postpartum depression (Segre et al., 2007). Domestic violence and marital maladjustment also increase the incidence of postpartum depression. The Centers for Disease Control and Prevention has recently completed a study of maternal recall of postpartum depressive symptoms at 6 months postpartum in 17 states during 2004–2005. The prevalence of self-reported postpartum depression ranged from 11.7 percent in Maine to 20.4 percent in New Mexico. The risk factors associated with reporting depressive symptoms included using tobacco during the last 3 months of pregnancy, physical abuse before or during pregnancy, partner-related stress during pregnancy, and financial stress during pregnancy (Pregnancy Risk Assessment Monitoring System Working Group and the Centers for Disease Control and Prevention Pregnancy Risk Assessment Monitoring System Team, 2008).

The studies of screening for postpartum depression often involve small study populations, and confirmation of a diagnosis of depression is limited. A careful meta-analysis has examined perinatal screening studies in which validation by psychiatric interview was available (Gaynes et al., 2005). The results show that women in the postpartum year were not at greater risk for a major depressive disorder than other women in their childbearing years. However, they did have higher rates of new-onset, subthreshold depressive symptoms in the first 3 months after birth. Gaynes et al. found that 14.5 percent of women had a new episode of major or minor depression during pregnancy and 14.5 percent of women in the first 3 months' postpartum. About half, or 7 percent, had major depression and half had subthreshold depressive symptoms. The evidence thus far shows that, in the postpartum period targeted by many programs, depressive symptoms, but not major depression, are more prevalent than at other times of parenthood.

Some public health programs have initiated comprehensive programs to address maternal depression. Several state health departments have programs that support screening, provider training, and parental supports. New Jersey, since 2006, has had a law requiring screening, education, and referral. Illinois provides additional clinician payment for conducting postpartum screening. Screening programs can have an educational role that decreases stigma as well as provides support to individuals in their parenting role. When screening is implemented the pressure to provide follow-up resources can stimulate treatment resources, such as depression support groups. In Washington state, with the advent of depression screening in the state's Maternal Support "First Steps" Program, the number of postpartum depression groups have more than doubled. In Australia, over 40,000 women have been screened antepartum or postpartum in a wide range of clinical and public health programs with the EPDS. Clinical outcomes from these public health–supported depression screening programs have not been published. This public momentum has emphasized women's increased risk for depression in this time period.

Despite the public attention to perinatal maternal depression, overall screening rates in both obstetrical and pediatric care settings are low. Formal screening during routine postpartum care is infrequent, with detection rates of 3.7 percent (Georgiopoulos et al., 2001) to 6.3 percent (Evins, Theofrastous, and Galvin, 2000). In a survey of obstetricians, 44 percent reported that they screened for depression, but less than a quarter used a validated written screen or interview (LaRocco-Cockburn et al., 2003). Among family physicians surveyed in one state, 31 percent self-reported that they always screen at postpartum visits and 13 percent always screen mothers at well-child visits. The use of written screening tools was rare, with 82 percent using an interview (Seehusen et al., 2005). Pediatricians report that observation or informal inquiry is the most common method of detecting maternal depression, and only 4 percent usually use a screening measure, despite recognizing the impact of maternal depression on children's health (Heneghan, Morton, and DeLeone, 2006; Olson et al., 2002).

Another approach is to extend screening beyond the initial postpartum visit and screen the parent during other child health visits. Thus far, there are only a few studies suggesting the yield and feasibility of this approach. A study in an urban primary care pediatric practice with primarily black, low-income mothers sought to screen at all infant well visits in the first year. Half of the mothers were screened, and 27 percent had an EPDS score greater than 10 (Chaudron et al., 2004). Maternal depression screening in a disadvantaged, urban, pediatric, clinic setting during well-child visits for children under age 6 showed that 27 percent of mothers screened positive using a yes or no response for the PHQ-2, and 12 percent screened positive with the Beck Depression Inventory (BDI) (Dubowitz et al., 2007). Mothers who presented their children for either acute care or well-child visits in an urban setting were screened with the PHQ-9; 9–10 percent screened positive for major depression, and 8 percent for subthreshold depression (Grupp-Phelan, Whitaker, and Naish, 2003). In pediatric practices in rural communities with predominantly white populations, routine brief parental screening conducted at all well-child visits showed that 17 percent of mothers screened positive on the PHQ-2 when scored with the method used by Dubowitz et al. There were substantially lower rates of positive depression screens (6 percent) using a newer PHQ-2 scoring, which determined severity of symptoms (Olson et al., 2006). Although these studies are limited to small populations, they show that a substantial number of mothers presenting at well-child visits have depressive symptoms when routine depression screening is conducted. The results vary by clinical settings, and sites taking care of primarily disadvantaged populations will have more mothers in need of further evaluation and assistance.

The current national recommendations for routine developmental screening of young children require clinical practices to develop organized systems to administer developmental screening measures during infancy and early childhood as well as to arrange appropriate follow-up. This provides the opportunity to target a high-risk population, children with developmental delays, for parental depression screening. Whether delays result from medical, social, or language conditions, coexisting maternal depression is likely to influence outcomes.

A recent analysis at the Child and Adolescent Health Measurement Initiative conducted for this report provides information about maternal depression screening in the context of childhood developmental screening (Bethell, Peck, and Schor, 2001). The Promoting Healthy Development Survey, which measures key aspects of the quality of delivery of preventive care for children under age 5 (Bethell, Peck, and Schor, 2001), was administered along with the Parents Evaluation of Developmental Status, a validated developmental and behavioral risk screener (Brothers, Glascoe, and Robertshaw, 2008), including a three-question maternal depression screen (Kemper and Babonis, 1992) to a sample of mothers of 4,654 Medicaid-insured children from seven states as well as a sample of mothers of 2,162 children receiving well-child care in the Kaiser Permanente Northwest health care system. Children were under 48 months of age.

Depression screens were positive in 20 percent of mothers in the Medicaid population and in 13.7 percent of mothers in the Kaiser Permanente population. Depression screen positive rates did not differ for different age subgroups (0–18 months, 19–36 months, and 37–48 months). These rates are similar to the smaller published screening studies in primary care and show that maternal depressive symptoms continue to be an issue beyond the postpartum period. Children who screened at risk for developmental or behavioral problems on the Parents' Evaluation of Developmental Status were 1.93 times more likely to have a mother who screened at risk for depression (28.5 versus 20.5 percent). Parents with a positive depression screen were no more likely to have their clinician ask about depression in the health visit than parents with normal depression screens (20.4 versus 20.8 percent).

These findings in the clinical setting are consistent with the research in Chapter 4 that shows increased developmental and behavioral consequences in young children with a depressed mother. A comprehensive approach that addresses both parental factors and child issues when developmental delays occur is appropriate. Targeting the population of children with developmental or behavioral problems for maternal depression screening is supported by these findings.

SCREENING IN OTHER SETTINGS

Parents, particularly women, with children who are at heightened risk for depression are served in other community programs that may provide the opportunity to screen for depression and offer further assessment and supports for treatment. Maternal depression is common among parents of Early Head Start programs, and depressive symptoms have been assessed as part of program evaluation. However, programs currently do not routinely screen mothers for depression. Mothers seen in programs for homeless families are at high risk for depression. Screening women served in homeless programs in western Massachusetts showed that 52 percent had depressive symptoms and received assistance (Weinreb et al., 2006). Promising new programs that are supported by the Commonwealth Fund's Assuring Better Child Health and Development project, better known as ABCD, and that assist state maternal and child health program are being established. As a result, a statewide public health approach to developmental screening that incorporates family mental health screening in Iowa (the 1 to 5 Initiative) links screening in either primary care or early childhood service agencies (e.g., the Special Supplemental Nutrition Program for Women, Infants, and Children; Visiting Nurse Associations) with a community-level care coordinator to address the entire range of child and family issues.

Screening in Substance Use Disorder Treatment Settings

Since 1995, there have been an increased awareness and emphasis on providing depression screening, assessment and diagnosis, and treatment to patients enrolled in treatment programs for substance use disorders (SUDs). Based on data reported to the Substance Abuse and Mental Health Services Administration from the National Survey of Substance Abuse Treatment Services in 2006, the most recent data available, 58 percent of programs provided screening for mental health disorders, 42 percent provided comprehensive assessment and diagnosis of mental health disorders, and 37 percent reported special programming for those with co-occurring disorders.

Women in their childbearing years with substance use disorders often have co-occurring disorders, including depression and experience with interpersonal violence that results in posttraumatic stress disorder. Data on parents with substance use disorders and depression and other mental health disorders are largely limited to comprehensive SUD treatment programs for women, mostly those who are perinatal. Among mothers, 83–88 percent screened positive for depressive symptoms at treatment entry (Conners et al., 2006; Lincoln et al., 2006). Of the women screening positive for depressive symptoms, 64 percent received a depressive disorder diagnosis using an independent diagnosis assessment (Lincoln et al., 2006). It has been estimated that, among pregnant women with a substance use disorder, 56 percent have depressive symptoms (e.g., Fitzsimons et al., 2007); 48 percent of pregnant, drug-dependent women enrolled in a comprehensive SUD treatment program have a current major depressive disorder; and 54 percent have major depressive disorder with a concurrent anxiety disorder (Fitzsimons et al., 2007). Mothers and fathers with substance use disorders often suffer from multiple and complex co-occurring disorders and environmental challenges, including poverty or deprivation, homelessness, inability to afford or access dental or medical care, unemployment, a lack of vocational skills, interpersonal violence, and ineffective parenting skills. As such, brief screening instruments, followed by assessment and treatment when needed, are urgently needed for front-line substance abuse treatment staff to quickly and easily administer, to interpret the results, and to refer their clients for further assessment for mental health treatment (Lincoln et al., 2006).

Although the rates of depression in parents who treated for substance use disorders are elusive, several promising programs that screen, assess, and treat depression in pregnant and parenting women who are also being treated for substance use disorders are highlighted below.

Specific to pregnant women, the Center for Addiction and Pregnancy, located in Baltimore City on the campus of the Johns Hopkins Bayview Medical Center, is a comprehensive care model (Jansson et al., 1996, 2007). The center provides treatment for substance use disorders while concurrently providing obstetrical, medical, and other psychiatric care to mothers and pediatric care to the children of patients. As a part of the center's comprehensive screening battery, a screen for mental health issues is included. Given the need to minimize paperwork and demands on patients and staff, a study comparing the utility of the Addiction Severity Index (ASI) to the BDI was conducted to see which instrument predicted mood disorders in this pregnant drug-dependent population. The ASI psychiatric severity rating by the interviewer was found to have better sensitivity and specificity than the BDI for predicting mood disorders (Chisolm et al., in press). The ASI, which is a required intake tool for substance abuse treatment programs in many states, is now used for screening patients for the need for further psychiatric assessment by the center psychiatrist. The center's research has also found that when using the Structured Clinical Interview for DSM Disorders, diagnosed depression in the absence of anxiety is especially prevalent (54 percent) in pregnant, drug-dependent patients (Fitzsimons et al., 2007).

Two promising programs described in Chapter 6 treat mental health, interpersonal violence, and substance use disorders in mothers and families. The first model is the Boston Consortium of Services for Families in Recovery Model, which under the Boston Public Health Commission has an active collaborative system of services for women with substance use disorders as well as mental health and trauma issues (Amaro et al., 2005). The system, which routinely screens all new patients for mental health disorders, found that 88 percent of patients reported experiencing mental health symptoms in the month before treatment entry (Lincoln et al., 2006). The other model is part of PROTOTYPES, which also provides services for women with substance use disorders as well as a variety of mental illnesses and trauma issues (Brown, Rechberger, and Bjelajec, 2005).

Screening in Home Visitation Programs

Home visitation programs potentially provide an important, large-scale context in which to identify and intervene in parental depression and associated parenting difficulties. Home visitation programs typically serve young, low-income families with high levels of stress, histories of trauma, and marital problems. These high-risk families typically have low utilization rates for traditional center-based mental health services. The high rate of depressed mothers encountered by home visitation programs and the negative impacts that maternal depression has on the effectiveness of home visitation has led to a number of home visitation–based treatment interventions, which are described in Chapter 6. Another intervention strategy that has been employed is screening by the home visitor with referral to community mental health services.

National home visiting models, such as the Nurse-Family Partnership, operating in 26 states, and Healthy Families America, operating in 440 communities, use a battery of parent-report and home visitor–administrated measures to determine the types and intensity of services required by the families. Standard depression screens, such as the EPDS or BDI-II, have been included at some sites of several major programs, but are not universally administered. In intervention studies reporting depression screening scores at baseline, positive screens occurred in 29 to 50 percent (Ammerman et al., 2009; Jacobs et al., 2005; Stevens et al., 2002). Thus, for mothers enrolled in home visiting programs, substantial numbers reported clinically significant depressive symptoms at entry to the study. Based on these rates of depression in the home visiting literature, routine screening can be expected to reach many high-risk families and to identify a large number of clinical cases.

Although no randomized clinical trial outcomes have been published for the strategy of screening all new mothers through home visitation, several state programs are conducting screening programs in which home visitors administer and score a standardized depression screen and then refer mothers (or fathers) scoring above a predetermined clinical threshold to community mental health services for further evaluation and treatment as indicated.

One promising example is the collaboration between the Ohio Department of Health's Help-Me-Grow statewide home visitation program, implemented at a county level, and the Ohio Department of Mental Health. Help-Me-Grow home visitors administer the EPDS to new mothers with infants ages 4 to 20 weeks. They enter the EPDS score and demographic data into a web-based data system that automatically scores the EPDS and prompts the home visitor to make a referral for mothers who score 12 or above or who endorse item 10 (a suicide question) at a level 2 or higher.

The database can email a copy of the client's EPDS and pertinent referral information, or the referral can be printed and mailed or faxed to the mental health agency. Once a referral is made, the database automatically prompts a monitor to contact the mental health agency at 30 and 90 days to see if an appointment was made and whether it was kept. This program is currently operating in 17 Ohio counties around the state and is slated to increase to 40 counties in 2010. Unpublished results indicate that 20 percent of screened mothers met the EPDS clinical threshold and 68 percent of positive screens accepted the home visitor's offer of a facilitated mental health referral. Follow-up at 30 days found that 37 percent of referred mothers had actually kept their mental health appointments. No data are collected on treatment outcomes.

CHALLENGES IN THE IMPLEMENTATION
OF SCREENING FOR DEPRESSION

For depression screening to be feasible in more primary care settings, more information about the details of implementing screening programs in different settings is needed for practices to plan for adequate time and support resources. For example, only one study provides information about the impact on the time spent by clinicians with routine depression screening (Olson et al., 2006). There has been little published evidence shedding light on the entire process of screening and systematic follow-up in different types of clinical settings. This is an issue for routine screening of adults in primary care and obstetric settings as well as pediatric health care settings (Chaudron et al., 2007).

The lack of information about the results of screening programs is another barrier to implementation. Data on program cost and effectiveness are rarely available. One example is a study in Florida (Gadsden County) that estimated a cost of $466 per client for 224 women screened. The number screening positive was 89 clients, or 36 percent. Since this county has a large number of families living in poverty, the rates of depression were higher. In all, 51 percent of the positive cases accepted treatment, and the average cost ($100 per treatment visit) was $2,229 for each client treated (Lynch and Harrington, 2003). This type of evaluation needs to occur in a variety of public and private health care settings.

A further barrier to implementation of screening programs for parental depression is that primary care providers report that they are not well enough prepared to deal with the mental health issue of depression, or they perceive inadequate resources in their community to provide treatment for clients. In a recent survey of pediatricians, those from the Midwest were five times more likely than in other regions to identify and manage mothers with depression. Michigan, Wisconsin, and Illinois have all implemented initiatives to increase public awareness about maternal depression (Heneghan et al., 2007). The state of Illinois has developed a comprehensive support system for providers dealing with perinatal clients. The system provides accessible information on the Internet and makes professional consultation easily accessible (Wiedmann and Garfield, 2007). Furthermore, there are challenges in screening in home visitation programs. The major problem raised by routine screening is how to provide effective services for the large number of depressed parents who are likely to be identified. In addition to needing local capacity to treat these newly recognized cases, several studies indicate that home visitors as a group are not good at connecting families with community-based services for depression, domestic violence, and substance abuse (Hebbeler and Gerlach-Downie, 2002; Tandon et al., 2005). Although there are no empirical studies of the reasons why this is so, it is thought in these programs that their concern about discussing sensitive issues may alienate families and undermine the effectiveness of the primary home visitation services.

It is challenging to implement depression screening and to ensure that individuals receive assistance. Although inadequacies of systems of care are often emphasized, there are other barriers at the patient level. Difficulty in engaging women to recognize and act on symptoms has been identified as a barrier to better outcomes. For example, in one study, when patients in perinatal care were willing to be screened for depression, many did not agree to further assessment or contact (Carter et al., 2005). In several studies, investigators have reported resistance to treatment services because of the stigma associated with mental illness and the fear of having their children removed because of the mother's function (Beeber, Perreira, and Schwartz, 2008; Lazear et al., 2008; Miranda et al., 2006). In addition, low-income and immigrant populations identified the following barriers to services: domestic violence; isolation; language problems; difficulties with public systems; lack of access to quality, culturally competent care; reliance primarily on informal systems of care; lack of insurance; and the attitudes of providers.

Engagement with a trusted clinician is important for mothers to discuss such issues as stress and depression (Heneghan, Mercer, and DeLeone, 2004). Screening in the child's health visit can provide a supportive setting for discussion, assistance, and referral. When screening occurred in the context of the infant's visit, Chaudron et al. reported that half of the depression screen positives were referred and 88 percent were seen by onsite social workers (Chaudron et al., 2004). In children's well-child visits, nearly half of the mothers with a positive depression screen thought they might be depressed and were willing to take action after discussion with the pediatrician (Olson et al., 2006). In clinical screening programs, it is desirable to also include an educational component. It is important to initiate a discussion of symptoms of depression that provides anticipatory guidance to help the child and motivates the parent to seek support and use existing resources. The educational role of screening linked with discussion is demonstrated in the Australian postpartum depression screening program, in which the women screened were more likely to identify symptoms as clinical depression when they had depression screening and discussion by health staff (Buist et al., 2006).

RESEARCH GAPS

Although evidence supports the effectiveness of brief screening measures for adult depression in clinical and community settings, there remain many unanswered questions. For example, more evidence is needed on the effectiveness of universal screening of parents with depression, including moving beyond the perinatal period. And, more research is needed to develop brief clinical screening measures for key parenting skills that relate to depression. More specifically, studies are needed that measure depression in parents with both diagnostic interviews and with symptom scales and that examine differences in parenting and in child functioning that might be related to measurement approach, severity, impairment, and other clinical characteristics of depression.

In terms of outcomes, research is lacking on the outcomes of screening parents as part of a two-generation comprehensive depression care program that addresses issues for both parent and child. The next stage is translational research to determine if comprehensive screening programs can ultimately influence parental mental health, parenting, or adverse outcomes in child development. More specifically, effectiveness of the implementation of programs, rather than efficacy studies, are needed in community and clinical settings. They should examine the impact of each step in the care process from screening, education, and parent engagement, through parent treatment preferences and choices made, to referrals made and completed, and to clinical outcomes.

More research is needed to determine the optimal ways to integrate parental depression screening with the assessment of parenting and child developmental and behavioral status for all children but especially in high-risk populations (i.e., with substance use disorders, low-income status, at risk for abuse).

CONCLUSION

Effective brief screening measures are available—and recommended—for recognizing depressed adults in a variety of clinical settings and existing community programs. However, depressive symptoms are more likely to improve when screening is accompanied by education and initiation of treatment. Most adult screening studies assess only changes in depressive symptoms and provide little information about patient or system variables that influence treatment choices or effectiveness. However, these screening studies do not inquire about parental status, do not examine how depression affects areas of functioning as a parent, and do not inquire about comorbid conditions (e.g., anxiety and substance use disorders). Rarely are screening programs integrated with service delivery. Mothers with elevated depressive symptoms as well as cases of clinical depression have been successfully identified primarily through screening programs in perinatal health care settings and, to a limited extent, in other private and public primary care settings. Depression in fathers has not been the focus of screening programs. Some programs providing early childhood services to high-risk populations have conducted screening and offer an opportunity to screen parents for depression and parenting function.

Despite the promise of screening programs, current approaches to parental depression screening have not been integrated with assessment of parental function or child development. As national initiatives by organizations and state agencies proceed to promote routine developmental and behavioral screening of young children, it is important to recognize that developmental or behavioral problems in this age group may be related to parenting difficulties and depression and should be assessed.

Furthermore, a number of barriers exist in implementing a comprehensive screening program. For screening to be effective, the paths to further care must be clear and accessible for both the providers who identify the depression and the families so that available clinical and community resources to address issues are used. Limited or poorly organized community resources, or lack of knowledge of existing resources, may decrease willingness to screen.

Linking depression screening to existing screening efforts—such as prenatal assessment during pregnancy and child developmental screening, at entry into programs serving high-risk parents (e.g., home visiting, homeless, and substance use programs), and other existing treatment or prevention programs—is a first step that could address depression in parents and its impact on their families.

REFERENCES

Abidin, R. (1995). *Parenting Stress Index: Professional Manual* (2nd ed.). Lutz, FL: Psychological Assessment Resources.

Amaro, H., McGraw, S., Larson, M.J., Lopez, L., Nieves, R., and Marshall, B. (2005). Boston Consortium of Services for Families in Recovery: A trauma-informed intervention model for women's alcohol and drug addiction treatment. *Alcoholism Treatment Quarterly, 22*, 95–119.

American Academy of Pediatrics and Council on Children with Disabilities. (2006). Identifying infants and young children with developmental disorders in the medical home: An algorithm for developmental surveillance and screening. *Pediatrics, 118,* 405–420.

Ammerman, R.T., Putnam, F.W., Altaye, M., Chen, L., Holleb, L.J., Steven, J., Short, J.A., and Van Ginkle, J.B. (2009). Changes in depressive symptoms in first-time mothers in home visitation. *Child Abuse and Neglect, 33,* 127–138.

Arroll, B., Goodyear-Smith, F., Kerse, N., Fishman, T., and Gunn, J. (2005). Effect of the addition of a help question to two screening questions on specificity of diagnosis of depression in general practice: Diagnostic validity study. *British Medical Journal, 331,* 884–888.

Beeber, L.S., Perreira, K.M., and Schwartz, T. (2008). Supporting the mental health of mothers raising children in poverty: How do we target them for intervention studies? *Annals of the New York Academy of Sciences, 1136,* 86–100.

Bethell, C., Peck, C., and Schor, E. (2001). Assessing health system provision of well-child care: The Promoting Healthy Development Survey. *Pediatrics, 107,* 1084–1094.

Boyd, R.C., Le, H.N., and Somberg, R. (2005). Review of screening instruments for postpartum depression. *Archives of Women's Mental Health, 8,* 141–153.

Brothers, K.B., Glascoe, F.P., and Robertshaw, N.S. (2008). PEDS: Developmental milestones—An accurate brief tool for surveillance and screening. *Clinical Pediatrics, 47,* 271–279.

Brown, V., Rechberger, E., and Bjelajac, P. (2005). A model for changing alcohol and other drug, mental health, and trauma services practice PROTOTYPES systems change center. *Alcoholism Treatment Quarterly, 22,* 81–94.

Buist, A., Condon, J., Brooks, J., Speelman, C., Milgrom, J., Hayes, B., Ellwood, D., Barnett, B., Kowalenko, N., Matthey, S., Austin, M.P., and Bilszta, J. (2006). Acceptability of routine screening for perinatal depression. *Journal of Affective Disorders, 93,* 233–237.

Burnam, M.A., Wells, K.B., Leake, B., and Landsverk, J. (1988). Development of a brief screening instrument for detecting depressive disorders. *Medical Care, 26,* 775–789.

Carter, F.A., Carter, J.D., Luty, S.E., Wilson, D.A., Frampton, C.M.A., and Joyce, P.R. (2005). Screening and treatment for depression during pregnancy: A cautionary note. *Australian and New Zealand Journal of Psychiatry, 39,* 255–261.

Chaudron, L.H., Szilagyi, P.G., Campbell, A.T., Mounts, K.O., and McInery, T.K. (2007). Legal and ethical considerations: Risks and benefits of postpartum depression screening at well-child visits. *Pediatrics, 119,* 123–128.

Chaudron, L.H., Szilagyi, P.G., Kitzman, H.J., Wadkins, H.I.M., and Conwell, Y. (2004). Detection of postpartum depressive symptoms by screening at well-child visits. *Pediatrics, 113,* 551–558.

Chisolm, M., Tuten, M., Strain, E.C., and Jones, H.E. (in press). Screening for mood disorder in pregnant substance dependent patients. *Addictive Disorders and Their Treatment.*

Conners, N.A., Grant, A., Crone, C.C., and Whiteside-Mansell, L. (2006). Substance abuse treatment for mothers: Treatment outcomes and the impact of length of stay. *Journal of Substance Abuse Treatment, 31,* 447–456.

Cutler, C.B., Legano, L.A., Dreyer, B.P., Fierman, A.H., Berkule, S.B., Lusskin, S.I., Tomopoulos, S., Roth, M., and Mendelsohn, A.L. (2007). Screening for maternal depression in a low education population using a two item questionnaire. *Archives of Women's Mental Health, 10,* 277–283.

Dubowitz, H., Feigelman, S., Lane, W., Prescott, L., Blackman, L.G., Meyer, W., and Tracy, K. (2007). Screening for depression in an urban pediatric primary care clinic. *Pediatrics, 119,* 435–443.

Evins, G.G., Theofrastous, J.P., and Galvin, S.L. (2000). Postpartum depression: A comparison of screening and routine clinical evaluation. *American Journal of Obstetrics and Gynecology, 182,* 1080–1082.

Fitzsimons, H.E., Tuten, M., Vaidya, V., and Jones, H.E. (2007). Mood disorders affect drug treatment success of drug-dependent pregnant women. *Journal of Substance Abuse Treatment*, 32, 19–25.

Gaynes, B.N., Gavin, N., Meltzer-Brody, S., Lohr, K.N., Swinson, T., Gartlehner, G., Brody, S., and Miller, W.C. (2005). Perinatal depression: Prevalence, screening accuracy, and screening outcomes. *Evidence Report/Technology Assessment (Summary)*, 119, 1–8.

Georgiopoulos, A.M., Bryan, T.L., Wollan, P., and Yawn, B.P. (2001). Routine screening for postpartum depression. *Journal of Family Practice*, 50, 117–122.

Grupp-Phelan, J., Whitaker, R.C., and Naish, A.B. (2003). Depression in mothers of children presenting for emergency and primary care: Impact on mothers' perceptions of caring for their children. *Ambulatory Pediatrics*, 3, 142–146.

Hagen, J.F., Shaw, J.S., and Duncan, P.M. (Eds.). (2008). *Bright Futures: Guidelines for Health Supervision of Infants, Children and Adolescents* (3rd ed.). Elk Grove, IL: American Academy of Pediatrics.

Hebbeler, K.M., and Gerlach-Downie, S. (2002). Inside the black box of home visiting: A qualitative analysis of why intended outcomes were not achieved. *Early Childhood Research Quarterly*, 17, 28–51.

Heneghan, A.M., Chaudron, L.H., Storfer-Isser, A., Kelleher, K.J., Hoagwood, K.E., O'Connor, K.G., and Horwitz, S.M. (2007). Factors associated with identification and management of maternal depression by pediatricians. *Pediatrics*, 119, 444–454.

Heneghan, A.M., Mercer, M., and DeLeone, N.L. (2004). Will mothers discuss parenting stress and depressive symptoms with their child's pediatrician? *Pediatrics*, 113, 460–467.

Heneghan, A.M., Morton, S., and DeLeone, N.L. (2006). Pediatricians' attitudes about discussing maternal depression during a paediatric primary care visit. *Child: Care, Health, and Development*, 33, 333–339.

Heneghan, A.M., Silver, E.J., Bauman, L.J., and Stein, R.E.K. (2000). Do pediatricians recognize mothers with depressive symptoms? *Pediatrics*, 106, 1367–1373.

Jacobs, F., Easterbrooks, M.A., Brady, A., and Mistry, J. (2005). *Healthy Families Massachusetts: Final Evaluation Report*. Medford, MA: Tufts University.

Jansson, L.M., Svikis, D., Lee, J., Paluzzi, P., Rutigliano, P., and Hackerman, F. (1996). Pregnancy and addiction. A comprehensive care model. *Journal of Substance Abuse Treatment*, 13, 321–329.

Jansson, L.M., Svikis, D.S., Velez, M., Fitzgerald, E., and Jones, H.E. (2007). The impact of managed care on drug-dependent pregnant and postpartum women and their children. *Substance Use and Misuse*, 42, 961–974.

Jellinek, M., Patel, B.P., and Froehle, M.C. (Eds.). (2002). *Bright Futures in Practice: Mental Health—Volume I. Practice Guide*. Arlington, VA: National Center for Education in Maternal and Child Health.

Kabir, K., Sheeder, J., and Kelly, L.S. (2008). Identifying postpartum depression: Are 3 questions as good as 10? *Pediatrics*, 122, e696–e702.

Kemper, K.J., and Babonis, T.R. (1992). Screening for maternal depression in pediatric clinics. *American Journal of Diseases of Children*, 146, 876–878.

Kroenke, K., Spitzer, R.L., and Williams, J.B. (2003). The Patient Health Questionnaire-2: Validity of a two-item depression screener. *Medical Care*, 41, 1284–1292.

LaRocco-Cockburn, A., Melville, J., Bell, M., and Katon, W. (2003). Depression screening attitudes and practices among obstetrician-gynecologists. *Obstetrics and Gynecology*, 101, 892–898.

Lazear, K.J., Pires, S.A., Isaacs, M.R., Chaulk, P., and Huang, L. (2008). Depression among low-income women of color: Qualitative findings from cross-cultural focus groups. *Journal of Immigrant and Minority Health*, 10, 127–133.

Lincoln, A.K., Liebschutz, J.M., Chernoff, M., Nguyen, D., and Amaro, H. (2006). Brief screening for co-occurring disorders among women entering substance abuse treatment. *Substance Abuse Treatment, Prevention, and Policy*, 7, 26.

Lynch, T., and Harrington, J. (2003). *Benefit Cost Analysis of the Maternal Depression Project in Gadsden County, Florida.* Tallahassee, FL: Center for Economic Forecasting and Analysis.

Miranda, J., Green, B.L., Krupnick, J.L., Chung, J., Siddique, J., Belin, T., and Revicki, D. (2006). One-year outcomes of a randomized clinical trial treating depression in low-income minority women. *Journal of Consulting and Clinical Psychology*, 74, 99–111.

O'Hara, M.W., and Swain, A.M. (1996). Rates and risk of postpartum depression—A meta-analysis. *International Review of Psychiatry*, 8, 37–54.

Olson, A.L., Dietrich, A.J., Prazar, G., and Hurley, J. (2006). Brief maternal depression screening at well-child visits. *Pediatrics*, 118, 207–216.

Olson, A., Dietrich, A.J., Prazar, G., Hurley, J., Tuddenham, A., Hedberg, V., and Naspinsky, D. (2005). Two approaches to maternal depression screening during well child visits. *Journal of Developmental and Behavioral Pediatrics*, 26, 169–175.

Olson, A.L., Kemper, K.J., Kelleher, K.J., Hammond, C.S., Zuckerman, B.S., and Dietrich, A.J. (2002). Primary care pediatricians' roles and perceived responsibilities in the identification and management of maternal depression. *Pediatrics*, 110, 1169–1176.

Pignone, M.P., Gaynes, B.N., Rushton, J.L., Burchell, C.M., Orleans, C.T., Mulrow, C.D., and Lohr, K.N. (2002). Screening for depression in adults: A summary of the evidence for the U.S. Preventive Services Task Force. *Annals of Internal Medicine*, 136, 765–776.

Pregnancy Risk Assessment Monitoring System Working Group and the Centers for Disease Control and Prevention Pregnancy Risk Assessment Monitoring System Team. (2008). Prevalence of self-reported postpartum depressive symptoms—17 states, 2004–2005. *Morbidity and Mortality Weekly Report*, 57, 361–366.

Seehusen, D.A., Baldwin, L.M., Runkle, G.P., and Clark, G. (2005). Are family physicians appropriately screening for postpartum depression? *Journal of the American Board of Family Practice*, 18, 104–112.

Segre, L.S., O'Hara, M.W., Arndt, S., and Stuart, S. (2007). The prevalence of postpartum depression: The relative significance of three social status indices. *Social Psychiatry and Psychiatric Epidemiology*, 42, 316–321.

Spitzer, R.L., Williams, J.B.W., Kroenke, K., Hornyak, R., and McMurray, J. (2000). Validity and utility of the PRIME-MD Patient Health Questionnaire in assessment of 3000 obstetric-gynecologic patients. *American Journal of Obstetrics and Gynecology*, 183, 759–769.

Stevens, J., Ammerman, R., Putnam, F., and Van Ginkel, J. (2002). Depression and trauma history in first-time mothers receiving home visitation. *Journal of Community Psychology*, 30, 551–564.

Tandon, S.D., Parillo, K.M., Jenkins, C., and Duggan A.K. (2005). Formative evaluation of home visitor's role in addressing poor mental health, domestic violence and substance abuse among low-income pregnant and parenting women. *Maternal and Child Health Journal*, 9, 273–283.

U.S. Preventive Services Task Force. (2002). *Screening for Depression: Recommendations and Rationale.* Available: http://www.ahrq.gov/clinic/3rduspstf/depression/ [accessed December 22, 2008].

Weinreb, L.F., Buckner, J.C., Williams, V., and Nicholson, J. (2006). A comparison of the health and mental health status of homeless mothers in Worchester, Massachusetts: 1993 and 2003. *American Journal of Public Health*, 96, 1444–1448.

Whooley, M.A., Avins, A.L., Miranda, J., and Bowner, W.S. (1997). Case finding instruments for depression: Two questions as good as many. *Journal of General Internal Medicine, 12,* 439–445.

Wiedmann, M., and Garfield, C. (2007). *Perinatal Maternal Depression and Child Development: Strategies for Primary Care Providers.* Available: http://www.iafp.com/pdfs/MaternalDepression.pdf [accessed January 22, 2009].

6

Treatment of Depression in Parents

SUMMARY

Treatment Rates

- Studies of community samples indicate that approximately 30 percent of depressed adults receive any treatment for their illness. Although limited, evidence suggests that treatment rates for mothers may be even lower than the general population.

Treatment Tools

- Evidence shows that a variety of safe and effective tools exist for treating adults with depression, including pharmacotherapies, psychotherapies, behavioral therapies, and alternative medicines.
- Studies of depression treatment tools in adults rarely measure outcomes that specifically affect parents, including parenting quality and impact of therapeutic treatments on children. Quality studies documenting the safety and efficacy of therapeutic treatments for perinatal depression are limited as well, although preliminary evidence and observational data are generally favorable.

Treatment Delivery Approaches

- A variety of approaches exist to deliver depression treatment in multiple settings, including primary and specialty care, web- and community-based. Evidence from primary care settings suggests that models of care that integrate multiple interventions (e.g., education, care management, frequent telephone follow-up) are clinically effective in reducing depressive symptoms in adults. Existing studies are relatively short term, however, and the cost-effectiveness and exportability of these models are not usually considered.

- Studies of approaches to effectively deliver treatment and to prevent relapse in adults with depression rarely target parents, especially in settings in which traditionally underserved populations of parents or their children are seen.

- Treatments that address individual patient preferences, concurrent conditions (such as medical comorbidities and substance abuse), overcoming depression-related stigma and mistrust, and health disparities tend to be better received and more effective than approaches that rely on health provider experience alone.

Depression is a common and recurrent disorder that can have profound effects on medical, social, and financial well-being, and a large body of literature documents safe and effective therapeutic strategies. In this chapter, we have divided these strategies into treatments (i.e., *tools*) and interventions (i.e., *approaches*). Standard treatments for depression include pharmacotherapy, psychotherapy and alternative remedies. Successful interventions have generally been more structured and comprehensive, often featuring multidisciplinary approaches that emphasize several treatment modalities (e.g., collaborative care).

Although the evidence base is rich for depression treatments and interventions in the general adult population, far fewer studies have analyzed outcomes in parents or families. For this reason, we have chosen to proceed in this chapter with a brief summary of treatment rates, therapeutic options, and interventions in the general adult population before focusing more intently on the body of literature specific to parents. Chapter 7 addresses the approaches to prevent adverse outcomes in depressed parents and the children of depressed parents, including the impact of treatment on families.

The committee reviewed the relevant literature in order to identify depression treatment rates, therapeutic options that are available to treat depression, and options for the delivery of depression treatment in the general adult population that address outcomes for depressed adults and then specifically in parents, as well as to identify areas in which relatively little research has been conducted. The committee did not seek to systematically identify every study on the evaluation of existing therapeutic tools or delivery interventions for treating depression in adults (and parents); instead, whenever possible, the committee drew on existing meta-analyses and systematic reviews. Whenever possible, the committee limited its review to interventions that have been evaluated in at least one randomized trial and presents a summary of the methodological details, study population demographics, and outcome measures (i.e., depressive symptoms or depression diagnosis) that were used for studies of treatment delivery interventions in a table that is described in the second part of this chapter.

TREATMENT RATES

General Population

More recent nationally representative work has illustrated that those in racial or ethnic minority populations with past-year depressive order are significantly more likely to go without mental health treatment than non-Hispanic whites (64 percent Hispanics, 69 percent Asians, 60 percent of African Americans, compared to 40 percent of non-Hispanic whites) Alegría et al., 2008). Disparities in the likelihood of both having access to and receiving adequate care for depression were significantly different for Asians and African Americans in contrast to non-Hispanic whites. Simply relying on present health care systems without consideration of the unique barriers to quality care that ethnic and racial minority populations face is unlikely to affect the pattern of disparities observed. Populations reluctant to visit a clinic for depression care may have correctly anticipated the limited quality of usual care.

The close association of depression with certain medical conditions (e.g., neurological, cardiovascular, and endocrine disorders) has inspired researchers to explore the feasibility of addressing this mental illness in specialty medical clinics. For example, recent investigations document higher treatment rates and superior outcomes among depressed patients identified at diabetes clinics (Simon et al., 2007).

Mothers with Depression

At the present time, there are no epidemiological data documenting treatment rates among depressed parents, although indirect evidence suggests that these figures are even lower than in the general population. In the Sequenced Treatment Alternatives to Relieve Depression (STAR*D) trial (a large national trial designed to identify depression treatment strategies), for example, only 22 percent of women seeking treatment had children living with them, implying that depressed mothers were underrepresented in this sample, perhaps owing to the perception of stigma or domestic responsibilities discouraging travel (Pilowsky et al., 2006). It is also documented that depressed people in the general population are at higher risk of having complex comorbid illnesses, including substance abuse and domestic violence (Regier et al., 1990). Exposure to interpersonal violence, for example, has been associated with poorer outcomes in mothers with substance use and mental health disorders (Amaro et al., 2005).

Mothers with Antepartum Depression

Treatment rates for pregnant women are believed to be considerably lower than the rest of the adult population, despite the fact that the risks of untreated antepartum depression usually outweigh any risks posed by psychotherapy or commonly prescribed antidepressants (see the discussion of the safety and efficacy of pharmacotherapy below). For example, Marcus et al. conducted a prospective study examining the incidence of antepartum depression in obstetric settings (Marcus et al., 2003). They reported that 20 percent of the women met a conventional threshold for significant depressive illness (they scored higher than 16 on the Center for Epidemiologic Studies Depression Scale, CESD), yet only 14 percent of these women ultimately received any treatment. Another study screened pregnant women and proceeded to conduct structured interviews to confirm the diagnosis and severity (Flynn, Blow, and Marcus, 2006). Among the pregnant women with a confirmed diagnosis of acute major depression, only 33 percent received any treatment. Another investigation was conducted using a large patient database in Canada (119,547 mothers; Oberlander et al., 2006). Approximately 15 percent of the population received a diagnostic code for depression within 4 months of delivery, yet less than 10 percent of this subset received a prescription for an antidepressant.

Mothers with Postpartum Depression

Data for the frequency of depression treatment during the postpartum period are scarce. One of the few investigations examined a secondary analysis of a mother-infant study that followed 117 mothers who were identified as depressed between 2 and 4 weeks postpartum. Three months after screening, only 14 women (12 percent) had received psychotherapy, and only 4 (3.4 percent) had received pharmacotherapy (Horowitz and Cousins, 2006).

Even when depression is addressed, the initiation of medication or counseling does not guarantee success. Insurance data claims and health maintenance organization (HMO) refill records suggest that approximately half of patients will stop their antidepressants during the first 3 months, and a vast majority do not complete the minimum recommended duration of 6 months. These figures are slightly higher among privately insured beneficiaries and somewhat lower in the public sector (National Committee on Quality Assurance, 2005). Data describing the percentage of parents who receive adequate treatment are not currently available. There is a growing awareness of the undertreatment of depression, including government efforts to improve medication adherence and treatment follow-up through such measures as Healthcare Effectiveness Data and Information Set (HEDIS), a tool created by the National Committee for Quality Assurance, to collect data about the quality of care, including depression care, provided by health plans. However, data from health care organizations do not indicate that significant improvement has transpired during the past decade (National Committee on Quality Assurance, 2008). Although depression treatment rates are low, there remains available a variety of safe and effective therapeutic interventions.

PHARMACOTHERAPY

General Population

Antidepressants are among the most commonly prescribed medications in health care today. Much of this popularity can be traced to the development of newer medications such as selective serotonin reuptake inhibitors (SSRI: fluoxetine, sertraline, paroxetine, citalopram), serotonin norepinephrine reuptake inhibitors (SNRI: venlafaxine, duloxetine), and norepinephrine reuptake inhibitors (NRI: bupropion), which are perceived to be safer than older antidepressants (Barbui et al., 2007). The enhanced utility of newer antidepressants may also add to their popularity as serotonergic agents (SSRI and SNRI) as they have proven to be very effective for anxiety disorders.

For the treatment of major depression, it is widely believed that roughly two-thirds of patients will respond to the first antidepressant that is initiated (Fava and Davidson, 1996). Data to support these response rates, however, have been gathered historically from randomized controlled trials conducted by pharmaceutical companies to demonstrate drug efficacy for regulatory bodies. Depressed subjects enrolled in such trials were usually young men with minimal medical and psychiatric comorbidity and do not necessarily represent the demographic characteristics of depressed parents. In the STAR*D trial, which attempted to examine antidepressant effects in a real-world setting, fewer than half of the subjects exhibited a clinical response after a full therapeutic trial of an SSRI (Trivedi et al., 2006).

Another notable development in research and clinical antidepressant trials has been a change in what is considered the ideal therapeutic endpoint. While a therapeutic response was the historic goal—defined as a greater than 50 percent decline on a given depression severity scale—experts have realized that patients who satisfied this criterion often had significant residual symptoms and fairly high relapse rates. Remission is now regarded as the desired therapeutic endpoint. In practical terms, remission is achieved when virtually all depressive symptoms are absent. Operationally, remission is usually defined as a depression severity score below an established threshold (e.g., a score of less than 7 on the Hamilton Depression Rating Scale). From recent research trials, the remission rates for antidepressants range from 30 to 40 percent (Thase, Entsuah, and Rudolph, 2001). Higher remission rates may be achieved through the addition of other antidepressant medications (i.e., augmentation) or concurrent psychotherapy (Keller et al., 2000).

Mothers with Antepartum Depression

The safety and efficacy of antidepressants during the antepartum period are a major concern from maternal, scientific, and health policy perspectives. Mothers, fathers, and health care providers must weigh the substantial risks of untreated antepartum depression against the potential risks of antidepressant exposure. When faced with this dilemma, many women have historically discontinued medications as soon as their pregnancy was confirmed, although a naturalistic investigation recently reported that women who stopped their antidepressants during the first trimester were much more likely to relapse before delivery than those who continued (68 versus 26 percent) (Cohen et al., 2006). And over half of these relapses actually occurred during the first trimester.

Prospective randomized studies of medications are rarely conducted on pregnant women in part because of ethical concerns. As a result, we have only retrospective or naturalistic data to consider when evaluating the efficacy and safety of antidepressants in the antepartum period. Since the effectiveness of antidepressants can be accurately assessed only through blinded, controlled trials, the literature summarizing the efficacy of antidepressants during pregnancy is nonexistent. The relative safety, however, can be inferred from a body of evidence that has grown remarkably in recent years.

As the SSRIs are currently the most popular class of antidepressants, most of the recent investigations have examined their relative safety. For the most part, it appears that SSRIs do not carry a significant risk for major congenital malformations. The only potential exception can be found in data suggesting that paroxetine may be associated with cardiovascular defects. A recent analysis of the Swedish Medical Birth Registry confirmed previous reports of this risk, citing an odds ratio of 1.81 (95 percent confidence interval, CI = 0.96–3.09) for ventricular and atrial defects (Kallen and Olausson, 2007). This finding was based on 13 cases among 959 exposures. A subsequent analysis of data pertaining to over 3,000 exposures was performed by the Motherisk Program in Canada, which found that paroxetine was associated with a *decreased* risk of malformations (0.7 percent versus an established population risk of 1.0 percent) (Einarson et al., 2008). On the basis of previous reports, however, the U.S. Food and Drug Administration (FDA) chose to demote paroxetine to Category D[1] status in pregnancy, discouraging its use unless absolutely necessary.

Other adverse outcomes associated with SSRI in pregnancy are worth considering, including persistent pulmonary hypertension, preterm labor, and neonatal adaptation syndrome. Persistent pulmonary hypertension (PPHN) is a relatively rare complication occurring shortly after delivery that has been associated with a 20 percent mortality rate (Hageman, Adams, and Gardner, 1984). Results of a case-control study identified 14 cases of SSRI-induced PPHN in the case group (n = 377) and 6 cases of PPHN among controls (n = 836) (Chambers et al., 2006). The risk appeared to be highest with exposure after 20 weeks gestation. While the SSRIs were associated with a sixfold increase in the relative risk of this serious phenomenon, it should also be remembered that the absolute risk remains quite low (6–12 cases per 1,000 exposures) and is probably not as serious as the risks posed by untreated depression on the mother and the infant alike.

Several studies have noted that SSRIs are associated with a decrease in gestational age, birth weight, or both. Although depression itself has been associated with these two effects, comparisons between SSRIs and other antidepressants and between SSRIs and matched controls appear to confirm these findings. For example, Suri et al. followed the outcomes of three different cohorts (antidepressants, depressed without antidepressants, nondepressed controls; n = 90) and reported significant differences in gestational age (38.5, 39.4, and 39.7 weeks, respectively), rates of preterm birth (14, 0, and 5 percent, respectively) and special care nursery admissions (21, 9, and 0 percent, respectively) (Suri et al., 2007). Results of this investigation were confirmed in the large retrospective study by Oberlander cited above. In comparison to depressed mothers not receiving pharmacotherapy, mothers who were prescribed SSRIs were much more likely to give birth before 37 weeks gestation (6 percent versus 9 percent; 95 percent CI = –0.009 to –0.04), and their infants were more likely to suffer respiratory distress

---

[1]For detailed description of U.S. Food and Drug Administration risk categories for drug use in pregnancy, see http://www.fda.gov/fdac/features/2001/301_preg.html#categories. Categories depend on the type of studies available and the risk of fetal abnormalities and include: A, B, C, D, and X.

(8 percent versus 14 percent; 95 percent CI = 0.042–0.079). These significant differences were upheld after propensity score matching as well.

Neonatal adaptation syndrome is a constellation of symptoms that have been attributed to third-trimester exposure of the fetus to concurrent SSRI or SNRI use. Symptoms include high-pitched crying, decreased appetite, tremor, hypertonicity, and respiratory distress. A prospective study used a scale created by Finnegan (1990) to measure these symptoms and concluded that the SSRIs were much more likely to be associated with this syndrome (Levinson-Castiel et al., 2006). In general, the symptoms peaked by day 2 after delivery and had remitted by the end of day 4. As neonatal adaptation syndrome has been implicated in a potential increase in the risk of admissions, some experts have recommended tapering mothers off antidepressants prior to delivery (U.S. Food and Drug Administration, 2004). This practice is somewhat controversial; however, opponents have pointed out that drug discontinuation would itself be associated with an increased risk for withdrawal symptoms in the mother, as well as an increased risk of relapse during the immediate postpartum period.

Adverse effects of SSRI antidepressants are a major concern in the parent and should be factored into the decision-making process as well. For instance, SSRIs have been associated with a 30–50 percent incidence of sexual dysfunction, which can impart considerable strain on a relationship regardless of the parent's reproductive status. Nausea is also common with SSRIs, which may diminish the mother's appetite, and sleep disturbances are frequently reported as well.

Data documenting the safety of other antidepressants in pregnancy is relatively limited. Bupropion was once considered the safest of the available antidepressants in pregnancy, but the FDA recently demoted it from Category B to Category C. This was based on a review of reproduction studies in rabbits, which found a slight increase in fetal malformations and skeletal variations with relatively low-dose exposure. Mirtazapine and venlafaxine have not been associated with major fetal malformations. As duloxetine was approved for use only recently, data regarding its safety in pregnancy are inconclusive. One theoretical concern found with duloxetine (as well as venlafaxine and bupropion) involves preeclampsia. As all three antidepressants have been shown to cause a small but significant increase in blood pressure and heart rate in adults, they may also predispose expectant mothers to this complication (Eli Lilly, 2009; GlaxoSmithKline, 2008; Wyeth Pharmaceuticals, 2008).

The long-term effects of in utero antidepressant exposure on the developing child have not been rigorously explored. Early studies reporting abnormal psychomotor development lacked sufficient control groups to separate the effects of the antidepressant from depression itself (i.e., the control groups were not depressed) (Mortensen et al., 2003). As untreated antepartum depression has been associated with deficits in IQ, language development, social functioning, and acceptable behavior, well-designed studies with matched controls would be required to distinguish the etiology of any detrimental effects. Two relatively small studies were unable to find an association between SSRI exposure and developmental abnormalities (Misri et al., 2006; Nulman et al., 2002). Another study concluded that externalizing behaviors in children were much more likely to be a reflection of the mother's current mood than exposure to antidepressants (Oberlander et al., 2007).

Mothers with Postpartum Depression

Untreated postpartum depression has been associated with serious consequences, most notably impaired mother-infant bonding and long-term effects on emotional behavior and cognitive skills. Although the risks of antidepressant transmission through breast milk are a common concern, it should be remembered that the risks of untreated depression are also readily transmitted to infants.

Studies examining the concentrations of antidepressants in breast milk have generally shown that the cumulative exposure of infants to antidepressants through lactation is low and the behavioral risks are minimal (Gentile, 2005). Until recently, the methodology employed in these investigations was quite diverse (or unknown), precluding any meaningful comparisons about the relative risk of various agents. In 2005, however, two comparative studies were published, both of which appeared to confirm that infant exposure was considerably lower than maternal exposure. In one study, the investigators compared the ratio of breast milk concentrations to maternal plasma concentrations among seven antidepressants, reporting values ranging from 0.021 (sertraline) to 0.33 (desipramine) (Whitby and Smith, 2005). In the other investigation, authors estimated the relative infant dose via breast milk for five antidepressants, with values ranging from 0.5 percent (sertraline) to 8.9 percent (fluoxetine) (Gentile, 2005), all of which were safely below the 10 percent threshold advocated by the American Academy of Pediatrics (Figure 6-1).

Prospective studies of adverse effects in infants receiving antidepressants through breast milk have not been numerous but generally support the relative safety of this exposure (Burt et al., 2001; Eberhard-Gran, Eskild, and Opjordsmoen, 2006).

A total of eight studies have been published, examining the impact of antidepressants on the treatment or prevention of postpartum depression. Only three of these investigations featured a randomized, double-blind design, but all reported positive findings. Appleby found that both fluoxetine and cognitive-behavioral therapy were significantly more effective than

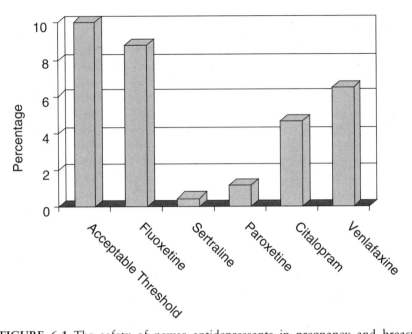

FIGURE 6-1 The safety of newer antidepressants in pregnancy and breast-feeding.
SOURCE: Adapted, with permission from data in Table II and Table III from Gentile (2005). Copyright (2005) by Wolters Kluwer.

placebo and that the combined treatment did not confer any additional benefits (Appleby et al., 1997). Similarly, Misri et al. (2004) found that paroxetine was associated with a highly significant treatment effect and that the combination of paroxetine plus cognitive-behavioral therapy was equally efficacious (versus monotherapy).

In the only head-to-head comparison of antidepressants, 95 women with postpartum depression were randomized to sertraline or nortriptyline (Wisner et al., 2006). Both medications improved psychosocial function, the only difference being an earlier separation of sertraline from baseline among responders (versus nortriptyline). Three small open-label trials with fluvoxamine, venlafaxine, and bupropion provide additional evidence for the effectiveness of antidepressants in relieving postpartum symptoms.

The data supporting the prevention of relapse of depression in women postpartum is limited. Two small randomized trials on prevention of relapse have also been published (Wisner et al., 2001, 2004). Patients given sertraline were much less likely to relapse than those randomized to placebo among nondepressed women with a history of perinatal depression (a relapse rate of 1 in 14 with active medication versus 4 in 8 with placebo). A similar investigation failed to find any difference between nortriptyline and placebo (a relapse rate of 6 in 26 versus 6 in 25 with placebo).

INTERPERSONAL PSYCHOTHERAPY AND COGNITIVE-BEHAVIORAL THERAPY

General Population

Multiple studies and meta-analyses provide evidence that cognitive-behavioral therapy (CBT) and interpersonal psychotherapy (IPT) are efficacious treatments for general depression (de Mello et al., 2005; Deckersbach, Gershuny, and Otto, 2000; Dobson, 1989). Cognitive-behavioral therapy is based on the idea that the way a person perceives an event determines how they will respond both affectively and behaviorally (Dennis and Hodnett, 2007). CBT helps patients identify and correct self-critical beliefs and distortions in thinking to reduce distress and enhance coping efforts. Interpersonal psychotherapy is a brief, highly structured, manual-based psychotherapy that addresses interpersonal issues in depression, such as role disputes, social isolation, or prolonged grief (Whooley and Simon, 2000). In summary, cognitive-behavioral therapy addresses distorted, negative thinking associated with depression, and interpersonal psychotherapy addresses stressful social and interpersonal relationships associated with the onset of depressive symptoms (Weissman, 2007).

Interpersonal psychotherapy is an accepted treatment for depression and has been found to be effective in multiple studies. A recent meta-analysis concluded that it was superior to placebo, similar to medication, and, when combined with medication, did not show an adjunctive effect compared with medication alone for acute treatment, maintenance treatment, or prophylactic treatment (de Mello et al., 2005). Although the meta-analysis found that IPT was more efficacious than CBT, other studies suggest that IPT is comparable to CBT in terms of outcomes. A recent review by Parker stated that IPT is unlikely to be the universal therapy for depression, given the heterogeneity of depressive disorders, but it may be appropriate therapy under specific circumstances (Parker et al., 2006).

Cognitive-behavioral therapy is widely used for the treatment of depression. Although earlier studies suggested that its use was less efficacious than medications for patients with severe depression (Elkin et al., 1995), more recent studies have found that CBT is as efficacious as medications for even severely depressed patients (DeRubeis et al., 2005). There is also evidence that the effects of CBT last beyond the end of treatment (Hollon, Stewart, and Strunk, 2006), and studies have shown that patients treated with CBT are less likely to relapse after treatment termination than are patients treated to remission with medications (Blackburn, Eunson, and Bishop, 1986; Gotlib and Hammen, 2008; Kovacs et al., 1981). In addition, studies suggest that CBT is effective for the prevention of depression in patients who are at risk but are not currently depressed (Seligman et al., 1999). Recent studies have suggested that, among the components of CBT, behavioral activation (i.e., getting patients to pleasurable and meaningful activities) may be even more effective than the cognitive restructuring component of CBT (Dimidjian et al., 2006). Because it is easy to teach patients and requires less therapist training than cognitive interventions, behavioral activation might extend the availability and effectiveness of psychotherapy for depression. However, strong empirical evidence is absent with regard to the efficacy of CBTs and other behavioral interventions among diverse racial and ethnic minority populations. Larger studies, including those examining adaptations of evidence-based treatments for diverse populations are needed. The use of race and/or ethnicity should be considered an integral part of the study methodology, data collection, and analyses, along with the utilization of culturally and linguistically appropriate instruments and measures (de Arellano et al., 2005). Studies examining disparities in depression treatment highlight the unique barriers that racial and ethnic minorities experience when seeking mental health care and quality of care remains a critical issue. Actually, having access to any mental health treatment remains a central point of concern for racial and ethnic minority groups (Alegría et al., 2008).

A new therapy, mindfulness-based cognitive therapy (MBCT), combines meditation with more conventional CBT (Segal, Williams, and Teasdale, 2002). MBCT is based on the Mindfulness-Based Stress Reduction Program developed by Jon Kabat-Zinn at the University of Massachusetts Medical Center. It integrates elements of CBT with components of Kabat-Zinn's mindfulness stress reduction program and "teaches patients to recognize and disengage from modes of mind characterized by negative and ruminative thinking and to access and use a new mode of mind characterized by acceptance and 'being'" (Coelho, Canter, and Ernst, 2007). Studies have demonstrated that MBCT is an effective therapy to prevent relapse or recurrence in recovered depressed patients with three or more previous episodes (Ma and Teasdale, 2004). It has also been shown to be an adjunct to the treatment of other psychological problems, including substance abuse, as well as changing behavior (Margolin et al., 2006; Witkiewitz and Marlatt, 2004). Multiple studies are currently investigating the effectiveness of MBCT for the treatment of current depression and prevention of relapse or recurrence. Furthermore, MBCT therapies have been effectively used in African American and Hispanic women to prevent relapse or recurrence of co-occurring disorders (i.e., substance use and trauma) (personal communication, H. Amaro, Northeastern University, February 13, 2009; Vallejo and Amaro, in press).

Mothers with Antepartum Depression

Given concerns over the safety of antidepressants during pregnancy and the postpartum period, psychological and psychosocial treatments for depression are an important alternative therapy for depression during this period. However, few studies have investigated whether cognitive-behavioral therapy or interpersonal psychotherapy are efficacious in the setting of antenatal depression. In fact, a recent Cochrane review (which are systematic reviews of health care interventions, see http://www.cochrane.org) found only one U.S. trial that met inclusion criteria to investigate the topic (Dennis, Ross, and Grigoriadis, 2007). One trial of 38 outpatient antenatal women who met criteria for major depression found that interpersonal psychotherapy compared with a parenting education program was associated with a reduction in the risk of depressive symptoms immediately following treatment. It also found that women who received 16 weeks of modified IPT were more likely to recover than controls (Spinelli and Endicott, 2003). Given the small size of the trial and the nongeneralizable sample, the Cochrane review concluded that the evidence was inconclusive regarding the effects of IPT for the treatment of antenatal depression.

Mothers with Postpartum Depression

Although the evidence is inconclusive in the setting of antepartum depression, a number of randomized trials have shown the benefit of psychological and psychosocial interventions to reduce postpartum depression diagnoses and symptoms. A recent review included nine trials of CBT, IPT, and psychodynamic therapy, as well as psychosocial interventions, such as peer support and nondirective counseling. The authors found that any psychosocial or psychological intervention, compared with usual postpartum care (variously defined), was associated with a reduction in the likelihood of depressive symptomatology at the final postpartum assessment (nine trials; n = 956, relative risk, RR = 0.70, 95 percent CI = 0.60–0.81) (Dennis and Hodnett, 2007).

ALTERNATIVE MEDICINE

Given the reluctance of many mothers to consume prescription antidepressants during pregnancy or breastfeeding, researchers have conducted several small studies examining alternative treatments. Results are very preliminary but encouraging.

Omega-3 Fatty Acids

Omega-3 fatty acid supplementation has been studied for the treatment and prevention of unipolar and bipolar depression in the general population with success reported for daily regimens of approximately 2–3g daily of eicosapentaenoic acid (EPA) plus docosahexaenoic acid (DHA) (Freeman et al., 2008; Su et al., 2008). As these two fatty acids are typically found in cold-water fish and many women avoid fish perinatally due to concerns over mercury exposure, supplementation would appear to be a prudent approach. Additional benefits of DHA in pregnant women would include decreasing the risks of preeclampsia and promoting healthy child development.

Following a small, open-label study documenting benefits among 15 women with antepartum depression, Freeman examined the benefit of omega-3 fatty acids among 59 women with perinatal depression (i.e., antepartum and postpartum subjects combined) (Freeman et al., 2006a, 2008). Subjects were randomized to 1.9g of omega-3 fatty acids daily (DHA + EPA) or placebo. At the end of the 8-week trial, both groups experienced substantial benefit, but the application of manualized CBT to both study groups may have prevented the authors from detecting a statistically significant difference.

Su et al. also conducted a small, randomized controlled trial of omega-3 fatty acids for antepartum depression, enrolling 33 subjects in their 8-week trial (Su et al., 2008). A total of 24 subjects completed the trial, with the group assigned to omega-3 fatty acids (3.4g daily) demonstrating superior response rates (62 versus 27 percent; p = 0.03) and remission rates (38 versus 18 percent; p = 0.28) in comparison to placebo controls.

While the favorable findings from these antepartum and other postpartum studies are encouraging, the investigations have been quite small, and little is known about the effective dosing range (Freeman et al., 2006b; Llorente et al., 2003). Omega-3 fatty acids have been very well tolerated, however. And given the fact that these naturally occurring compounds may impart additional benefits to adults (e.g., anti-inflammatory effects) and pregnant women in particular (decreased risks of complications), further studies are clearly warranted.

St. John's Wort

St. John's wort, an herbal remedy from the *Hypericum perforatum* plant, has been used to treat major depression for many years (Maurer and Colt, 2006). An initial Cochrane review investigated 37 randomized trials and concluded that the evidence for the use of St. John's wort for depression was confusing and inconsistent (Linde et al., 2005). However, a more recent review of 29 studies concluded that St. John's wort was more effective than placebo, comparable in effectiveness to standard antidepressants, and appeared to cause fewer side effects than prescription remedies (Linde, Berner, and Kriston, 2008). Authors did note that St. John's wort appeared to be more effective in studies conducted in German-speaking countries, owing perhaps due to the greater potency of preparations administered. An additional review of 13 studies comparing St. John's wort to SSRIs reported that the two treatments were equivalent in efficacy and adverse effects but that St. John's wort was associated with lower dropout rates (Rahimi, Nikfar, and Abdollahi, 2009). An additional systematic review investigated whether St. John's wort was safe during pregnancy and breast-feeding. It reported that there is very weak evidence that St. John's wort is safe during pregnancy and lactation and concluded that more research is needed (Dugoua et al., 2006). In addition, it should be noted that St. John's wort is a potent inducer of several liver enzymes, potentially interacting with many prescription and nonprescription drugs (e.g., birth control pills, antibiotics) (Weier and Beal, 2004).

Phototherapy

Bright light therapy or phototherapy has been used with some success for seasonal affective disorder, but there is less evidence supporting its use in major depression. A Cochrane review analyzed 20 studies and found the results of its use for the treatment of nonseasonal depression to be modest but promising (Tuunainen, Kripke, and Endo, 2004). Light therapy has also been proposed as a safe and effective intervention for perinatal depression, which can be safely and conveniently administered in one's home. The rationale for this approach to perinatal depression may stem from the fact that pregnant and postpartum women are often deficient in exposure to natural sunlight. Small open-label trials have featured 7,000–10,000 lux of bright light for up to 1 hour daily with generally favorable results; these should serve as a stimulus for more rigorous investigations (Corral, Kuan, and Kostaras, 2000; Epperson et al., 2004; Oren et al., 2002).

Exercise

Exercise has long been promoted as an alternative to prescription antidepressants in the postpartum period as well. For the general population of depressed adults, a wide variety of studies have reported therapeutic benefits with exercise regimens, although the number of large, randomized investigations with appropriate controls is very limited (Stathopoulou et al., 2006). Frequent modest cardiovascular workouts impart a wide variety of benefits to depressed people, including appetite regulation, sleep and energy improvements, an enhanced sense of well-being, and observed increases in plasma serotonin concentrations.

A 2007 review of the literature identified a total of two small, randomized controlled trials of pram (baby carriage) walking in postnatal mothers, both of which reported significant benefit (Armstrong and Edwards, 2003, 2004; Daley, Macarthur, and Winter, 2007). However, the authors were not able to control for the confounding influence of concurrent medications. A variety of other uncontrolled or observational studies for postpartum depression have reported similar positive preliminary findings.

Yoga

Yoga consists of a complex system of spiritual, moral, and physical practices aimed at raising self-awareness (Pilkington, Rampes, and Richardson, 2006). It has been studied for the treatment of depression. Five randomized controlled trials evaluating the efficacy of yoga in the treatment of depression were identified in a systematic review (Pilkington et al., 2005). Different forms of yoga were used. All trials reported positive findings, but poor study quality limited the usefulness of their results. Yoga is a particularly interesting therapy during pregnancy and the postpartum period, given the other physical and emotional symptoms women experience (such as back pain, anxiety) at this time. Yoga programs for perinatal women are widely available throughout the country, and further research of this intervention appears warranted.

Acupuncture

Acupuncture has been used in China and other Asian countries for thousands of years. Acupuncture is generally safe, and studies suggest that it may be an effective treatment for psychological problems, including depression (Weier and Beal, 2004). A Cochrane review that examined the efficacy of acupuncture for depression included seven trials: five trials compared acupuncture with medication, and two trials compared acupuncture with a wait-list control of sham acupuncture (Smith and Hay, 2005). There was no evidence that medication was better than acupuncture in reducing the severity of depression or in improving depression. Given the small sample sizes and poor quality of the studies, the authors concluded that there was insufficient evidence to determine the efficacy of acupuncture compared with medication for depression. There are no randomized trials evaluating the use of acupuncture for depression during pregnancy or for postpartum depression.

Other therapies, such as aromatherapy, massage therapy, and reflexology, have also been investigated as adjunctive therapies for depression. The evidence is inconclusive, and further research is needed.

IMPACT OF TREATMENT OF DEPRESSED PARENTS AND THEIR CHILDREN

While the benefits and risks of antidepressants for adult depression have been widely studied, very few investigations have examined the use of antidepressants, interpersonal psychotherapy, or cognitive-behavioral therapy by parents and its role in the prevention of adverse outcomes in their children. The treatment of parents' depression to remission and to prevent relapse reduces or removes exposure to this risk factor for their children. Chapter 7 reviews preventive interventions and programs that investigate the role of treatment of a parent's depression in the prevention of adverse outcomes for children as well as approaches that target intermediate mechanisms (i.e., parenting, social support). In general, successful treatment of a parent's depression has been associated with improvement in children's symptoms of emotional and behavioral problems, academic and global functioning, and parent-children interactions, but it may not be sufficient for improving some other aspects of their cognitive development and functioning (Gunlicks and Weissman, 2008). The systematic review by Gunlicks and Weissman (2008) found no studies of the effects on children of treating depressed fathers.

INTERVENTIONS

Depression is best viewed as a chronic illness, with most patients suffering multiple episodes over the course of a lifetime. Thus, the treatments used acutely to relieve depressive symptoms are best viewed as tools, whereas interventions may be analogous to comprehensive approaches to delivering treatments and preventing relapse. In response, researchers have answered this challenge by applying structured and comprehensive treatment strategies inspired by Wagner's chronic illness model. Most of these interventions are consistent with this model to the extent that they feature (1) frequent, scheduled follow-up, (2) efficient information systems, (3) decision support trees, and (4) emphasis on self-management. By individualizing the management of a patient's depression in this stepped care approach, researchers have been able to demonstrate very positive outcomes, but the preponderance of these studies have been conducted in primary care settings.

As with the previous section on treatments, the body of literature on interventions for parents, specifically, is quite thin. It is also site specific. Thus, we have provided a brief summary of interventions in the general depressed population (which has been studied almost exclusively in primary care) to take a closer look at interventions for parental depression (which have occurred in a variety of clinical and community settings). Within these sites, we have summarized the specific interventions, beginning with monotherapeutic approaches (e.g., emphasizing education, providing telephone support) and progressing to programs that incorporate several of these elements (e.g., collaborative care). These studies are summarized in Table 6-1.

Primary Care Practices

For adults, the medical management of depressive illness has ordinarily fallen under the purview of primary care providers, as over 70 percent of patients receive treatment in this setting (Katon and Schulberg, 1992). Under the influence of managed care, this trend has been further accentuated in the United States, placing greater emphasis on the diagnostic and therapeutic skills of the primary care provider to facilitate recovery from mental illness. A significant body of evidence has accumulated in the past decade strongly suggesting that outcomes for depressed patients in this health service model are suboptimal (Kessler et al., 2003).

Inefficiencies with health care delivery for depressed individuals have inspired a wide variety of interventions targeting the primary care setting. They have ranged from didactic educational programs to web-based monitoring and counseling to a complete restructuring of health service delivery, mandating the integration of mental health professionals—that is, collaborative care. Health policy experts and researchers have come to a general consensus that collaborative care models are the most efficacious approach to managing depression, incorporating several specific interventions within respective protocols. The relative merits of these interventions, as well as a review of evidence supporting the collaborative care approach, are found below.

Education

Many efforts have been made to improve the basic understanding of patients and providers toward depression and the effectiveness of treatments. Two pivotal trials strongly suggest that these training programs are effective only in the context of systemic changes to care delivery and follow-up (Lin et al., 2001; Thompson et al., 2000).

In the first study, known as the Hampshire Project, 59 primary care practices in England were randomized to two conditions: enhanced education focused on practice guidelines (in the form of a 4-hour seminar for physicians) and the control group (Lin et al., 1997). At endpoint, there were no apparent improvements in detection (39 percent sensitivity to diagnosing depression in the intervention group versus 36 percent in the control group) or in rates of recovery at 6 weeks or 6 months. In the second study, researchers examined the impact of enhanced education of provider performance in two staff model HMOs. Physicians in the intervention group received a 2-hour training session from psychiatrists (didactic presentations as well as role playing) and then met with them on several other occasions to discuss patient welfare for the first 3 months of the study. One year later, there were no statistically significant differences between groups in regard to detection rates, new prescriptions for antidepressants, or adherence to medication guidelines. This investigation confirmed the results of a previous study by this same research group, which failed to find any persistent benefits to provider training.

Although these studies demonstrate that education alone is not a sufficient and enduring approach to improving outcomes, there is still a widely held belief that education should be an important ingredient in any systematic intervention. Several meta-analyses of collaborative care interventions have been published recently (see collaborative care section below) that have attempted to determine which aspect of this approach was most influential in improving medication adherence or depressive symptoms (Bower et al., 2006; Craven and Bland, 2006; Gilbody et al., 2006). Bower et al. (2006) were unable to show that physician training improved outcomes significantly for either of these outcome measures ($p = 0.194$ and 0.237, respectively). Craven and Bland (2006) did not conduct this type of statistical analysis but did note that the most successful interventions contained an educational component. An interesting body of literature has also emerged that takes the analysis a step further, attempting to identify the most important aspects of efficient patient-provider communication (Nolan and Badger, 2005).

Guideline-Based Treatment

Many of the educational efforts targeting primary care providers have used guideline-based treatments to improve outcomes. Some have analyzed the impact of guidelines specifically as the primary intervention, and results have not been favorable (Linden and Schotte, 2007; Thompson et al., 2000). One investigation compared the impact of guideline-based treatment, enhanced physician communication skills, and the combination of the two; it concluded that both components are required to witness significant change in depressive symptoms (van Os et al., 2005). As the content and recommendations in guidelines may vary widely, Hepner et al. (2007) looked at 20 different indicators found in guidelines and examined their impact on clinical outcomes. Overall, they reported that adherence to treatment guidelines was associated with a significant decrease in depressive

TABLE 6-1 Detailed Summary of the Approaches to Delivering Treatment and Preventing Relapse in Adults and Parents with Depression

Primary Intervention	Citation	Populations and Demographics Studied	Settings
Education (of health professional)	Bower et al. (2006) Lin et al. (1997) Thompson et al. (2000) Rost, Smith, and Dickinson (2004)	Adults with major depression and depressive symptoms Mothers with depression	Primary care
Education (of the patient)	Christensen, Griffiths, and Jorm (2004) Craven and Bland (2006) Hayes and Muller (2004) Jorm et al. (2003) Lumley et al. (2006) Tam et al., (2003)	Adults with depression and depressive symptoms Mothers with depression	Pregnancy/ postpartum Primary care Community Web-based
Guideline-Based Treatment	Flynn et al. (2006) Hepner et al. (2007) Linden and Schotte (2007) Miranda et al. (2003, 2006) Revicki et al. (2005) Thompson et al. (2000) Trivedi et al. (2004) Van Os et al. (2005)	Adults Adults with ICD-9 clinical depression Mothers (some minority and low-income) Adults with major depressive disorder (some with alcohol or drug problems)	Community Mental health Primary care Pregnancy/ postpartum
Self-Help (written and computer-assisted)	Clarke et al. (2002) Gellatly et al. (2007) Wright et al. (2005)	Adults (some at risk for and some with clinical depression)	Primary care Mental health Web-based

Outcomes/Follow-up	Research Method
No significant improvements in depression detection or treatment outcomes in adults, except in one study in adults beginning new treatment As a component of collaborative care, the physician training component was not most influential in improving depressive symptoms and medication adherence in adults	Randomized experimental
No difference in depressive outcomes in adults and mothers Enhanced patient education along with provider education in addition to usual care in existing community and primary care services did not significantly improve identification of depression in women postpartum As a component of collaborative care, most successful interventions contained an enhanced patient education component Useful in changing attitudes about treatment Literacy website effective in reducing symptoms of depression in adults	Randomized experimental
Greater clinician adherence of guidelines is associated with significant decrease in depressive symptoms Combined with enhanced communication skills found significant improvements in depressive symptoms In pregnancy/postpartum settings, screening combined with clinician notification and follow-up showed only modest short-term impact on depressive symptoms in mothers In community settings, guideline-based care with case management and referral was more effective in reducing depressive symptoms at 6 months and 1 year than those only referred to community care among minority and low-income mothers In mental health setting, combined with clinical support and patient and family education, algorithm-based approach significantly reduced depressive symptoms and overall mental functioning at 1 year	Observational Randomized experimental
Cognitive-based therapy reduced depressive symptoms for adults with major depressive disorder in mental health specialty settings and at 6 month follow-up, reduced therapist time Meta-analysis revealed reduction of depressive symptoms were associated with self-help models that recruit participants from nonclinical settings, included participants who had an existing mood disorder (not prevention), featured some sort of expert guidance, and used CBT principles with adults In addition to usual care, Internet-based self-help program was effective in reducing depressive symptoms in adults only with follow-up reminders	Randomized experimental

continued

TABLE 6-1 Continued

Primary Intervention	Citation	Populations and Demographics Studied	Settings
Telecare	Bullock et al. (1995) Dennis and Kingston (2008) Hunkeler et al. (2000) Wang et al. (2007)	Adults with depression Antenatal women Postpartum women	Primary care Workplace Pregnancy/ postpartum
Collaborative Care	Bower et al. (2006) Craven and Bland (2006) Dietrich et al. (2004b) Gilbody et al. (2006) Rojas et al. (2007) Wang et al. (2007)	Adults with depression	Primary care Pregnancy/ postpartum Workplace
Problem Solving	Dowrick et al. (2000)	Adults with depression	Community (home)
Group Psychoeducation	Brown et al. (2004) Christensen, Griffiths, and Jorm (2004) Dowrick et al. (2000) Rojas et al. (2007) Spek et al. (2007)	Adults with depression Mothers with postpartum depression (low-income)	Community sites Pregnancy/ postpartum Web-based
Home Visitation	Ammerman et al. (2005) Barnet et al. (2007) Lagerberg (2000) Navaie-Waliser et al. (2000)	Mothers with postpartum depression (some defined as at higher risk, first time mothers) Pregnant adolescents	Home
Culturally Enhanced	Grote et al. (2009)	Low-income pregnant/ postpartum women	Pregnancy/ postpartum

NOTES: The committee did not seek to systematically identify every study on the evaluation of delivery interventions for treating depression in adults (and parents); instead, whenever possible, the committee drew on existing meta-analyses and systematic reviews and lim-

Outcomes/Follow-up	Research Method
Compared with usual pharmacotherapy care, telecare in addition to usual care significantly improved depressive symptoms at 6 weeks and 6 months for adults in primary care and at 4–8 weeks for mothers considered at high risk for postpartum depression Telephone outreach and care management significantly improved self-reported depressive symptoms and some indicators of work performance in adults Telephone support for women throughout pregnancy was associated with lower depressed mood, stress, and anxiety scores compared with controls	Randomized experimental
Compared with usual care, multidisciplinary models of care significantly improved depressive symptoms in adults Increased antidepressant use and adherence in adults Use of mental health specialists as care managers is associated with improved depressive symptoms in adults Structured follow-up improves depressive symptoms in adults Care management and referral using telephone outreach significantly improved self-reported depressive symptoms and some indicators of work performance in adults	Randomized experimental
Compared with usual care, delivering problem-solving techniques at home significantly improved depressive symptoms at 6 months	Randomized experimental
Compared with usual care, group psychoeducation significantly decreased depressive episodes and symptoms at 3 and 6 months (not at 1 year) for adults Interventions that included psychoeducational groups, treatment adherence support, and pharmacotherapy if needed significantly lowered depressive scores at 3 months (not at 6 months) for low-income mothers postpartum Web-based psychoeducational and CBT with therapist support significantly reduced symptoms of depression in adults	Randomized experimental
Compared with controls, treatment through a support and counseling program or CBT improved postpartum depression symptoms at 1 year after treatment but not for pregnant adolescents	Randomized experimental
Culturally enhanced psychotherapy reduced depression diagnosis and symptoms	Randomized experimental

ited its review to interventions that have been evaluated in at least one randomized trial. CBT = cognitive-behavioral therapy; ICD-9 = International Classification of Diseases, ninth revision.

symptoms. They also reported that adherence to guideline treatment was fairly high for certain factors—such as patient education, disease detection, and acute care treatment—but low for many others—such as inquiry into suicide assessment, alcohol abuse, previous history of depression, as well as subsequent medication adjustment. In summary, guidelines for the management of depressed patients in primary care may be very influential in facilitating recovery. Adherence to accepted guidelines should be widely encouraged. The ultimate impact of guideline-based treatment cannot be observed, however, unless this approach is embedded in protocols featuring multiple interventions, as guideline adherence alone has not been demonstrated to improve depression outcomes.

Self-Help

As many clients have difficulty accessing the services of therapists or care managers, investigators have begun to look at methods to improve treatment of depressive illness through remote technology or self-guided protocols (e.g., bibliotherapy, computer programs). Theoretically, these approaches may be more cost-effective and promote a broader dissemination of interventions, but clients must also be sufficiently motivated and educated to persist with treatment.

Previous investigations of various self-help models for depression have met with varying degrees of success. A recent meta-analysis was conducted in an attempt to determine which moderators were associated with positive outcomes. The authors found that there were considerable differences in study methodology (i.e., heterogeneity) among the 34 investigations that were identified (Gellatly et al., 2007). The analysis featured 29 interventions with written materials of which 10 were computer-assisted (e.g., web-based). The researchers concluded that the following moderators were associated with superior outcomes: (1) recruitment of participants from nonclinical settings, (2) inclusion of participants who had an existing mood disorder at baseline (as opposed to prevention), and (3) some sort of expert "guidance." CBT principles appeared to be more effective than education alone. No significant associations were demonstrated based on the duration of the intervention, the delivery mode, or the therapists' background.

Telecare

Telecare involves extensive telephone follow-up, often delivered by trained care managers (e.g., nurses or pharmacists) who relay treatment outcomes and recommendations to referring providers. This type of intervention is relatively inexpensive and can be implemented fairly easily. Theoretically, it may be performed by adequately trained paraprofessionals at remote sites (e.g., administrative assistants), rendering the model even more cost-effective. Most of the investigations employing telecare have done so in combination with other systematic improvements, and systematic reviews examining the impact of telecare alone have not been published.

Two investigations emphasized telecare as the primary intervention for depressed patients. In the first study, Hunkeler et al. (2000) demonstrated an improvement in depression scores among primary care patients at an HMO, despite the fact that the model had no significant impact on medication adherence. As a result, the authors theorized that the protocol may have effectively delivered more of a psychosocial intervention. More recently, Wang et al. (2007) examined the impact of telephone outreach and associated care management on clinical parameters and work performance. After 6 and 12 months of treatment, employees demonstrated significantly more clinical improvement, as well as higher job retention and measured work productivity.

The popularity of telecare can be traced to the relative simplicity of this approach, but the inclusion of this component in highly successful models suggests that regularly scheduled telephone follow-up is conducive to therapeutic success. As many experts have emphasized the importance of a therapeutic alliance in optimizing depression outcomes (developed, presumably, through face-to-face contact with case managers), it would appear that telecare would be most effective after a relationship with individual clients has been forged. Given the fact that meta-analyses of collaborative care models have consistently demonstrated superior outcomes with case managers from the mental health sector, it also remains to be seen how effective telecare can be when delivered by paraprofessionals who lack this training.

Mailed Reminders

Insurance companies and health care organizations have relied on mailed reminders as a means for improving medication adherence for many years. This would appear to be an inexpensive approach to improving adherence to depression measures from the Healthcare Effectiveness Data and Information Set, although the lack of individualized follow-up is less than ideal, particularly when one considers that most patients started on antidepressants may eventually require medication adjustment to achieve remission (Trivedi et al., 2006). As with the other interventions discussed, there is little evidence suggesting that this approach alone would suffice in optimizing outcomes. And mailed reminders have generally been just one component of a system-wide intervention. Although the authors are aware of several pilot projects or programs that have emphasized mailed reminders, there are no randomized controlled trials of this intervention for depression in the medical literature.

Collaborative Care

Collaborative care is the most comprehensive of primary care interventions and often incorporates several of the other interventions discussed above. The development of collaborative care models is consistent with the principles laid out by Wagner in his seminal papers on the management of chronic illness, emphasizing close follow-up, efficient information systems, self-management, and decision support (Wagner, Austin, and VonKorff, 1996). For the management of depression in primary care, investigators have applied these concepts, with three essential components noted: a prepared practice (i.e., with providers and support staff suitably trained), care management, and a mental health interface (Oxman et al., 2002; Wells et al., 2000). Although no consensus exists as to what constitutes collaborative care, the most common components include the following:

- Advanced training provided to the primary care provider regarding guideline-based care
- Enhanced patient education
- Skilled medication management and/or brief psychotherapy
- Increased duration and/or number of clinic visits
- Routine surveillance of progress (featuring validated instruments)
- Integration of the mental health specialist into the primary care setting for care management, clinical consultation, or supervision
- Feedback/recommendations provided to the primary care provider by care managers

Collaborative care is probably the most extensively studied of primary care interventions, and a reasonably strong body of evidence to encourage integrated care, at least for depression, have been published. Numerous systematic reviews are currently available in the literature, most recently by Bower et al. (2006), Butler et al. (2008), Craven and Bland (2006), and Gilbody et al. (2006). Results of these reviews are fairly consistent in regard to (1) collaborative care results in superior clinical outcomes (e.g., 0.25 standardized mean difference in outcomes with 95 percent CI = 0.18–0.32 in the Gilbody analysis), (2) collaborative care results in greater antidepressant medication use or adherence, (3) the use of mental health specialists as care managesr/supervisors is associated with better outcomes, and (4) structured follow-up improves outcomes.

Racial and ethnic minority populations appear to utilize the primary care setting more often for mental health interventions. Simultaneously, research indicates that dramatic differences in the utilization of mental health services for minority groups are not due to differences in rates of mental illnesses (Alegría et al., 2007, 2008; Takeuchi et al., 2007). Therefore, employing treatments for depression in primary care settings may be more advantageous for minority populations and a more viable approach to reducing and ultimately eliminating mental health disparities (Chapa, 2009). Exemplar studies in these systematic reviews and others are further detailed in Table 6-2.

The therapeutic modalities employed in the collaborative care studies ordinarily feature pharmacotherapy (either prescribed independently by the provider or based on the recommendations of care managers) or psychotherapy (most often manualized cognitive-behavioral therapy) or both. The informed choice of preferred treatments by participants appears to be a common feature of successful models and has been widely advocated in both adolescents and adults with depression (Asarnow et al., 2005; Rost et al., 2001). As mentioned above, meta-analyses of collaborative care models have demonstrated a positive impact on clinical outcomes and on medication adherence. Interestingly, medication adherence has not always been associated with superior clinical responses in individual studies or quantitative reviews (Bower et al., 2006; Craven and Bland, 2006). Meta-analyses have also examined the influence of counseling or CBT alone on depression outcomes and failed to demonstrate clinical benefit with brief psychotherapy in multicomponent models (Gilbody et al., 2006). Furthermore, attempts to demonstrate an association between the number and duration of psychotherapy sessions with clinical response have met with equivocal results in collaborative care models (Bower et al., 2006).

Although randomized controlled trials of collaborative care interventions have consistently reported positive findings, the cost-effectiveness of these relatively intensive multidisciplinary models is not clear. Most collaborative care studies for depression have been conducted in the primary care settings of academic centers or HMOs, and the generalizability of these results to real-world settings has been questioned (Gilbody, Bower, and Whitty, 2006). From these investigations, collaborative care interventions appear to be most cost-effective for new episodes of depression, severe depression, or high users of health care resources, but the relative cost-effectiveness of systematic interventions for mild to moderate depression or subsyndromal depression have been either inconclusive or not adequately studied.

Critical issues persist in regard to the exportability and sustainability of the various collaborative care models. Consequently, recent efforts have been made to examine the impact of collaborative care on populations rather than individuals, the implication being that most health care systems and settings have limited resources, and financial incentives are not always

TABLE 6-2 Detailed Summary of Exemplar Collaborative Care Studies
Delivering Treatments and Preventing Relapse in Adults with Depression

Study	Setting	Patient Population	Study Design	Study Duration
Asarnow et al. (2005)	Primary care clinics Practices affiliated with 5 different health care organizations (includes managed care, public-sector, and academia) managed care settings	Adolescents between ages 13 and 21 Average age: 17 years 78% female 56% Hispanic	Randomized after screening Intervention (n = 211) Usual care (n = 207)	6 months
Dietrich et al. (2004b)	Primary care practices Practices affiliated with 5 different health care organizations Nonacademic	81% female Average age: 42 years 57% married 34% ethnic minority	Randomized 60 practices Intervention (n = 177) Usual care (n = 146)	6 months
Rojas et al. (2007)	Primary care practices	100% female Average age = 27 years 65% married or cohabitating All treatment-naïve at baseline	Randomized	6 months

Intervention	Outcomes	Comments
Care managers were psychotherapists Subjects and clinicians had treatment choice of medications (QI-meds), psychotherapy (QI-therapy), or both (QI-both) For QI-meds, care managers followed guideline-based algorithms For QI-therapy, care managers provided weekly sessions of manualized CBT (group or individual)	Statistically significant difference of intervention compared to control at 6 months for the following outcomes: • depressive symptoms (CESD = 19.0 vs 21.4; p = 0.02) • quality of life scores (SF-12-MCS = 44.6 versus 42.8; p = 0.03) Nonsignificant improvements seen in greater decrease of suicide attempts among intervention subjects versus controls (14.2% to 6.4% versus 11.6% to 9.5%)	Greater emphasis placed on psychotherapy, particularly in intervention group Unclear as to what interface was between primary care physicians and care managers Degree of improvement consistent with previous studies among adults and elderly conducted by same research group (Partners in Care)
Centrally located care managers contacted subjects after 1 week and monthly thereafter to assess response, promote adherence, and endorse self-help practices Providers were contacted with treatment updates and recommendations Psychiatrists supervised care managers on weekly basis via telephone	Statistically significant difference of intervention compared to control in depressive symptoms, remission rates, and at least one follow-up visit at 3 and 6 months Not significantly different on antidepressant adherence and specialty counseling	Subsequent analysis demonstrated that high fidelity with chronic care model associated with better outcomes (e.g., education of subjects, regular contact with care managers, interface with mental health)
Intervention group received psychoeducation (hour-long session weekly × 8 weeks), adherence monitoring and advice from "nonprofessional" care managers Providers for intervention subjects received training in pharmacotherapy (5 hours) plus weekly supervision by research psychiatrist	Statistically significant difference of intervention compared to control in depressive symptoms (EPDS), social function, and vitality (SF-36) at 3 months Increase in antidepressant adherence	Psychoeducation attendance very low (2.7 visits of 8 possible) Authors attribute failure to sustain response due to decrease medication adherence over time (68% relapse rate if medication discontinued during first 3 months versus 26% relapse if medication continued)

continued

TABLE 6-2 Continued

Study	Setting	Patient Population	Study Design	Study Duration
Rost et al. (2001)	Primary care practices Recruited from practice networks Nonacademic Practices not permitted to have mental health specialist on site	84% female Average age: 43 years 47% married 83% had health insurance 16% minority	12 clinics randomized Intervention (n = 221) Usual care (n = 240)	24 months
Miranda et al. (2003)	Women screened at food subsidy programs and family planning clinics Nonacademic	100% female Average age: 29 years 46% married or living with partner "Vast majority" living with children (average = 2.3)	Randomized Medications (n = 88) Psychotherapy (n = 90) Usual care (referral to community mental health services (n = 89)	6 months (subsequent 12-month follow-up)

Intervention	Outcomes	Comments
Two physicians and one nurse at each intervention site received training consistent with AHCPR treatment guidelines Subjects encouraged by clinicians to seek their treatment of choice Nurses called subjects weekly × first 5–8 weeks, assessing symptoms and promoting medication adherence If suboptimal response, subjects encouraged by nurse to contact provider Otherwise, providers contacted subjects on monthly basis to adjust treatment	Statistically significant difference of intervention compared to control in the following: • antidepressant adherence • percentage receiving specialty counseling • remission rates at 24 months (74% versus 41%) • physical functioning (61 points versus 44 points on SF-36)	Effects most pronounced in subjects willing to accept pharmacotherapy or if newly diagnosed episode Intervention also noted to improve physical functioning (61 points versus 44 points), and 35% of improvement over baseline attributable to intervention
Subjects assigned to medication were treated by nurse practitioners supervised by a psychiatrist They received an empiric paroxetine trial and were switched to bupropion if unsuccessful Psychotherapy group received 8 weekly sessions of manualized CBT (group or individual) delivered by psychotherapist supervised by clinical psychologist	Statistically significant difference of intervention compared to control in depressive symptoms (HRSD), social functioning, and instrumental role (medication therapy only) all at 6 months	Subjects randomized to psychotherapy much less likely to complete protocol in spite of extensive outreach (e.g., childcare, transportation)

continued

TABLE 6-2 Continued

Study	Setting	Patient Population	Study Design	Study Duration
Wang et al. (2007)	Employees identified through health screening and referred to behavioral health management company Employees from 16 large companies	74% female Average age: 42 years 41% college educated	Eligible subjects had to have at least moderate depression (QIDS-SR > 7) Randomized Intervention (n = 304) Usual care (n = 300)	12 months
Wells et al. (2000)	Primary care, managed care settings Nonacademic	71% female Average age = 44 years 55% married 57% White 30% Hispanic	Group level randomized of 30 clinics Randomized 14 to intervention (n = 913) 16 to usual care (n = 44)	12 months

NOTES: AHCPR = Agency for Health Care Policy and Research; CBT = cognitive behavioral therapy; CESD = Center for Epidemiologic Studies Depression Scale; EPDS = Edinburg Postnatal Scale; HRSD = Hamilton Rating Scale for Depression; QI = quality improvement; QIDS-SR = Quick Inventory of Depressive Symptomatology-Self-report; SF-12-MCS = Short-Form Survey-12-Mental Component Score; SF-36 = Short-Form Survey-36.

Intervention	Outcomes	Comments
Intervention group received in-person treatment via care manager referral (psychotherapy or pharmacotherapy) or manualized CBT over phone If suboptimal response after 2 months, weekly CBT program × 8 weeks All received self-help manuals Care managers assessed response and adherence, and delivered treatment recommendations to provider	Statistically significant difference of intervention compared to control in depressive symptoms (QIDS-SR) at 12 months; remission rates at 6 and 12 months; work productivity and job retention at 6 and 12 months	Very modest clinical improvements Intervention patients 70% more likely to receive mental health specialty care (OR = 1.6; CI = 1.1–2.3). Authors also reported decrease in presenteeism and stated that cost savings were much greater than investment in outreach and care management
Patients and providers had choice of either medications (QI-meds) or psychotherapy (QI-therapy) For QI-meds, subjects contacted by nurses monthly to assess clinical outcomes and promote adherence Subjects had access to usual care counseling but not to study CBT For QI-therapy, psychotherapists provided 12–16 sessions of manualized CBT (group or individual)	Statistically significant difference of intervention compared to control at 6 months and 12 months for the following: • depressive symptoms (CESD), • antidepressant adherence • use of specialty counseling Also, job retention rates higher in intervention than control after 12 months	Rates of subjects receiving appropriate care higher in QI-med group than QI-therapy (14% higher than control versus 8% higher than control) QI-therapy group less likely to be diagnosed as depressed upon follow-up (vs. QI-med; p = 0.05) Benefits of intervention not sustained after conclusion of study Relative cost-effectiveness of intervention unknown

aligned in a manner consistent with HMO practices (Katon and Seelig, 2008). As with earlier collaborative care models, the population-based interventions are multidisciplinary and multimodal, but the emphasis is on more of a stepped approach (i.e., intensity of treatment based on the severity and complexity of the depressive illness). These models emphasize flexibility and sustainability, as care managers and behavioral health specialists are often centrally located away from the primary care setting.

For example, Dietrich and colleagues designed an intervention whereby care managers contacted patients over the phone, monitoring their progress on a monthly basis and relaying their outcomes and treatment recommendations to primary care providers (Dietrich et al., 2004b). Psychiatrists supervised these care managers and were available for consultation with the primary care provider as well. Clearly, the emphasis in this intervention was on creating a practical and exportable model, but, given issues surrounding the reimbursement of mental health specialists, the relative cost-effectiveness of this approach can vary with the treatment setting (Dietrich et al., 2004a).

Wang et al. conducted a collaborative care study of depression from a slightly different perspective, analyzing the impact of successful treatment on productivity (as well as clinical outcomes) (Wang et al., 2007). Depressed employees were identified through a behavioral health management company, which used care managers to discuss treatment options. Care managers authorized psychotherapy referrals or pharmacological management services or both for participants willing to pursue in-person treatment. Others received manualized CBT over the telephone from the care managers, and all employees were encouraged to incorporate self-help practices to promote recovery. Those given the intervention had significantly different (lower) depressive scores and significantly higher job retention and more hours worked. While benefits of this trial may not be generalizable to unemployed or marginally employed individuals, it is certainly applicable to many real-world settings in which employers experience much of the economic impact of decreased productivity among depressed employees.

Pregnancy and Postpartum Settings

Fewer data are available on interventions targeting depression during and after pregnancy. Although collaborative care for depression has been extensively studied in the primary care setting, there are few data examining the effectiveness of large-scale, systems-based approaches to antepartum or postpartum depression care (Gjerdingen, Katon, and Rich, 2008). The majority of depression cases during and after pregnancy are not recognized, and even more are not treated or are inadequately treated (Evins, Theofrastous, and Galvin, 2000; Georgiopoulos et al., 2001).

The vast majority of studies on the treatment of antepartum and postpartum depression investigate single-treatment modalities rather than multicomponent interventions or systems-based approaches. Strategies to improve antepartum and postpartum depression care range from screening and education to support. Few studies have rigorously evaluated these strategies. There have been a few multidisciplinary interventions, and a number of promising interventions to treat maternal depression in the setting of antepartum and postpartum care are now under evaluation. The merits and limitations of each of these strategies are described below.

Patient Education

As in the primary care setting, evidence for the use of education to prevent or treat perinatal depression suggests that education is effective only in the context of multicomponent care. A few studies have evaluated interventions aimed at educating pregnant or postpartum mothers about postpartum depression. Hayes and Muller (2004) conducted a randomized controlled trial to evaluate an education intervention to reduce antenatal depression. They distributed an educational package and assessed women once antenatally (at 12–28 weeks) and twice postnatally (at 8–12 and 16–24 weeks). They found that the women in both the study and the control groups were more depressed antenatally than postnatally. There was no difference detected when comparing the intervention group with the control group. Another randomized controlled trial of educational counseling on the management of women who suffered suboptimal outcomes in pregnancy found that educational counseling, given on top of routine clinical care, did not impart any additional beneficial effects on the women's psychological well-being or quality of life (Tam et al., 2003). Although nonrandomized studies that utilize community health worker models, such as Promotoras de Salud, appear to be highly effective educational models for minority, monolingual or non-English proficient, and rural populations (Getrich, 2007; Ro, Treadwell, and Northridge, 2003).

Guideline-Based Treatment

Guidelines of the American College of Obstetricians and Gynecologists for perinatal depression address the safety of pharmacological agents during pregnancy and the postpartum period (American College of Obstetricians and Gynecologists, 2007). They recommend multidisciplinary care and individualization of a patient's treatment. Few, if any, studies have investigated whether guideline-based care improves outcomes in the perinatal setting. One study investigated the impact of prenatal depression screening and obstetrical clinician notification procedures with depression treatment (Flynn et al., 2006). The researchers found that depression screening combined with systematic clinician follow-up showed a modest short-term impact on depression treatment rates for perinatal depression, but it did not affect depression treatment rates postpartum. The majority of women with major depression were not engaged in treatment throughout the follow-up period despite the interventions.

Telephone Support

Telecare as the primary intervention for perinatal depression has not been investigated. However, telephone support has been evaluated in a few studies. Bullock et al. (1995) conducted a randomized controlled trial of antenatal women at less than 20 weeks gestation. The women in the intervention group received weekly telephone calls throughout their pregnancy. Women were interviewed initially and at 34 weeks gestation. The intervention group at 34 weeks had lower depressed mood, lower stress scores, and lower trait anxiety compared with the control group.

A recent systematic review found only one study aimed at investigating the effect of telephone peer support on postpartum depression. It was a small study to evaluate the effect of peer support (mother-to-mother) on depressive symptoms among mothers identified as at high risk for postpartum depression (Dennis and Kingston, 2008). A total of 42 mothers were randomly assigned to either a control group or an experimental group. The experimental group received standard care plus telephone-based peer support, initiated within 48–72 hours of randomization, from a mother who previously experienced postpartum depression and attended a 4-hour training session. Follow-up assessments were conducted at 4 and 8 weeks after randomization. At the 4-week assessment, 41 percent (n = 9) of the mothers in the control group scored higher than 12 on the Edinburgh Postnatal Depression Scale (EPDS), compared with only 10 percent (n = 2) in the experimental group. Similar findings were found at the 8-week assessment. Of the 16 mothers in the experimental group who evaluated the intervention, 87.5 percent were satisfied with their peer-support experience.

Multidisciplinary Models of Care

The American College of Obstetricians and Gynecologists recommends multidisciplinary care for the treatment of antepartum and postpartum depression. Few if any studies have evaluated multidisciplinary care for depression treatment in the obstetrics and gynecology (ob-gyn) setting. A few studies of maternal depression have been instituted in other primary care settings.

In Australia, Lumley et al. (2006) conducted a community-randomized trial to reduce depression and improve women's physical health 6 months after birth. Primary care and community-based strategies embedded in existing services were implemented in a cluster-randomized trial involving 16 rural and metropolitan communities, pair matched, in the state of Victoria. Intervention areas were also provided with a community development officer for 2 years. The intervention strategy was to develop multifaceted educational training programs for general practitioners, including workshops, simulated patients, clinical practice audits, and evidence-based guidelines. Patient education was given in the form of a listing of local services for mothers and babies, two booklets outlining common physical and emotional health issues for mothers, a booklet for fathers, a package of free or discounted service vouchers, and a range of mother-to-mother support strategies. Primary outcomes were obtained by postal questionnaires and intent-to-treat analysis (i.e., based on initial treatment intent, not what was administered) was performed. Women's mental health scores or probable diagnosis for depression were not significantly different in the intervention and the comparison components. They did not investigate the impact of the intervention on child outcomes.

A multicomponent intervention for postpartum depression treatment was evaluated in 230 low-income mothers with major depression attending postnatal clinics in Chile to improve the recognition and treatment of postnatal depression (Rojas et al., 2007). Mothers were randomized to either a multicomponent intervention (n = 114) or usual care (n = 116). The multicomponent intervention included a psychoeducational group, treatment adherence support, and pharmacotherapy if needed. Usual care included all services normally available in the clinics (i.e., therapeutic and psychotherapeutic interventions, medical consultations, and external referral). Using intent-to-treat analysis, the crude mean EPDS score was significantly lower for the multicomponent intervention group than for the usual care group at 3 months (–4.5 on this 10-item scale, 95 percent CI = –6.3 to –2.7, p < 0.0001) and 6 months, although the differences between groups decreased by 6 months. Box 6-1 describes other multicomponent treatment models that are currently being evaluated for treatment of perinatal depression.

As multidisciplinary care and new models of care are evaluated for the treatment of antepartum and postpartum depression, respect for patient preferences should be an integral component of any intervention. Studies have shown that pregnant women have preferences for type of treatment (Sleath et al., 2005). Delivering mental health care treatment in a nonstigmatizing environment, respecting patient choice, and using a multidisciplinary framework for the delivery of depression care are all likely to be essential components for effective depression treatment in the perinatal period.

BOX 6-1
Examples of Existing Multicomponent
Treatment Models in Perinatal Care

A number of other multicomponent interventions and models of care are currently being evaluated for treatment of perinatal depression.

- The UIC Perinatal Mental Health Project is a program at the University of Illinois at Chicago (Miller, 2008). The program includes provider training and consultation, stepped-care models for perinatal clinics, and MotherCare (guided self-care) as part of the perinatal care. The provider training includes basic education, screening assessment, perinatal psychopharmacology, and detection/intervention for mother-infant relationship problems. The program also provides consultation services via a telephone line with experts in postpartum depression. This comprehensive program's preliminary findings are promising, but there are no published data yet (Miller, 2008).
- The Olmstead Medical Center in Minnesota is currently conducting a randomized controlled trial (Yawn, 2008) to test the impact of translation of a universal screening and follow-up program for postpartum depression versus usual care in family physician's offices. The study, which includes 28 family practices in the United States, uses the EPDS for screening and evidence-based tools developed for primary care follow-up of major depression that have been modified for management of postpartum depression (Yawn, 2008).
- Collaborative care in the primary care setting has been extensively studied for the treatment of depression and has consistently been associated with improved outcomes. The collaborative care model has not been studied in the perinatal setting. However, recently Gjerdingen, Katon, and Rich (2008) describe a type of collaborative care model, Stepped Care Treatment of Postpartum Depression, which is being evaluated at seven sites and is sponsored by the National Institute of Mental Health. Mothers from seven family medicine and pediatric clinics are screened for depression during their infants' 0–9 month well-child visits, and depressed women are randomized to usual care or stepped care. Stepped-care patients receive patient education and team-based management, involving a primary care provider, a case manager, and a mental health specialist as needed. Both treatment arms are advised to see their primary care providers for initial depression care (medications and/or psychotherapy).

Specialty Mental Health Settings

Although treatments have been found effective for those in specialty mental health care settings, little has been done to understand the most effective ways to deliver these treatments. Such settings include mental health clinics, psychiatric hospitals, rehabilitation and reintegration, and mental health–related departments in institutions. Recently one study investigated the effectiveness of using cognitive therapy to treat depression in adults in a clinical setting—in this case a community mental health setting (Merrill, Tolbert, and Wade, 2003). Compared with two benchmark randomized controlled trials of cognitive therapy, delivering the cognitive-behavioral therapy in a community mental health setting found similar results in effectively reducing depressive symptoms. Individual characteristics that led to more favorable outcomes included having less severe depression, having more therapy sessions and more years of education, and having an absence of a comorbid personality disorder.

The delivery mechanisms that have been studied to increase the effectiveness of treatment in these settings include an algorithm-based disease management program, computer-assisted therapies, and more accessible settings for follow-on treatment.

One study used an algorithm-based disease management approach, which involves a sequence of treatment steps to increase the likelihood of response or remission of persistently and severely mentally ill patients (i.e., major depressive disorder) in the public mental health system (Trivedi et al., 2004). This type of delivery holds the promise of consistency of treatment and more efficient use of health care resources. Combined with clinical support and a patient and family educational package, the algorithm approach was found to significantly reduce clinician-rated and self-reported symptoms and overall mental functioning at 1 year compared with usual treatment. The participants included a mix of racial and ethnic groups and were mostly women. Of importance to note is that one-third of the participants had a current alcohol or drug problem, and the treatment-as-usual group had a significantly higher percentage receiving financial assistance. The only exclusion criteria were other mental health–related disorders or being hospitalized for detoxification.

Another study used a computer-assisted cognitive therapy approach in delivering treatment of major depressive disorder in a psychiatric center (Wright et al., 2005). This approach could decrease costs and improve access to cognitive therapy for depression. In the computer-assisted therapy, therapist time was reduced after the first visit from 50-minute to 25-minute sessions. Both computer-assisted and standard therapy reduced depression in the medication-free patients and maintained this result in 6-month follow-up evaluations. Exclusion criteria included those with other mental health disorders, including substance abuse and chronic major depression, and those with a history of past treatment using cognitive therapy.

Another small, pilot study looked to provide follow-up psychotherapy of women diagnosed with depression in rural, community, mental health clinics in a supermarket rather than in the clinic (Swartz et al., 2002). This approach, in a novel setting, aimed to reduce barriers and the stigma of receiving treatment for low-income women and mothers. This study found significant improvement on standardized depression and anxiety scores. Although this study was small, it shows that alternative follow-up sessions may hold promise for specific vulnerable populations that have barriers to care.

Community-Based Settings

There is little information available on effective interventions targeting depressed parents in community-based settings as alternatives to traditional primary care settings. However, such interventions hold promise to reach individuals who would not generally seek treatment because of a variety of individual, community, and system barriers. These settings include family planning clinics, child care programs, food subsidy programs, schools, and community centers. The majority of studies found during a literature search on the treatment of depression in alternative community settings target adults rather than multiple generations. Strategies to improve the effectiveness of the treatment of depression in these settings have incorporated additional approaches to usual care (e.g., CBT, pharmacotherapy), including social support, problem solving, and referral. A number of promising interventions to treat depressed parents in alternative community-based settings are just beginning to be evaluated. The merits and limitations of each of these strategies are described below.

Problem Solving

Problem solving has been found to be as effective as pharmacotherapy for major depression in primary care (Mynors-Wallis et al., 1995, 2000). Researchers have investigated the acceptability and effectiveness of problem solving to treat depression in community settings, since it is easily taught to a range of health professionals. Problem solving links depressive symptoms to problems, the problems are clearly defined, and a structured attempt is made to solve the problems. One randomized controlled study in an international multicenter found that using problem-solving techniques delivered at home to treat adults with depression was acceptable and effective in treating depression in comparison to a group that was not given the intervention at 6 month follow-up (Dowrick et al., 2000). Such differences were not seen at 1-year follow-up. Concurrent treatment using antidepressants and diagnosis category (i.e., single episode, recurrent episode) did not affect the results.

Group Psychoeducation

Group psychoeducation emphasizes instruction and promotes relaxation, positive thinking, and general coping and social skills. It has been used in primary care settings and seems effective in preventing depression and improving quality of life. Researchers have investigated the role of adapting cognitive-behavioral techniques to a group educational approach in treating adults with depression in alternative settings. Using community centers or other local places, researchers have found that this approach significantly reduced depressive episodes and increased other social functioning in adults diagnosed with a depressive episode at 6 months follow-up, but not significantly so at 1 year (Brown et al., 2004; Dowrick et al., 2000).

Researchers have also investigated the role of social support and coping skills in the mental health of those taking care of chronically ill family members in community-based family support interventions. Using a variety of approaches, (e.g., linking the parents of children with similar chronic illnesses with family-led educational approaches involving problem solving, communication skills training, and family support) researchers demonstrated improvements in the parent's or caretaker's psychological well-being (i.e., anxiety, depressive symptoms) that were sustained for 6 months after the intervention phase (Ireys et al., 2001; Pickett-Schenk et al., 2006).

Although the evaluation literature is limited, group psychoeducation holds promise in alternative community settings. Researchers note the ease of training diverse health professionals and the limited infrastructural needs in implementing this approach. In addition, psychoeducation in these alternative community settings may reach out to individuals who never sought treatment before. One researcher noted that 40 percent of the experimental group (i.e., those diagnosed with a depressive episode) had never seen a health practitioner for their depression (Brown et al., 2004).

Health Communication

Health communication is one tool for promoting or improving health. It can increase knowledge, influence or reinforce perception, beliefs, and attitudes, and increase demand or support for health services. Combined with other strategies, it can overcome barriers or system issues. However, health communication alone cannot compensate for inadequate health care or access to health care (Loughery et al., 2001). Australian researchers developed an evidence-based consumer guide about effective depression treatment options to change attitudes and take actions to reduce depression in adults. In a randomized controlled study, this evidence-based guide was found to be useful in changing attitudes about treatment, but it did not significantly change depressive symptoms compared with a general informational brochure (Jorm et al., 2003). This study illustrates a promising opportunity to increase the knowledge and attitudes of individuals with depressive symptoms.

Web-Based Interventions

The rapid expansion of the Internet into the homes of a large segment of the population offers new treatment opportunities. Women, minorities, and the elderly are increasingly using the Internet, and its use continues to rise, particularly among ethnic minority individuals. In 2005, the Pew Internet and American Life Project reported that 79 percent of web users reported using the Internet to obtain health information, with 23 percent searching for specific information related to depression, anxiety, and other mental health issues (Fox, 2005). Internet-based interventions are particularly attractive in the setting of depression treatment. The Internet offers anonymity, avoids the stigma of seeing a therapist, offers the maximum flexibility in terms of access to treatment (access in one's home, in the office, in the middle of the night, etc.), allows for monitoring and feedback, and has the potential to provide treatment to patients who do not seek help for depression (Christensen, Griffiths, and Jorm, 2004; Spek et al., 2007).

One treatment, cognitive-behavioral therapy, is a structured treatment approach that has been adapted to a computer format. Previous studies have demonstrated that computerized cognitive-behavioral therapy is effective for the treatment of depression (Kaltenthaler et al., 2002). CBT has also been found to be effective when provided over the Internet (Christensen, Griffiths, and Jorm, 2004; Clarke et al., 2005). Christensen, Griffiths, and Jorm (2004) tested the efficacy of a psychoeducational website offering information about depression and an interactive website offering CBT to reduce symptoms of depression. They recruited by survey 525 community residents with increased depressive symptoms and randomized them into three groups: psychoeducation, CBT, and attention placebo. For the first two intervention groups, lay interviewers contacted participants weekly by phone to direct their use of the websites. Participants were given guides outlining the weekly assignments and details about the websites. The placebo participants were phoned weekly by the interviewers to discuss lifestyle and environmental factors. Both interventions delivered via the Internet were more effective in reducing symptoms of depression than the control intervention. CBT reduced dysfunctional thinking, and the psychoeducation group had an improved understanding of effective evidence-based treatments for depression (Christensen, Griffiths, and Jorm, 2004). There is also evidence that these benefits were sustained at 6 and 12 months (MacKinnon, Griffiths, and Christensen, 2008).

Successful programs that use Internet-based treatment approaches (including CBT) incorporate some telephone or e-mail contact, and adherence to Internet treatment programs is better when an interviewer or counselor provides tracking, contact, or support (Christensen et al., 2006). A meta-analysis on the use of Internet-based CBT for depression and anxiety found that the study with the highest effect size in depression treatment was an Internet-based intervention with therapist support (Spek et al., 2007). It was not the type of problem (anxiety or depression) that explained the effect size but rather whether support was added or not.

Clarke et al. (2002) conducted two randomized trials to test whether an Internet-based cognitive therapy, self-help program was effective in reducing depression. In the first trial, they randomized 299 adults with highly elevated depressive symptoms to either access or no access to the Overcoming Depression on the Internet (ODIN) website. Subjects were free to receive treatment as part of usual care. Participants in the intervention group infrequently used the website, and they found no effect of the Internet program on the reduction of depressive symptoms. In their second trial, they randomized 255 persons to either usual control group without access to the Internet site, ODIN program group with postcard reminders, or ODIN program group with telephone reminders. Intervention participants had a significantly greater reduction in depression compared with the control group. There was no difference in the reduction in depression between the intervention group with telephone reminders and the intervention group with postcard reminders (Clarke et al., 2005).

Studies have shown that online, brief, CBT-based interventions are not as effective as extended CBT (Christensen et al., 2006). Other studies confirm that web-based interventions with support or contact (e.g., minimal therapist contact, e-mail contact, e-mail feedback) are effective for reducing depressive symptoms (Andersson et al., 2005; van Straten, Cuijpers, and Smits, 2008). Interestingly, while the majority of Internet-based programs use CBT or problem-solving strategies, a trial that tested a depression literacy website (offering evidence-based information on depression and its treatment) was also effective in reducing symptoms of depression (Christensen, Griffiths, and Jorm, 2004).

Web-based perinatal and postpartum depression treatment and intervention programs are well suited for the everyday lives of expectant and new mothers. Internet-based programs are accessible to individuals who are less inclined to seek psychological services (Bai et al., 2001; Christensen and Griffiths, 2002), such as women suffering from perinatal and postpartum depression. Pregnant women screening positive for depression can be encouraged to seek medical and psychological consultation for this condition so it can be treated prior to delivery, which will have an immediate and long-term desired impact on both the mother and her newborn baby. Thus, health-related websites have the potential of functioning as viable resources to eliminate disparities in service availability or access to care. There are a number of examples of educational or support websites or community programs that have not been evaluated but may be helpful to parents and families experiencing depression. A few examples of such programs are Postpartum Support International,[2] Postpartum Dads,[3] Bootcamp for New Dads,[4] Heartstrings (postpartum depression),[5] Families First,[6] and Postpartum Education for Parents.[7]

Workplace Interventions

Depression significantly impacts an employee's ability to work (Rost, Smith, and Dickinson, 2004). Multiple studies have demonstrated that depression is associated with increased absenteeism and reduced productivity during days at work (Rost, Smith, and Dickinson, 2004). Depression has been found to be the most common "severe"[8] mental health diagnosis encountered in employee assistance programs (Conti and Burton, 1994) and is one of the most costly of all health problems for employers (Stewart et al., 2003). Stewart et al. (2003) estimated the impact of depression on labor costs (work absence and reduced performance while at work) in the U.S. workforce to be $44 billion per year, not including costs for short-term and long-term disability (Stewart et al., 2003). In their study, workers with depression reported significantly more total health-related lost productive time than those without depression (mean, 5.6 hours per week versus an expected 1.5 hour per week), and 81 percent of the lost productive time costs were explained by reduced performance while at work.

Given the large economic burden of depressive illness, it is important to evaluate the impact of depression treatment programs on work outcomes. Studies in the primary care setting have evaluated the impact of enhanced depression treatment programs on work outcomes. Rost, Smith, and Dickinson (2004) randomized 12 primary care practices to enhanced or usual care. Enhanced care clinicians and care managers received brief training on high-quality depression care (i.e., guideline-based pharmacotherapy or psychotherapy during the acute phase of treatment) for depressed pa-

---

[2] See http://postpartum.net/.

[3] See http://postpartumdads.wordpress.com/.

[4] See http://www.bootcampfornewdads.org/.

[5] See http://postpartum.net/resources/women-mothers/heartstrings/.

[6] See http://www.familiesfirstri.org/index.html.

[7] See http://www.sbpep.org/.

[8] Axis I Level: According to the definitions and criteria of the *International Statistical Classification of Diseases and Related Health Problems*, 10th revision, and the *Diagnostic and Statistical Manual of Mental Disorders*, 4th edition.

tients during treatment. Care managers followed patients and encouraged treatment adherence. Employed patients in the enhanced care condition reported 6.1 percent greater productivity and 22.8 percent less absenteeism over 2 years.

Despite the large cost to employers, studies evaluating employer-based programs for screening, outreach, and disease management efforts are scarce (Stewart et al., 2003). A recent study evaluated the impact of an employer-based depression care management system (Wang et al., 2007). A randomized controlled trial of 604 employees with depression covered by a behavioral health plan tested whether telephone screening, outreach, and care management for depressed workers had any impact on clinical outcomes and work productivity (Wang et al., 2007). The program encouraged workers to enter outpatient treatment psychotherapy and/or use antidepressant medications, monitored treatment quality continuity, and attempted to improve treatment by giving recommendations to providers. The outcomes of interest were depression severity and work performance at 6 and 12 months. The intervention group had significantly lower Quick Inventory of Depressive scores (RR of recovery = 1.4, 95 percent CI = 1.1–2.0, p = 0.009) and significantly higher job retention (RR = 1.7, 95 percent CI = 1.1–3.3, p = 0.02).

Workplace initiatives to screen and treat depression are increasing, although evaluations of these programs have not been published. For example, the MidAmerica Coalition on Health Care collaborated with the city of Kansas City, Missouri, and 15 large area employers to develop the Community Initiative on Depression (CID) in 2000 (Mid-America Coalition on Health Care, 2009). The project was designed to reduce community and workplace depression by raising awareness, reducing stigma, and improving depression care quality for depressed employees and their dependents. It is a multiphase project with a projected timeline of 3 to 5 years. Phase I included a multilevel needs assessment among employees and employers regarding knowledge, attitudes, health care use, and the costs of depression and depression care among 13 of the 15 CID-partnered work sites. It also included extensive educational programs for employers, employees, providers, and health plans. These educational efforts were continued in Phase II, along with a series of work site and clinical research projects, including a study of employer benefit design practices, and a health plan–medical office manager collaboration to reduce outpatient coding barriers for depression care. Phase III will include a community public relations campaign to increase depression awareness and reduce stigma, a postintervention reassessment of depression help-seeking behavior among employees, and depression care quality profiling of onsite occupational health care providers.

Given the enormous costs of depression in the workplace, investment in enhanced depression care is essential. Enhanced depression care improves absenteeism and productivity among employees. Accumulating evidence suggests that improvements in depression management in employed work-forces offset the costs of such programs. Wang et al. (2006) estimated the costs and benefits of enhanced depression care for workers from the societal and employer-purchaser perspectives in a recent study. They found that screening and depression care management for workers result in an incremental cost-effectiveness ratio of $19,976 per quality-adjusted life year relative to usual care, and, from the employer's perspective, enhanced depression care yielded a net cumulative benefit of $2,895 after 5 years.

The case for the cost-effectiveness of enhanced depression care for workers would probably be even stronger if the costs of parental depression on children and families were fully captured in these analyses from the societal perspective. A human capital development and household production economic model of the impact of parental depression on children highlights the costs of depression on parents individually and on their children and families, as well as the longer term economic consequences of parental depression on children. The evidence demonstrates that parental depression is associated with reduced family resources; increased child health risks; negative human capital outcomes in children, such as poorer cognitive and behavioral outcomes (Farahati, Marcotte, and Wilcox-Gök, 2003; Meara and Frank, 2008); poorer academic performance; and poor social outcomes in children such as impairment in marital and work relationships (Weissman et al., 2006). The costs of such negative outcomes are rarely included in cost-effectiveness models evaluating the impact of depression treatment.

Furthermore, the longer-term costs of parental depression are not included in cost-effectiveness models. Exposure to parental depression in childhood leads to increased rates of work difficulty, health problems, and health service use. Additional studies have linked negative school and social outcomes with negative outcomes in adulthood, such as reduced levels of employment, greater contact with the justice system, and increased use of public services (Fronstin, 2005; Haveman and Wolfe, 1995; Trostel, Walker, and Woolley, 2002). The economic costs of parental depression on parents, children, families, and society are enormous, and the case for cost-effectiveness of depression treatment may be much stronger when cost models include a comprehensive assessment of the costs of depression on parents, children, and families.

Home Visitation

A wide range of exclusively home visiting programs and programs that included home visiting among their interventions have been fielded, although only a few were rigorously evaluated. The number of home visiting–based programs in the United States has been estimated in the thousands (Gomby, Culross, and Behrman, 1999). The Parents as Teachers model has over 3,000 sites alone. At any given time, an estimated half-million families are receiving some form of home visitation services, ranging from a single postpartum "welcome home" visit by a public health nurse to multiyear intensive services (Gomby, Culross, and Behrman, 1999). Initially formulated to prevent child maltreatment, home visiting programs also seek to promote optimal child development and improve maternal well-being. Home visits can begin prenatally and may continue until the child is 2 to 5 years of age, depending on the model. Programs typically target parenting skills, the mother-child relationship, home safety, maternal health and educational/occupational attainment, and infant health, especially immunization and nutrition.

Many of the correlates and predictors of maternal depression, such as low self-esteem, stress related to child care, low social support, and poor marital relationships (Goodman and Gotlib, 1999), are at least partly addressed by the major home visiting models, such as the Nurse-Family Partnership and Healthy Families America. Observational studies suggest that, for some mothers, participation in a home visitation program reduces scores on standard depression measures, but they may not be clinically significant. A review of a diverse set of European home visitation programs for new mothers identified the reduction of maternal depression as the most robust outcome common for many of them (Lagerberg, 2000). Investigating the impact of a paraprofessional home visitation model on maternal depression, Navaie-Waliser et al. (2000) found that, after 1 year, home-visited mothers reported a decrease in depression compared with a demographically similar control group. A community-based, paraprofessional home visitation program did not, however, have any effect relative to a matched comparison group on CESD scores for pregnant adolescents (Barnet et al., 2007). Over 30 percent of both the intervention and control groups scored 22 or higher on the CESD. The Ammerman et al. (2009) study of over 800 mothers found only a minimal average decrease of about two points (12.29 ± 8.9 to 10.12 ± 8.9, statistically significantly different [p < .001], but not clinically significant) on the Beck Depression Inventory (BDI-II) over a 9-month period for the sample as a whole. The evaluation of Healthy Families Massachusetts (Jacobs et al., 2005) concluded that approximately half of the mothers scoring in the depressed range were chronically depressed. In the aggregate, the extant data suggest that home visiting alone has a relatively minimal, nonclinical impact on maternal depressive symptoms.

Home visitation programs potentially provide an important context in which to identify and intervene in parental depression and associated parenting difficulties. The high rate of depressed mothers encountered by home visitation programs, together with the negative impacts that maternal depression has on the effectiveness of home visitation, has led to a number of home visitation–based interventions. These can be categorized into three basic strategies: (1) screening by the home visitor with referral to community mental health services (discussed in Chapter 5); (2) mental health consultation provided to home visitors, who in turn are expected to deliver an intervention to depressed mothers; and (3) in-home treatment provided by mental health specialists in addition to the standard home visitation services. Examples of strategies 2 and 3 are described below.

No randomized clinical trial outcomes have yet been published for any of these strategies. Thus, at this time, these strategies should be regarded as promising but unproven. However, studies are under way to investigate the effectiveness of the latter two strategies, which embed depression treatment services in home visiting programs instead of depending on referrals to the community for treatment. This approach is warranted on the basis of several studies that indicate that home visitors as a group are not good at connecting families with community-based services for depression, domestic violence, or substance abuse (Hebbeler and Gerlach-Downie, 2002; Tandon et al., 2005). These integrated treatment models, however, face the daunting task not only of providing effective depression treatments but also of addressing the often considerable psychiatric and social comorbidity found in the families served by home visitation programs.

Mental Health Consultants to Home Visitors

Boris et al. (2006) provided a qualitative description of the incorporation of mental health consultants into nurse home visitation teams in Louisiana. The mental health consultants first received 4 months of training in infant mental health and then provided consultation and support to the home visiting nurses. They conducted ongoing case conferences with the nursing team and provided additional one-on-one consultation for nurses with difficult cases. Telephone consultations proved to be the most effective. Initially some of the nurses expressed concern or skepticism about the role of the mental health consultant, and it took approximately a year for them to be integrated into the team. Some nurses reported feeling overwhelmed by the recommendations of the mental health consultant in addition to fulfilling their own duties. The mental health consultants, who were primarily experienced with adults, reported feeling like novices with some of the infant mental health issues. Boris et al. (2006) concluded that adding a mental health consultant to a team of nurse home visitors is complex but offers promise in reaching a large number of families with mental health needs.

Depression Treatment Delivered in Home Visitation

Efforts have been made to adapt cognitive-behavioral therapy, a well-established office-based treatment for depression, for delivery in the context of a home visitation program. Ammerman et al. (2005) conducted an open trial of in-home cognitive-behavioral therapy with 26 first-time mothers in a home visitation program. Subjects scored 20 or higher on the screening BDI-II and were diagnosed with major depression on the Primary Care Evaluation of Mental Disorders (PRIME-MD), a semistructured diagnostic interview designed for clinical settings using DSM-IV criteria for common mental disorders. A total of 24 mothers received the full course of 15 in-home CBT sessions, and 2 received partial treatments of 11 and 8 sessions, respectively. An intent-to-treat analysis found that 84 percent of the mothers had either fully (69 percent) or partially (15 percent) remitted major depressive disorder on the PRIME-MD. There was a significant reduction (p < 0.001) in BDI-II scores from a pretreatment mean of 30.4 ($\pm$ 8.2) to a posttreatment mean of 13.7 ($\pm$ 9.4). Maternal function as measured by the Brief Patient Health Questionnaire was significantly improved, as was self-reported maternal parenting satisfaction as measured by the Maternal Attitudes Questionnaire. In-home CBT is currently undergoing a randomized clinical trial funded by the National Institute of Mental Health.

Substance Use Disorder Treatment Setting

Evidence has repeatedly supported the link between substance use disorders (SUDs) and depression and the finding that the combination of these disorders can negatively impact the course of each illness, its treatment, and long-term outcomes (Dodge, Sindelar, and Sinha, 2005; Quello, Brady, and Sonne, 2005). Adequate treatment for depression reduces substance use disorders, and treatment of substance use disorders has been found to reduce depression (Davis et al., 2008). Among individuals seeking treatment for illicit substance use disorders, 30.5 percent met criteria for at least one major depressive episode in their lifetime (Rounsaville et al., 1991) and 60 percent had a comorbid mood disorder (Grant et al., 2004). Among alcohol treatment seekers, 40 percent had a co-occurring mood disorder (Grant et al., 2004). One of the most serious consequences of the combination of a substance use disorder and depression was found in a study showing that among patients with major depressive disorder, those with a substance use disorder were at greatest risk for suicide (Young et al., 1994), and over 66 percent of those who committed suicide had a substance use disorder (Rounsaville et al., 1991).

The diagnosis of a mood disorder in the presence of an active SUD is challenging owing to the fact that recent cessation of drug use can produce depressive mood states. The presence of a mood disorder may be mistakenly concluded if the patient is evaluated under the influence of or during active withdrawal from certain substances (Quello, Brady, and Sonne, 2005). For example, a patient under the influence of alcohol can manifest symptoms of mania or hypomania. In contrast, symptoms of alcohol (and/or cocaine) withdrawal may appear as dysphoria and depression (DSM-IV). While screening for depression typically occurs at SUD treatment intake, assessment and diagnosis are most accurately determined after withdrawal is complete and abstinence has been achieved (Brown and Schuckit, 1988). However, it is recognized that the severity of depressive symptoms must be carefully assessed, and immediate treatment may be required for severe depression and in order to initiate treatment (Quello, Brady, and Sonne, 2005).

Behavioral Treatments

Recent efforts to treat depression and substance use disorders have focused on integrated treatments (Brown et al., 1997; Weiss et al., 2000). As described above, CBT is among the most powerful behavioral treatments for depression and also has proven efficacy for substance use disorders. A manual for CBT with substance use disorders is available from the National Institute on Drug Abuse (Carroll, 1998). Only one study has compared CBT for depression with a relaxation training control, i.e., condition plus treatment as usual for alcohol in patients who are currently alcohol dependent and with elevated depressive symptoms (BDI score > 9). CBT participants showed, on average, significant improvements in depressive symptoms relative to participants in the control condition. The average effect size was 0.85. CBT participants showed, on average, more abstinence and reduced drinking at 3- and 6-month follow-up. Changes in depressive symptoms were reported to mediate the number of drinks ingested daily (Brown et al., 1997).

More recently, a comparison of LETS Act!, a manual-based intervention modification of the Behavioral Activation Treatment for Depression for the SUD inpatient population, was compared with a control group of usual treatment. The results showed that, on average, LETS Act! participants had greater reductions in depressive symptoms compared with the usual treatment group. This potentially promising treatment is unique in that it provides initial data in the development of a specialized depression-centered treatment for SUD patients with depressive symptoms (Daughters et al., 2008).

Box 6-2 describes other integrated treatment models of care that have been used in substance abuse disorder settings. Both of these models were sites for the Substance Abuse and Mental Health Services Administration's Women, Co-Occurring Disorders Study. Results from this study provided

---

BOX 6-2
Example Treatment Models in Substance
Abuse Disorder Settings

Specific to parenting women and families, two integrated models of care are promising programs with strong clinical services and initial evidence to support their use.

- The **Boston Consortium of Services for Families in Recovery Model**, under the Boston Public Health Commission, has an active collaborative system of services for women with SUDs as well as mental health and trauma issues (Amaro et al., 2005). The system includes not only outpatient treatment but also residential treatment programs that serve women and their children, focusing on culturally specific approaches to provide trauma-informed substance abuse treatment, parenting training, case management, and coordination of mental health services through partner providers.
- **PROTOYPES:** The Centers for Innovation in Health, Mental Health, and Social Services is a nonprofit corporation in California that provides substance abuse and mental health treatment through a variety of programs, as well as additional services, such as housing and domestic violence programs (Brown et al., 2004). The PROTOTYPES Women's Center is a residential treatment program for women and their children with a special focus on women with co-occurring disorders, such as mental illness, trauma, and HIV/AIDS. The residential program provides onsite comprehensive services that include substance abuse treatment, mental health services for women and their children, medical care, educational programs and vocational training, case management, parenting training, and programs for children, including child care and Head Start.

Both of these programs participated in the Co-Occurring Disorders and Violence study funded by the Substance Abuse and Mental Health Services Administration. This quasi-experimental treatment outcome study showed that, on average, compared with usual care, more integrated treatment for substance use disorders, mental health, and interpersonal trauma was associated with modest yet greater improvements in women's interpersonal violence and mental health symptoms when examined at 12 months (Morrissey et al., 2005). These programs have also shown that treatment retention is greater for the integrated model of care compared with treatment as usual (Amaro et al., 2007a).

---

evidence that integrated treatment for mental illness, trauma, and addiction produced better outcomes than did standard substance abuse treatment. Together these findings show that integrated treatment produced better outcomes with respect to drug use and mental health symptoms—including depression—and trauma symptoms (Amaro et al., 2007b; Morrissey et al., 2005); treatment retention (Amaro et al., 2007a) and HIV risk behaviors (Amaro et al., 2007c).

Medications

Compared with behavioral treatments, a somewhat larger body of work exists that examines medications to treat depression in SUD patients, including a meta-analysis (Nunes and Levin, 2004) and a recent review (Tiet and Mausbach, 2007). Nunes and Levin (2004) identified 14 studies from 300 studies examining the issue of treating depression with medication in SUD patients. Tricyclic antidepressants and selective serotonin reuptake inhibitors (SSRIs) were the most common agents examined. Of the 14 studies, 57 percent (n = 8) reported a modest effect of medications to treat depression in this population. The pooled effect size from the random-effects model was 0.38 (95 percent CI = 0.18–0.58). The results appeared to be more robust in alcohol-dependent patients than drug-dependent patients. It should be noted that the heterogeneity of effects on the measure of depression (HRSD) was significant (p < 0.02) and related to the placebo response.

Overall, the results suggested that when medication effectively treats depression, it also appears to help reduce the use of substances (Nunes and Levin, 2004). The SSRIs were concluded to be first-line medications based on their tolerability and low toxicity relative to tricyclic antidepressants. The review concluded that existing treatments for reducing depressive symptoms also work in depressed SUD patients, and efficacious treatments of SUDs also reduce substance use in depressed SUD patients. However, the efficacy of integrated treatments remains uncertain given the limited data in this area and the methodological challenges that limit confidence in strong conclusions from the existing data (Tiet and Mausbach, 2007). Knowledge is clearly lacking in the interaction that depression medications and substance use may have on patients. While recent research is focused on developing and examining behavioral and pharmacotherapies in depressed SUD patients, to the best of our knowledge no studies have examined these interventions specifically in parents with depression and SUDs or examined the parenting outcomes that these treatments may help improve. Furthermore, while effective treatments exist for depressed patients with SUD comorbidities, the current systems of SUD treatment and mental health treatment often operate in parallel rather than in integration, making optimal care a continuing challenge (Quello, Brady, and Sonne, 2005).

VULNERABLE POPULATIONS

Low-Income and Minority Mothers

The impact of treatment interventions and, more specifically, collaborative care models on parental depression has not been rigorously studied in vulnerable populations. Previous investigations of collaborative care models in the general depressed population have featured a preponderance of female subjects, most of whom were of childbearing age and many, presumably, were mothers. Few if any of these studies conducted a subgroup analysis of parents or looked explicitly at the impact of interventions on the functioning and well-being of the family unit.

Interest in increasing the engagement and treatment of depression in minority or low-income individuals has led researchers to study effective strategies to deliver treatment to these specific groups (see Ward, 2007). One randomized controlled study compared guideline-based treatments with case management and referral to community care (i.e., education about treatment in the community) in minority and low-income mothers with major depression recruited from public clinics (Special Supplemental Nutrition Program for Women, Infants, and Children, Title X family planning). Overall, this study found that guideline-based treatment with case management was more effective for reducing depressive symptoms at 6 months than was referral to community care (Miranda et al., 2003). Results also suggest that pharmacotherapy interventions may be more effective than psychotherapy. Although those with current substance or alcohol abuse were excluded, more than one-third reported trauma, including rape or child abuse victimization, and half reported domestic violence and posttraumatic stress disorder. Long-term follow-up revealed similar results after 1 year and have similar cost-effectiveness ratios compared with those in advantaged populations (Miranda et al., 2006; Revicki et al., 2005).

Although the research is limited, this study found that evidence-based interventions appear effective for poor and minority women if the treatment scenario was culturally and linguistically appropriate, and if supports to overcome barriers to care (i.e., transportation and child care) were provided. Interventions were appropriately tailored within a cultural context and provided in the patient's preferred language (i.e., providing care in Spanish). Finally, professionals keenly sensitive to low-income and minority populations were employed in this study (Miranda et al., 2003). A small study by Grote et al. (2009) tested whether culturally enhanced brief interpersonal psychotherapy (enhanced IPT-B) was effective in reducing depression among low-income women attending a large, urban ob-gyn clinic. Enhanced IPT-B consisted of an engagement session, eight acute IPT-B sessions before the birth, and maintenance IPT up to 6 months postpartum and was specifically enhanced to make it culturally relevant to low-income and minority women. They conducted a randomized controlled trial with 53 pregnant patients and found significant reductions in depression diagnoses and symptoms and significant improvements in social functioning before childbirth and at 6 months postpartum in the IPT-B participants compared with the enhanced usual care group. This study lends support to the notion that evidence-based therapies for depression can be effective when appropriately tailored for ethnic and disadvantaged populations.

BARRIERS TO TREATMENT

Despite the efficacy of depression treatments, this disorder is undertreated. Adults experiencing major depression are often not inclined to seek treatment for their illness. Barriers for pregnant and postpartum mothers with depression are similar to those in the general population, as described in Chapter 1, but they also include the tendency to normalize depressive symptoms and to dismiss them as self-limiting and the fear of losing one's baby (Dennis and Chung-Lee, 2006). The diagnosis of postpartum depression is also complicated by the overlap of common postpartum symptoms with symptoms of depression (e.g., lack of sleep, change in eating). And, racial, ethnic, and non-English speakers are also less likely to seek or receive quality interventions (see Alegría et al., 2008).

Furthermore, the lack of insurance or underinsurance, in which the benefit package lacks comprehensive insurance, limits the access and use of mental health services for those seeking depression care. Often those with coverage are limited because of high cost-sharing methods (i.e., copayments, premiums) and benefit restrictions (i.e., annual or lifetime limits) (U.S. Surgeon General, 1999). However, recent efforts regarding mental health parity have picked up momentum at the federal level, with cooperation by state agencies. For example, the passage of the Paul Wellstone and Pete Domenici Mental Health Parity and Addiction Equity Act of 2008 (P.L. 110-343) requires employers with 50 or more employees to offer health plans with mental health and substance abuse disorders coverage equal to all other medical and surgical benefits covered by the plan.

Barriers to treatment operate at both institutional level and sociocultural levels. This categorization is not mutually exclusive, however, and there exists substantial mutual influence and interaction between the two realms. At the institutional level, lack of health insurance overall and lack of insurance coverage (and the associated high cost of care) for mental health services, referral system fragmentation, and the limited availability of mental health specialists are the primary factors limiting vulnerable populations' access to depression treatment (Das et al., 2006; Kung, 2004; Lazear et al., 2008; Thompson, Bazile, and Akbar, 2004; Van Voorhees et al., 2007; Wong et al., 2006). When they do receive depression treatment, racial and ethnic minority groups are more likely to seek and receive mental health care from the primary care setting. However, primary care physicians are not typically trained in the intricacies of diagnosing depression or any other mental illnesses, resulting in the underrecognition, diagnosis, and treatment of depression (Van Voorhees et al., 2007). The lack of appropriate language services further limits access and quality treatment to the already limited number of mental health services for those with limited English proficiency (Center for Reducing Health Disparities, 2007; Kung, 2004; Lazear et al., 2008; Scuglik et al., 2007; Wong et al., 2006).

Differential access to insurance and providers does not account for all the disparities in rates of depression treatment, however. A study by Padgett and colleagues found that even in an insured population of federal employees, whites were 1.7 times more likely to visit outpatient mental health providers and make 2.6 more mental health visits per year compared with their African American and Hispanic counterparts (Padgett et al., 1994). Moreover, after accounting for differences at the institutional level, there remain differences in treatment-seeking behaviors between non-Hispanic whites and minority populations. Disparities are likely to be attributable to sociocultural barriers and social determinants of health (World Health Organization, 2008), which operate at the level of both the community and the individual patient.

According to the Surgeon General's assessment, stigma plays a key role in shaping barriers to treatment that operate at the sociocultural level (U.S. Department of Health and Human Services, 2001), which manifest themselves in underutilization of mental health services, particularly among racial and ethnic minorities. Communities have different norms and beliefs surrounding depression, which include differential definitions of the illness and varying views on appropriateness of treatment options (Cooper et al., 2003; Givens et al., 2007; Scuglik et al., 2007; U.S. Department of Health and Human Services, 2001). These beliefs can be associated with stigmatizing attitudes toward and privacy concerns among those manifesting symptoms of or seeking treatment for depression, thus acting as sources of denial in recognizing symptoms and as barriers to seeking and adhering to treatment (Ayalon and Alvidrez, 2007; Das et al., 2006; Grandbois, 2005; Interian et al., 2007; Nadeem et al., 2007; Sanchez and Gaw, 2007; Scuglik et al., 2007; Van Voorhees et al., 2007). Moreover, in some close-knit communities, where "boundary maintenance" is perceived as a necessity for maintaining community cohesion, those who "leave the community" to seek mental health services may be subjected to severe negativity (Van Voorhees et al., 2007). This problem is further compounded by low levels of mental health literacy found in many communities, especially as it relates to mainstream definitions, availability, and effectiveness of treatments for depression (Ayalon and Alvidrez, 2007; Corrigan et al., 2004; Jorm et al., 2003; Kung, 2004; Thompson, Bazile, and Akbar, 2004). The mental health encounter is unique, requiring a higher level of understanding, empathy, and sensitivity. Racial and ethnic minorities experience issues of trust and linguistic barriers and emphasize a greater need for provider cultural and linguistic sensitivity (Chapa, 2009).

In many minority communities, there is an additional layer of mistrust of government agencies. This can be traced to historical and ongoing experience of oppression and marginalization (Center for Reducing Health Disparities, 2007; Grandbois, 2005). Such "mistrust may include stories of how governmental agencies have determined 'needs' of a community without consulting with the community being served, promised particular services that were never delivered, or come into a community with a service or program that was not sustained" (Center for Reducing Health Disparities, 2007, p. 10).

For example, American Indian communities have been found to avoid accessing mental health treatment because traditional healing practices are often not equally afforded the attention or respect given to mental health treatments implemented by Western psychology theory, which further exacerbates mistrust, perpetuates marginalization, and impedes depression treatment (Center for Reducing Health Disparities, 2007). Additionally, the sense of mistrust extends beyond government agencies to include a mistrust of Western models of care or mainstream mental health services altogether (Jesse, Dolbier, and Blanchard, 2008; Whaley, 2004; Wong et al., 2006). The limited number of racial and ethnic minority providers has resulted in a large proportion of race-discordant patient-provider relationships, often leading to adverse mental health treatment experiences, like miscommunication and diagnostic bias, thus creating adverse treatment experiences, further eroding trust, reinforcing stigma, and perpetuating treatment and service underutilization (Ayalon and Alvidrez, 2007; Das et al., 2006; Lazear et al., 2008; Thompson, Bazile, and Akbar, 2004; Van Voorhees et al., 2007).

Simple variation in treatment preferences among different populations and between individuals—which may be, at least partially, the result of experiences with stigma and mistrust—further affect their utilization of mental health services and the appropriateness of the care they receive (Jesse, Dolbier, and Blanchard, 2008; Van Voorhees et al., 2007). Studies have found that community-based resources (such as ethnicity-specific community agencies and churches) may be the preferred sources of depression-related support and care for minority communities, even though many such institutions may not be adequately equipped to provide psychiatric services (Brown, 2004; Sadavoy, Meier, and Ong, 2004; Sleath and Rubin, 2002). Yet others may seek primarily alternative sources of treatment, such as informal systems of care (Lazear et al., 2008) or non-Western approaches (Sanchez and Gaw, 2007; Wong et al., 2006), because of either cultural or personal preferences, stigma, negative experiences with the mental health care system, or alternative explanatory models of healing precluding their contact with the formal health care system (Shin, 2002; Van Voorhees et al., 2007).

Studies have shown that cultural factors may be protective of mental health status. When comparing Mexican immigrants with U.S. born Mexican Americans, researchers found that Mexican Americans and non-Hispanic whites born in the United States have a higher risk (a ratio of 2–3 to 1) for developing psychiatric disorders including major depressive episode than their foreign-born counterparts who have emigrated to the United States (Grant et al., 2004; Vega et al., 1998).

ENGAGING VULNERABLE POPULATIONS

The relationship between mental health disparities, access to care, and quality of care is complex. Behavioral health care in the United States is fragmented and fraught with barriers, regardless of the point of entry. For racial and ethnic minority populations it includes poor quality, limited access to care, and a lack of utilization and little care coordination—often leading to more chronic and disabling mental health conditions (Chapa, 2009; U.S. Department of Health and Human Services, 2003). Furthermore, the existing knowledge on the interrelationship of these three areas has not been translated into specific programs (Aguilar-Gaxiola et al., 2002).

When seeking to eliminate mental health disparities, treatment interventions and single-component interventions, such as physician education, depression screening (Gilbody et al., 2003), and facilitated access to care (Brown et al., 1999), alone are not effective at reducing disparity gaps. Poor treatment rates and outcomes may be due to a lack of minority representation in the mental health provider workforce. Research suggests that enhancing quality in mental health care could potentially lead to the elimination of mental health disparities (Miranda et al., 2008). A culturally respectful environment coupled with culturally and linguistically competent providers may be a key to disparities elimination, along with numerous, systemic, multicomponent, chronic disease management interventions.

Targeting the health care system was found to be effective at reducing disparities. One highly effective approach is clinical case management. This patient-focused strategy may be particularly beneficial for ethnic minorities because it assists patients unfamiliar with and at the margins of the traditional mental health care system to navigate the already fragmented health care system. Moreover, case managers contribute to mental health literacy, helping to assuage adverse attitudes toward depression treatment protocols and stigma, alternative explanatory models, and variations in symptom descriptions. Case managers assists marginalized groups, such as racial and ethnic minorities, throughout their involvement in depression treatment, maintenance, and completion.

The case managers' specialized work involves serial conversations to address incremental barriers and provide ongoing guidance that is outside the scope of time-short physician encounters. This may be critical to aid minorities and/or persons with limited English proficiency in circumnavigating the interrelated web of barriers. In addition, the relationship-building aspect of case management may enhance trust and address negative attitudes toward treatment and alternative, culturally based explanatory models, thus acting to incrementally break down stigma-related barriers.

Culturally focused and culturally appropriate community-based interventions are additionally important approaches not evaluated by Van Voorhees and colleagues, but highlighted by them and others (Aguilar-Gaxiola et al., 2008; Gilmer et al., 2007; Grandbois, 2005; Miranda, 2008; Park and Bernstein, 2008; Scuglik et al., 2007; Shin, 2002) as critical in improving depression interventions for racial and ethnic minorities. Succinctly summarizing the extensive literature on this topic, Van Voorhees and colleagues state that "ethnic minorities have unique vulnerabilities (e.g., immigration, racism), protective factors (social support), and adverse events (stressors such as 'daily hassles') that must be simultaneously considered in treatment and prevention programs" (2007, p. 162S). Further work by the Hogg Foundation for Mental Health through the University of Texas at Austin has been devoted to collect and highlight approaches to help assess, develop, and implement research-informed practices to racial and ethnic minorities, termed cultural adaptation (Hogg Foundation of Mental Health, 2006).

Pescosolido (1996) formalized this insight—that the social structure that systematically influences individuals' health behavior and outcomes is the influence of personal, organizational, and community network ties—into a network-episode model of care use. This model acknowledges the importance of community factors in influencing care utilization and posits that it is necessary to adopt a network-focused approach to understanding treatment entry and outcome at the individual, organizational, and system levels (Miranda, 2008). As Miranda states, "combining information from clients, their families and support networks, treatment providers, and bureaucratic officers is necessary to understand client episodes of treatment and outcomes of care" (2008, p. 229). More generally, the importance of adapting a community-based approach has been emphasized as a key factor in developing culturally sensitive interventions aimed at encouraging appropriate use of mental health services that will simultaneously act to overcome stigma and build trust from the perspective of the targeted communities (Bernal and Sáez-Santiago, 2006; Center for Reducing Health Disparities, 2007; Miranda, 2008; Shin, 2002).

A report by the Center for Reducing Health Disparities at the University of California, Davis, *Building Partnerships: Key Considerations When Engaging Underserved Communities Under the MHSA*, states the key principles and strategies for community engagement to facilitate mental health system transformation in underserved communities: paying attention to histories of discrimination and marginalization; engaging in transparent discussions of power dynamics; documenting community strengths and local knowledge; cooperating with key informants in communities; creating forums for communities to teach county providers about social networks, traditions, concepts of prevention, and community assets and needs; building capacity; focusing on systems development and sustainability; and upholding ethics of engagement (Center for Reducing Health Disparities, 2007).

In summary, the concept of vulnerability has important research and policy implications for two main reasons. First, risks may accumulate additively or multiplicatively, depending on the number of high-risk groups to which an individual or family belongs. Second, compared with their normative counterparts, vulnerable populations may require additional medical and social services to meet their multiple coinciding physical and mental health needs, as well as their children's developmental needs. Depression has been shown to adversely impact factors critical to establishing and maintaining social inclusion and functioning, such as educational attainment, productivity, and employment, and it may therefore be particularly damaging to socioeconomically disadvantaged ethnic minorities and other marginalized populations (Van Voorhees et al., 2007).

Bearing in mind such vulnerability-related considerations is of particular importance in the context of depression, because it is precisely those social environments and characteristics in which depression most commonly occurs—such as poverty, unmarried status, or disadvantage because of gender, race, or ethnicity, immigrant and/or refugee status—that are themselves factors likely to exacerbate or prolong depression. Because of their typically stressful and enduring nature, these conditions may create a constellation of vulnerabilities that overwhelm the person's coping capabilities and diminish the effectiveness of treatments that have proven successful under less challenging circumstances. Moreover, given the disproportionate prevalence of depression among women in their prime childbearing and child rearing years, particularly those who are young, poor, and single, depression poses a concern because of its potential for impairing affected mothers' parenting effectiveness.

Community-based approaches to depression screening and treatment among vulnerable populations are highlighted in the literature as critical for overcoming depression-related stigma and mistrust and reducing health disparities. One key conclusion from our review is that stigma, which is often mentioned as one of many barriers to depression care and treatment among vulnerable populations, appears to have a far more pervasive role. In fact, the Surgeon General links stigma-related considerations to many, if not most, of the barriers enumerated in the research literature (U.S. Department of Health and Human Services, 2001). Accordingly, stigma should be integrated into culturally and linguistically appropriate depression interventions; it may even lend itself to being addressed as a factor in its own right (Givens et al., 2007; Link et al., 1997).

RESEARCH GAPS

Although there is evidence available on the safety and efficacy of therapeutic and delivery approaches to treating depression and preventing relapse in adults, little is known about the impact of the successful treatment of depression for (1) adults who are parents and its effects on the functioning and well-being of their children (e.g., prevention of adverse outcomes), (2) racial and ethnic minority populations, and (3) non-English or limited English speakers.

In order to maintain a variety of therapeutic treatments to choose from to satisfy patient preference, further research is needed on the safety and efficacy of therapeutic treatments specifically for depressed parents (e.g., anti-depressants, therapy, alternative medicine). Specifically, research is needed on culturally and linguistically competent evidenced-based models; the appropriate duration of perinatal depression interventions, including indications for prophylactic treatment; the long-term effects of antidepressants on the growth and development of children exposed in utero; and further studies on the safety and efficacy of alternative treatments for perinatal depression (e.g., herbal medications or supplements, ultraviolet light).

With regard to delivery approaches for parents with depression, more research is needed to understand the effectiveness of certain settings in which parents and their children are regularly seen (i.e., pediatric, obstetric, gynecological settings, community-based centers, home); the effectiveness of alternative delivery mechanisms that can reduce barriers in receiving needed treatment (e.g., web-based therapy and follow-up for depressed parents, especially during pregnancy and postpartum periods); as well as the effectiveness of integrating treatment for depression and substance abuse disorders.

CONCLUSION

Although data specific to parents with depression are scarce, available evidence suggests that detection and treatment rates are even lower among mothers and fathers than rates reported for the general adult population. A variety of effective tools and approaches to delivery of treatment for depressed adults exist; however, studies rarely measure the effects of these tools that are important in depressed adults who are parents, including parenting quality and prevention of adverse child outcomes, nor do they account for delivery approaches in settings in which traditionally underserved populations of parents are seen.

Regarding the therapeutic interventions provided to depressed parents, it appears to be vital that individuals have an informed choice in treatment modalities (e.g., antidepressant medications, counseling, other alternatives). They should also be provided with the necessary resources and encouragement to pursue self-help options, and efforts should be made to tailor these interventions to accommodate the entire family.

Despite the lack of research documenting the effectiveness of interventions for depression specifically in *parents*, collaborative care models, (i.e., those that incorporate multiple interventions) appear to be a reasonable approach to delivering care for depression, providing that treatment models are flexible, efficient, inexpensive, and, above all, acceptable to the participants in a wide variety of community and clinical settings. At a minimum, the pivotal ingredients of collaborative care models have historically been (1) frequent client contact and follow-up, (2) stepped care tailored to the stage and severity of illness, (3) an active role for care managers and/or mental health specialists in orchestrating recovery or being accessible for questions and concerns, (4) the involvement of mental health specialists for treatment or consultation, and (5) community-based. Providers should consider taking advantage of technology-based (e.g., Internet) resources to assist and explore with depressed patients alternative and adjunct tools to traditional treatment modalities. For example, health providers servicing traditionally underserved populations (e.g., immigrant, limited or non-English proficient, rural) can help eliminate health disparities by accessing online health information for patients or using printed materials as adjunct tools in the treatment of depression and other psychological problems. Further, community-based approaches to depression screening and treatment among vulnerable populations are highlighted in the literature as critical for overcoming depression-related stigma and mistrust and in reducing health disparities.

REFERENCES

Aguilar-Gaxiola, S., Elliott, K., Debb-Sossa, N., King, R.T., Magaña, C.G., Miller, E., Sala, M., Sribney, W.M., and Breslau, J. (2008). *Engaging the Underserved: Personal Accounts of Communities on Mental Health Needs for Prevention and Early Intervention Strategies.* Center for Reducing Health Disparities, Monograph No. 1. Sacramento: University of California, Davis.

Aguilar-Gaxiola, S.A., Zelezny, L., Garcia, B., Edmonson, C., Alejo-Garcia, C., and Vega, W.A. (2002). Translating research into action: Reducing disparities in mental health care for Mexican Americans. *Psychiatric Services, 53,* 1563–1568.

Alegría, M., Chatterji, C., Wells, W., Cao, Z., Chen, C., Takeuchi, D., Jackson, J., and Meng, X. (2008). Disparity in depression treatment among racial and ethnic minority populations in the United States. *Psychiatric Services*, *59*, 1264–1272.

Alegría, M., Mulvaney-Day, N., Woo, M., Torres, M., Gao, S., and Oddo, V. (2007). Correlates of past-year mental health service use among Latinos: Results from the National Latino and Asian American Study. *American Journal of Public Health*, *97*, 1–8.

Amaro, H., Chernoff, M., Brown, V., Arévalo, S., and Gatz, M. (2007a). Does integrated trauma-informed substance abuse treatment increase treatment retention? *Journal of Community Psychology*, *35*, 845–862.

Amaro, H., Dai, J., Arevalo, S., Acevedo, A., Matsumoto, A., and Nieves, R. (2007b). Effects of integrated trauma treatment on outcomes in a racially/ethnically diverse sample of women in urban community-based substance abuse treatment. *Journal of Urban Health*, *84*, 508–522.

Amaro, H., Larson, M.J., Zhang, A., Acevedo, D., Dai, J., and Matsumoto, A. (2007c). Effects of trauma intervention on HIV sexual risk behaviors among women with co-occurring disorders in substance abuse treatment. *Journal of Community Psychology*, *35*, 895–908.

Amaro, H., McGraw, S., Larson, M.J., Lopez, L., Nieves, R., and Marshall, B. (2005). Boston Consortium of Services for Families in Recovery: A trauma-informed intervention model for women's alcohol and drug addiction treatment. *Alcoholism Treatment Quarterly*, *22*, 95–119.

American College of Obstetricians and Gynecologists. (2007). Use of psychiatric medications during pregnancy and lactation. Clinical Management Guidelines for Obstetrician-Gynecologists. *ACOG Practice Bulletin*, *87*.

Ammerman, R.T., Putnam, F.W., Altaye, M., Chen, L., Holleb, L.J., Stevens, J., Short, J.A., and Van Gingel, J.B. (2009). Changes in depressive symptoms in first time mothers in home visitation. *Child Abuse and Neglect*, *33*, 127–138.

Ammerman, R.T., Putnam, F.W., Stevens, J., Holleb, L.J., Novack, A.L., and Van Ginkel, J.B. (2005). In-home cognitive-behavior therapy for depression: An adapted treatment for first-time mothers in home visitation. *Best Practices in Mental Health*, *1*, 1–14.

Andersson, G., Bergstrom, J., Hollandare, F., Carlbring, P., Kaldo, V., and Ekselius, L. (2005). Internet-based self-help for depression: Randomised controlled trial. *British Journal of Psychiatry*, *187*, 456–461.

Appleby, L., Warner, R., Whitton, A., and Faragher, B. (1997). A controlled study of fluoxetine and cognitive-behavioural counseling in the treatment of postnatal depression. *British Medical Journal*, *314*, 932–936.

Armstrong, K., and Edwards, H. (2003). The effects of exercise and social support on mothers reporting depressive symptoms: A pilot randomized controlled trial. *International Journal of Mental Health Nursing*, *12*, 130–138.

Armstrong, K., and Edwards, H. (2004). The effectiveness of pram-walking exercising programme in reducing depressive symptomatology for postnatal women. *International Journal of Nursing Practice*, *10*, 177–194.

Asarnow, J.R., Jaycox, L.H., Duan, N., LaBorde, A.P., Rea, M.M., Murray, P., Anderson, M., Landon, C., Tang, L., and Wells, K.B. (2005). Effectiveness of a quality improvement intervention for adolescent depression in primary care clinics. *Journal of the American Medical Association*, *293*, 311–319.

Ayalon, L., and Alvidrez, J. (2007). The experience of black consumers in the mental health system: Identifying barriers to and facilitators of mental health treatment using the consumers' perspectives. *Issues in Mental Health Nursing*, *28*, 1323–1340.

Bai, Y.M., Lin, C.C., Chen, J.Y., and Liu, W.C. (2001). Virtual psychiatric clinics. *American Journal of Psychiatry*, *158*, 1160–1161.

Barbui, C., Hotopf, M., Freemantle, N., Boynton, J., Churchill, R., Eccles, M.P., Geddes, J.R., Hardy, R., Lewis, G., and Mason, J.M. (2007). Treatment discontinuation with selective serotonin reuptake inhibitors versus tricyclic antidepressants. *Cochrane Database of Systematic Reviews*, 3, CD002791.

Barnet, B., Liu, J., DeVoe, M., Alperovitz-Bichell, K., and Duggan, A.K. (2007). Home visiting for adolescent mothers: Effects on parenting, maternal life course, and primary care linkage. *Annals of Family Medicine*, 5, 224–232.

Bernal, G., and Sáez-Santiago, E. (2006). Culturally centered psychosocial interventions. *Journal of Community Psychology*, 34, 121–132.

Blackburn, I.M., Eunson, K.M., and Bishop, S. (1986). A two-year naturalistic follow-up of depressed patients treated with cognitive therapy, pharmacotherapy and a combination of both. *Journal of Affective Disorders*, 10, 67–75.

Boris, N.W., Larrieu, J.A., Zeanah, P.D., Nagle, G.A., Steier, A., and McNeill, P. (2006). The process and promise of mental health augmentation of nurse home-visiting programs: Data from the Louisiana Nurse-Family Partnership. *Infant Mental Health Journal*, 27, 26–40.

Bower, P., Gilbody, S., Richards, D., Fletcher, J., and Sutton, A. (2006). Collaborative care for depression in primary care—making sense of a complex intervention: Systematic review and meta-regression. *British Journal of Psychiatry*, 189, 484–493.

Brown, C., Schulberg, C.H., Sacco, D., Perel, J.M., and Houck, P.R. (1999). Effectiveness of treatments for major depression in primary medical care practice: A post hoc analysis of outcomes for African American and white patients. *Journal of Affective Disorders*, 53, 185–192.

Brown, J.A. (2004). *African American Church Goers' Attitudes Toward Treatment Seeking from Mental Health and Religious Sources. The Role Of Spirituality, Cultural Mistrust, and Stigma Toward Mental Illness*. (UMI No. 3129678.) Chapel Hill: University of North Carolina.

Brown, J.S., Elliott, S.A., Boardman, J., Ferns, J., and Morrison, J. (2004). Meeting the unmet need for depression services with psycho-educational self-confidence workshops: Preliminary report. *British Journal of Psychiatry*, 185, 511–515.

Brown, R.A., Evans, D.M., Miller, I.W., Burgess, E.S., and Mueller, T.I. (1997). Cognitive-behavioral treatment for depression in alcoholism. *Journal of Consulting and Clinical Psychology*, 65, 715–726.

Brown, S.A., and Schuckit, M.A. (1988). Changes in depression among abstinent alcoholics. *Journal of Studies of Alcohol*, 49, 412–417.

Bullock, L.F., Wells, J.E., Duff, G.B., and Hornblow, A.R. (1995). Telephone support for pregnant women: Outcome in late pregnancy. *New Zealand Medical Journal*, 108, 476–478.

Burt, V.K., Suri, R., Altshuler, L., Stowe, Z., Hendrick, V.C., and Muntean, E. (2001). The use of psychotropic medications during breast-feeding. *American Journal of Psychiatry*, 158, 1001–1009.

Butler, M., Kane, R.L., McAlpine, D., Kathol, R.G., Fu, S.S., Hagedorn, H., and Wilt, T.J. (2008). *Integration of Mental Health/Substance Abuse and Primary Care*. (No. 173 AHRQ Publication No. 09-E003.) Rockville, MD: Agency for Healthcare Research and Quality.

Carroll, K. (1998). *A Cognitive-Behavioral Approach: Treating Cocaine Addiction*. National Institute on Drug Abuse. NIH Publication No. 98-4308. Rockville, MD: National Institutes of Health.

Center for Reducing Health Disparities. (2007). *Building Partnerships: Key Considerations When Engaging Underserved Communities Under the MHSA*. Monograph No. 2, Center for Reducing Health Disparities. Sacramento: University of California, Davis.

Chambers, C.D., Hernandez-Diaz, S., Van Marter, L.J., Werler, M.M., Louik, C., Jones, K.L., and Mitchell, A.A. (2006). Selective serotonin-reuptake inhibitors and risk of persistent pulmonary hypertension of the newborn. *New England Journal of Medicine, 354,* 579–587.

Chapa, T. (2009). Eliminating mental health disparities in racial and ethnic minority populations through the integration of behavioral and primary healthcare: Recommendations and strategies. *American Psychological Association, Communique, 32–36.*

Christensen, H., and Griffiths, K.M. (2002). The prevention of depression using the Internet. *Medical Journal of Australia, 7,* S122–S125.

Christensen, H., Griffiths, K.M., and Jorm, A.F. (2004). Delivering interventions for depression by using the Internet: Randomized controlled trial. *British Medical Journal, 328,* 265–268A.

Christensen, H., Griffiths, K.M., MacKinnon, A.J., and Brittliffe, K. (2006). Online randomized controlled trial of brief and full cognitive behaviour therapy for depression. *Psychological Medicine, 36,* 1737–1746.

Clarke, G., Eubanks, D., Reid, E., Kelleher, C., O'Connor, E., DeBar, L.L., Lynch, F., Nunley, S., and Gullion, C. (2005). Overcoming depression on the Internet (ODIN) (2): A randomized trial of a self-help depression skills program with reminders. *Journal of Medical Internet Research, 7,* e16.

Clarke, G., Reid, E., Eubanks, D., O'Connor, E., DeBar, L.L., Kelleher, C., Lynch, F., and Nunley, S. (2002). Overcoming depression on the Internet (ODIN): A randomized controlled trial of an Internet depression skills intervention program. *Journal of Medical Internet Research, 4,* E14.

Coelho, H.F., Canter, P.H., and Ernst, E. (2007). Mindfulness-based cognitive therapy: Evaluating current evidence and informing future research. *Journal of Consulting and Clinical Psychology, 75,* 1000–1005.

Cohen, L.S., Altshuler, L.L., Harlow, B.L., Nonacs, R., Newport, D.J., Viguera, A.C., Suri, R., Burt, V.K., Hendrick, V., Reminick, A.M., Loughead, A., Vitonis, A.F., and Stowe, Z.N. (2006). Relapse of major depression during pregnancy in women who maintain or discontinue antidepressant treatment. *Journal of the American Medical Association, 295,* 499–507.

Conti, D.J., and Burton, W.N. (1994). The economic impact of depression in a workplace. *Journal of Occupational Medicine, 36,* 983–988.

Cooper, L.A., Gonzales, J.J., Gallo, J.J., Rost, K.M., Meredith, L.S., Rubenstein, L.V., Wang, N.Y., and Ford, D.E. (2003). The acceptability of treatment for depression among African American, Hispanic, and white primary care patients. *Medical Care, 41,* 479–489.

Corral, M., Kuan, A., and Kostaras, D. (2000). Bright light therapy's effect on postpartum depression. *American Journal of Psychiatry, 157,* 303–304.

Corrigan, P.W., Watson, A.C., Warpinski, A.C., and Gracia, G. (2004). Implications of educating the public on mental illness, violence, and stigma. *Psychiatric Services, 55,* 577–580.

Coyne, J.C., Schwenk, T.L., and Fechner-Bates, S. (1995). Nondetection of depression by primary care physicians reconsidered. *General Hospital and Psychiatry, 17,* 3–12.

Craven, M.A., and Bland, R. (2006). Better practices in collaborative mental health care: An analysis of the evidence base. *Canadian Journal of Psychiatry, 51*(Suppl. 1), 1–72.

Daley, A.J., Macarthur, C., and Winter, H. (2007). The role of exercise in treating postpartum depression: A review of the literature. *Journal of Midwifery and Women's Health, 52,* 56–62.

Das, A.K., Olfson, M., McCurtis, H.L., and Weissman, M.M. (2006). Depression in African Americans: Breaking barriers to detection and treatment. *Journal of Family Practice, 55,* 30–39.

Daughters, S.B., Braun, A.R., Sargeant, M.N., Reynolds, E.K., Hopko, D.R., Blanco, C., and Lejuez, C.W. (2008). Effectiveness of a brief behavioral treatment for inner-city illicit drug users with elevated depressive symptoms: The life enhancement treatment for substance use (LETS Act!). *Journal of Clinical Psychiatry, 69,* 122–129.

Davis, L., Uezato, A., Newell, J.M., and Frazier, E. (2008). Major depression and comorbid substance use disorders. *Current Opinions in Psychiatry, 21,* 14–18.

de Arellano, M.A., Waldrop, A.E., Deblinger, E., Cohen, J.A., Danielson, C.K., and Mannarino, A.P. (2005). Community outreach program for child victims of traumatic events: A community-based project for underserved populations. *Behavior Modification, 29,* 130–155.

de Mello, M.F., de Jesus Mari, J., Bacaltchuk, J., Verdeli, H., and Neugebaur, R. (2005). A systematic review of research findings on the efficacy of interpersonal therapy for depressive disorders. *European Archives of Psychiatry and Clinical Neuroscience, 255,* 75–82.

Deckersbach, T., Gershuny, B.S., and Otto, M.W. (2000). Cognitive-behavioral therapy for depression: Applications and outcome. *Psychiatric Clinics of North America, 23,* 795–809.

Dennis, C.L., and Chung-Lee, L. (2006). Postpartum depression help-seeking barriers and maternal treatment preferences: A qualitative systematic review. *Birth, 33,* 323–331.

Dennis, C.L., and Hodnett, E. (2007). Psychosocial and psychological interventions for treating postpartum depression. *Cochrane Database Systemic Reviews,* (4), CD006116.

Dennis, C.L., and Kingston, D. (2008). A systematic review of telephone support for women during pregnancy and the early postpartum period. *Journal of Obstetrics and Gynecological Neonatal Nursing, 37,* 301–314.

Dennis, C.L., Ross, L.E., and Grigoriadis, S. (2007). Psychosocial and psychological interventions for treating antenatal depression. *Cochrane Database Systemic Reviews,* (3), CD006309.

DeRubeis, R.J., Hollon, S.D., Amsterdam, J.D., Shelton, R.C., Young, P.R., Salomon, R.M., O'Reardon, J.P., Lovett, M.L., Gladis, M.M., Brown, L.L., and Gallop, R. (2005). Cognitive therapy vs. medications in the treatment of moderate to severe depression. *Archives of General Psychiatry, 62,* 409–416.

Dietrich, A.J., Oxman, T.E., Williams, J.W., Kroenke, K., Schulberg, H.C., Bruce, M., and Barry, S.L. (2004a). Going to scale: Re-engineering systems for primary care treatment of depression. *Annals of Family Medicine, 2,* 301–304.

Dietrich, A.J., Oxman, T.E., Williams, J.W., Schulberg, H.C., Bruce, M.L., Lee, P.W., Barry, S., Raue, P.J., Lefever, J.J., Heo, M., Rost, K., Kroenke, K., Gerrity, M., and Nutting, P.A. (2004b). Re-engineering systems for the treatment of depression in primary care: Cluster randomized controlled trial. *British Medical Journal, 329,* 602–605.

Dimidjian, S., Hollon, S.D., Dobson, K.S., Schmaling, K.B., Kohlenberg, R.J., Addis, M.E., Gallop, R., McGlinchey, J.B., Markley, D.K., Gollan, J.K., Atkins, D.C., Dunner, D.L., and Jacobson, N.S. (2006). Randomized trial of behavioral activation, cognitive therapy, and antidepressant medication in the acute treatment of major depression. *Journal of Consulting and Clinical Psychology, 74,* 658–670.

Dobson, K.S. (1989). A meta-analysis of the efficacy of cognitive therapy for depression. *Journal of Consulting and Clinical Psychology, 57,* 414–419.

Dodge, R., Sindelar, J., and Sinha, R. (2005). The role of depression symptoms in predicting drug abstinence in outpatient substance abuse treatment. *Journal of Substance Abuse Treatment, 28,* 189–196.

Dowrick, C., Dunn, G., Ayuso-Mateos, J.L., Dalgard, O.S., Page, H., Lehtinen, V., Casey, P., Wilkinson, C., Vazquez-Barquero, J.L., and Wilkinson, G. (2000). Problem-solving treatment and group psychoeducation for depression: Multicentre randomised controlled trial. Outcomes of Depression International Network (ODIN) Group. *British Medical Journal, 321,* 1450–1454.

Dugoua, J.J., Mills, E., Perri, D., and Korem, G. (2006). Safety and efficacy of St. John's wort (hypericum) during pregnancy and lactation. *Canadian Journal of Clinical Pharmacology, 13,* e268–e276.

Eberhard-Gran, M., Eskild, A., and Opjordsmoen, S. (2006). Use of psychotropic medications in treating mood disorders during lactation: Practical recommendations. *CNS Drugs, 20,* 187–198.

Einarson, A., Pistelli, A., Desantis, M., Malm, H., Paulus, W.D., Panchaud, A., Kennedy, D., Einarson, T.R., and Koren, G. (2008). Evaluation of the risk of congenital cardiovascular defects associated with use of paroxetine during pregnancy. *American Journal of Psychiatry, 165,* 749–752.

Eli Lilly. (2009). *Highlights of Prescribing Information Cymbalta® (duloxetine HCl).* Available: http://pi.lilly.com/us/cymbalta-pi.pdf [accessed March 9, 2009].

Elkin, I., Gibbons, R.D., Shea, T., Sotsky, S.M., Watkins, J.T., Pilkonis, P.A., and Hedeker, D. (1995). Initial severity and differential treatment outcome in the National Institutes of Mental Health Treatment of Depression Collaborative Research Program. *Journal of Consulting and Clinical Psychology, 63,* 841–847.

Epperson, C.N., Terman, M., Terman, J.S., Hanusa, B.H., Oren, D.A., Peindl, K.S., and Wisner, K.L. (2004). Randomized clinical trial of bright light therapy for antepartum depression: Preliminary findings. *Journal of Clinical Psychiatry, 65,* 421–425.

Evins, G.G., Theofrastous, J.P., and Galvin, S.L. (2000). Postpartum depression: A comparison of screening and routine clinical evaluation. *American Journal of Obstetrics and Gynecology, 182,* 1080–1082.

Farahati, F., Marcotte, D.E., and Wilcox-Gök, V.L. (2003). The effects of parents' psychiatric disorders on children's high school dropout. *Economics of Education Review, 22(2),* 167–178.

Fava, M., and Davidson, K.G. (1996). Definition and epidemiology of treatment resistant depression. *Psychiatric Clinics of North America, 19,* 179–200.

Finnegan, L.P. (1990). Current therapy in neonatal perinatal medicine-2. In N. Nelson (Ed.), *Neonatal Abstinence Syndrome* (pp. 314–320). Toronto: BC Decker.

Flynn, H.A., Blow, F.C., and Marcus, S.M. (2006). Rates and predictors of depression treatment among pregnant women in hospital-affiliated obstetrics practices. *General Hospital Psychiatry, 28,* 289–295.

Flynn, H.A., O'Mahen, H.A., Massey, L., and Marcus, S. (2006). The impact of a brief obstetrics clinic-based intervention on treatment use for perinatal depression. *Journal of Women's Health, 15,* 1195–1204.

Fox, S. (2005). *Health Information Online: Eight in Ten Internet Users Have Looked for Health Information Online, with Increased Interest in Diet, Fitness, Drugs, Health Insurance, Experimental Treatments, and Particular Doctors and Hospitals.* Washington, DC: Pew Internet and American Life Project.

Freeman, M.P., Davis, M., Sinha, P., Wisner, K.L., Hibbeln, J.R., and Gelenberg, A.J. (2008). Omega-3 fatty acids and supportive psychotherapy for perinatal depression: A randomized placebo-controlled study. *Journal of Affective Disorders, 110,* 142–148.

Freeman, M.P., Hibbeln, J.R., Wisner, K.L., Brumbach, B.H., Watchman, M., and Gelenberg, A.J. (2006a). Randomized dose-ranging pilot trial of omega-3 fatty acids for postpartum depression. *Acta Psychiatria Scandinavia, 113,* 31–35.

Freeman, M.P., Hibbeln, J.R., Wisner, K.L., Watchman, M., and Gelenberg, A.J. (2006b). An open trial of omega-3 fatty acids for depression in pregnancy. *Acta Neuropsychiatrica, 18,* 21–24.

Fronstin, P. (2005). *Sources of Coverage and Characteristics of the Uninsured: Analysis of the March 2005 Current Population Survey.* (EBRI Issue Brief No. 287.) Washington, DC: Employee Benefit Research Institute.

Gellatly, J., Bower, P., Hennessy, S., Richards, D., Gilbody, S., and Lovell, K. (2007). What makes self-help interventions effective in the management of depressive symptoms? Meta-analysis and meta-regression. *Psychological Medicine, 37,* 1217–1228.

Gentile, S. (2005). The safety of newer antidepressants in pregnancy and breastfeeding. *Drug Safety, 28,* 137–152.

Georgiopoulos, A.M., Bryan, T.L., Wollan, P., and Yawn, B.P. (2001). Routine screening for postpartum depression. *Journal of Family Practice, 50,* 117–122.

Getrich, C., Heying, S., Willging, C., and Waitzkin, H. (2007). An ethnography of clinic "noise" in a community-based, promotora-centered mental health intervention. *Social Science & Medicine, 65,* 319–330.

Gilbody, S., Bower, P., and Whitty, P. (2006). Costs and consequences of enhanced primary care for depression: Systematic review of randomised economic evaluations. *British Journal of Psychiatry, 189,* 297–308.

Gilbody, S., Whitty, P., Grimshaw, J., and Thomas, R. (2003). Educational and organizational interventions to improve the management of depression in primary care: A systematic review. *Journal of the American Medical Association, 289,* 3145–3151.

Gilmer, T.P., Ojeda, V.D., Folsom, D.P., Fuentes, D., Garcia, P., and Jeste, D.V. (2007). Initiation and use of public mental health services by persons with severe mental illness and limited English proficiency. *Psychiatric Services, 58,* 1555–1562.

Givens, J.L., Houston, T.K., Van Voorhees, B.W., Ford, D.E., and Cooper, L.A. (2007). Ethnicity and preferences for depression treatment. *General Hospital Psychiatry, 29,* 182–191.

Gjerdingen, D., Katon, W., and Rich, D.E. (2008). Stepped care treatment of postpartum depression: A primary care-based management model. *Women's Health Issues, 18,* 44–52.

GlaxoSmithKline. (2008). *Prescribing Information. Wellbutrin XL® (bupropion hydrochloride extended-release tablets).* Available: tp://us.gsk.com/products/assets/us_wellbutrinXL.pdf [accessed March 9, 2009].

Gomby, D., Culross, P., and Behrman, R. (1999). Home visiting: Recent program evaluations-analysis and recommendations. *Future of Children, 9,* 5–25.

Goodman, S., and Gotlib, I. (1999). Risk for psychopathology in the children of depressed mothers: A developmental model for understanding mechanisms of transmission. *Psychology Review, 106,* 458–490.

Gotlib, I.H., and Hammen, C.L. (Eds.). (2008). *Handbook of Depression* (2nd ed.). New York: Guilford Press.

Grandbois, D. (2005). Stigma of mental illness among American Indian and Alaska Native nations: Historical and contemporary perspectives. *Issues in Mental Health Nursing, 26,* 1001–1024.

Grant, B.F., Stinson, F.S., Hasin, D.S., Dawson, D.A., Chou, S.P., and Anderson, K. (2004). Immigration and lifetime prevalence of DSM-IV psychiatric disorders among Mexican Americans and non-Hispanic whites in the United States: Results from the National Epidemiologic Survey on Alcohol and Related Conditions. *Archives of General Psychiatry, 61,* 1226–1233.

Grote, N.K., Swartz, H.A., Geibel, S.L., Zuckoff, A., Houck, P.R., and Frank, E. (2009). A randomized controlled trial of culturally relevant, brief interpersonal psychotherapy for perinatal depression. *Psychiatric Services, 60,* 313–321.

Gunlicks, M.L., and Weissman, M.M. (2008). Change in child psychopathology with improvement in parental depression: A systematic review. *Journal of the American Academy of Child and Adolescent Psychiatry, 47*, 379–389.

Hageman, J.R., Adams, M.A., and Gardner, T.H. (1984). Persistent pulmonary hypertension of the newborn: Trends in incidence diagnosis and management. *Archives of Pediatric and Adolescent Medicine, 138*, 592–595.

Haveman, R., and Wolfe B. (1995). The determinants of children's attainments: A review of methods and findings. *Journal of Economic Literature, 33*, 1829–1878.

Hayes, B.A., and Muller, R. (2004). Prenatal depression: A randomized controlled trial in the emotional health of primiparous women. *Research and Theory for Nursing Practice, 18*, 165–183.

Hebbeler, K.M., and Gerlach-Downie, S. (2002). Inside the black box of home visiting: A quantitative analysis of why intended outcomes were not achieved. *Early Childhood Research Quarterly, 17*, 28–51.

Hepner, A.J., Rowe, M., Rost, K., Hickey, S.C., Sherbourne, C.D., Ford, D.E., Meredith, L.S., and Rubenstein, L.V. (2007). The effect of adherence to practice guidelines on depression outcomes. *Annals of Internal Medicine, 147*, 320–329.

Hogg Foundation for Mental Health. (2006). *Cultural Adaptation: Providing Evidence-Based Practices to Populations of Color.* Available: http://www.hogg.utexas.edu/programs_cc.html [accessed April 2, 2009].

Hollon, S.D., Stewart, M.O., and Strunk, D. (2006). Cognitive behavior therapy has enduring effects in the treatment of depression and anxiety. *Annual Review of Psychology, 57*, 285–315.

Horowitz, J.A., and Cousins, A. (2006). Postpartum depression treatment rates for at-risk women. *Nursing Research, 55*, S23–S27.

Hunkeler, E., Meresman, J.F., Hargreaves, W.A., Fireman, B., Berman, W.H., Kirsch, A.J., Groebe, J., Hurt, S.W., Braden, P., Getzell, M., Feigenbaum, P.A., Peng, T., and Salzer, M. (2000). Efficacy of nurse telehealth and peer support in augmenting treatment of depression in primary care. *Archives of Family Medicine, 9*, 700–708.

Interian, A., Martinez, I.E., Guarnaccia, P.J., Vega, W.A., and Escobar, J.I. (2007). A qualitative analysis of the perception of stigma among Latinos receiving antidepressants. *Psychiatric Services, 58*, 1591–1594.

Ireys, H.T., Chernoff, R., DeVet, K.A., and Kim, Y. (2001). Maternal outcomes of a randomized controlled trial of a community-based support program for families of children with chronic illnesses. *Archives of Pediatrics and Adolescent Medicine, 155*, 771–777.

Jacobs, F., Easterbrooks, M.A., Brady, A., and Mistry, J. (2005). *Healthy Families Massachusetts: Final Evaluation Report.* Medford, MA: Tufts University.

Jesse, D.E., Dolbier, C.L., and Blanchard, A. (2008). Barriers to seeking help and treatment suggestions for prenatal depressive symptoms: Focus groups with rural low-income women. *Issues in Mental Health Nursing, 29*, 3–19.

Jorm, A.F., Griffiths, K.M., Christensen, H., Korten, A.E., Parslow, R.A., and Rodgers, B. (2003). Providing information about the effectiveness of treatment options to depressed people in the community: A randomized controlled trial of effects on mental health literacy, help-seeking and symptoms. *Psychological Medicine, 33*, 1071–1079.

Kallen, B.A., and Olausson, P.O. (2007). Maternal use of selective serotonin re-uptake inhibitors in early pregnancy and infant congenital malformations. *Birth Defects Research, 79*, 301–308.

Kaltenthaler, E., Shackley, P., Stevens, K., Beverley, C., Parry, G., and Chilcott, J. (2002). A systematic review and economic evaluation of computerised cognitive behaviour therapy for depression and anxiety. *Health Technology Assessment, 6*, 1–89.

Katon, W., and Schulberg, H. (1992). Epidemiology of depression in primary care. *General Hospital Psychiatry, 14*, 237–247.

Katon, W.J., and Seelig, M. (2008). Population-based care of depression: Team care approaches to improving outcomes. *Journal of Occupational and Environmental Medicine, 50*, 459–467.

Keller, M.B., McCullough, J.P., Klein, D.N., Arnow, B., Dunner, D.L., Gelenberg, A.J., Markowitz, J.C., Nemeroff, C.B., Russell, J.M., Thase, M.E., Trivedi, M.H., and Zajecka, J. (2000). A comparison of nefazodone, the cognitive behavioral analysis system of psychotherapy, and their combination for the treatment of chronic depression. *New England Journal of Medicine, 342*, 1462–1470.

Kessler, R.C., Berglund, P., Demler, O., Jin, R., Koretz, D., Merikangas, K.R., Rush, A.J., Walters, E.E., and Wang, P.S. (2003). The epidemiology of major depressive disorder. *Journal of the American Medical Association, 289*, 3095–3105.

Kovacs, M., Rush, A.J., Beck, A.T., and Hollon, S.D. (1981). Depressed outpatients treated with cognitive therapy or pharmacotherapy. A one year follow-up. *Archives of General Psychiatry, 38*, 33–39.

Kung, W.W. (2004). Cultural and practical barriers to seeking mental health treatment for Chinese Americans. *Journal of Community Psychology, 32*, 27–43.

Lagerberg, D. (2000). Secondary prevention in child health: Effects of psychological intervention, particularly home visitation, on children's development and other outcome variables. *Acta Paediatric Supplement, 434*, 43–52.

Lazear, K.J., Pires, S.A., Isaacs, M.R., Chaulk, P., and Huang, L. (2008). Depression among low-income women of color: Qualitative findings from cross-cultural focus groups. *Journal of Immigrant and Minority Health, 10*, 127–133.

Levinson-Castiel, R., Merlob, P., Linder, N., Sirota, L., and Klinger, G. (2006). Neonatal abstinence syndrome after in utero exposure to selective serotonin reuptake inhibitors in term infants. *Archives of Pediatric and Adolescent Medicine, 160*, 173–176.

Lin, E.H., Katon, W.J., Simon, G.E., Von Korff, M., Bush, T.M., Rutter, C.M., Saunders, K.W., and Walker, E.A. (1997). Achieving guidelines for the treatment of depression in primary care: Is physician education enough? *Medical Care, 35*, 831–842.

Lin, E.H., Simon, G.E., Katzelnick, D.J., and Pearson, S.D. (2001). Does physician education on depression management improve treatment in primary care? *Journal of General Internal Medicine, 16*, 614–619.

Linde, K., Berner, M.M., and Kriston, L. (2008). St Johns wort for major depression. *Cochrane Database Systematic Reviews*, (4), CD000448.

Linde, K., Mulrow, C.D., Berner, M., and Egger, M. (2005). St John's wort for depression. *Cochrane Database Systematic Reviews*, (2), CD000448.

Linden, M., and Schotte, K. (2007). A randomized controlled trial comparing guideline-exposed and guideline-naïve physicians in respect to dosage selection and treatment outcome with doxpein with depressive disorders. *Pharmacopsychiatry, 40*, 77–81.

Link, B.G., Struening, E., Rahav, M., Phelan, J., and Nuttbrock, L. (1997). On stigma and its consequences: Evidence from a longitudinal study of men with dual diagnoses of mental illness and substance abuse. *Journal of Health and Social Behavior, 38*, 177–190.

Llorente, A.M., Jensen, C.L., Voigt, R.G., Fraley, J.K., Berretta, M.C., and Heird, W.C. (2003). Effect of maternal docosahexanoic acid supplementation on postpartum depression and information processing. *American Journal of Obstetrics and Gynecology, 188*, 1348–1353.

Loughrey, K., Maloney, K.K., Mara, J.R., McGrath, J., Miller, D., Rabin, K., Ratzan, S.C., Rimer, B.K., Strecher, V.J., and Tinker, T.L. (2001). *Making Health Communication Programs Work*. Washington, DC: U.S. Department of Health and Human Services.

Lumley, J., Watson, L., Small, R., Brown, S., Mitchell, C., and Gunn, J. (2006). PRISM (Program of Resources, Information, and Support for others): A community-randomized trial to reduce depression and improve women's physical health six months after birth [ISRCTN03464021]. BMC Public Health, 6, 37.

Ma, S.H., and Teasdale, J.D. (2004). Mindfulness-based cognitive therapy for depression: Replication and exploration of differential relapse prevention effects. Journal of Consulting and Clinical Psychology, 72, 31–40.

MacKinnon, A., Griffiths, K.M., and Christensen, H. (2008). Comparative randomized trial of online cognitive-behavioural therapy and an information website for depression: 12-month outcomes. British Journal of Psychiatry, 192, 130–134.

Marcus, S.M., Flynn, H.A., Blow, F.C., and Barry, K. (2003). Depressive symptoms among pregnant women screened in obstetrics settings. Journal of Women's Health, 12, 373–380.

Margolin, A., Beitel, M., Schuman-Olivier, Z., and Avants, S.K. (2006). A controlled study of a spirituality focused intervention for increasing motivation for HIV prevention among drug users. AIDS Education Prevention, 18, 311–322.

Maurer, D., and Colt, R. (2006). An evidence-based approach to the management of depression. Primary Care, 33, 923–941, vii.

Meara, E., and Frank, R. (2008). Impacts of Maternal Depression and Substance Abuse on the Development of Children's Human Capital. Presentation at the American Society of Health Economists, June 24, Duke University, Durham NC.

Merrill, K.A., Tolbert, V.E., and Wade, W.A. (2003). Effectiveness of cognitive therapy for depression in a community mental health center: A benchmarking study. Journal of Consulting and Clinical Psychology, 71, 404–409.

Mid-America Coalition on Health Care. (2009). Mid-America Coalition on Health Care: Community Initiative on Depression. Available: http://www.machc.org/documents/CID%20 Overview%20-%208-05%20BB.doc [accessed March 19, 2009].

Miller, L.J. (2008). The UIC Perinatal Mental Health Project. Workshop on Depression and Parenting, Committee on Depression, Parenting Practices, and the Healthy Development of Children, Irvine, CA.

Miranda, J. (2008). Community-based interventions for depression. In S. Aguilar-Gaxiola and T. Gullotta (Eds.), Depression in Latinos: Assessment, Treatment, and Prevention (pp. 225–236). New York: Springer.

Miranda, J., Chung, J.Y., Green, B.L., Krupnick, J., Siddique, J., Revicki, D.A., and Belin, T. (2003). Treating depression in predominantly low-income young minority women: A randomized controlled trial. Journal of the American Medical Association, 290, 57–65.

Miranda, J., Green, B.L., Krupnick, J.L., Chung, J., Siddique, J., Belin, T., and Revicki, D.A. (2006). One-year outcomes of a randomized clinical trial treating depression in low-income minority women. Journal of Consult Clinical Psychology, 74, 99–111.

Miranda, J., McGuire, T.G., Williams, D.R., and Wang, P. (2008). Mental health in the context of health disparities. American Journal of Psychiatry, 165, 1102–1108.

Misri, S., Reebye, P., Corral, M., and Millis, L. (2004). The use of paroxetine and cognitive-behavioral therapy in postpartum depression and anxiety: A randomized-controlled trial. Journal of Clinical Psychiatry, 65, 1236–1241.

Misri, S., Reebye, P., Kendrick, K., Carter, D., Ryan, D., Grunau, R.E., and Oberlander, T.F. (2006). Internalizing behaviors in 4–year-old children exposed in utero to psychotropic medications. American Journal of Psychiatry, 163, 1026–1032.

Morrissey, J.P, Jackson, E.W., Ellis, A.R., Amaro, H., Brown, V.B., and Najavits, L.M. (2005). Twelve-month outcomes of trauma-informed interventions for women with co-occurring disorders. Psychiatric Services, 56, 1213–1222.

Mortensen, J.T., Olsen, J., Larsen, H., Bendsen, J., Obel, C., and Sorensen, H.T. (2003). Psychomotor development in children exposed in utero to benzodiazepines, antidepressants, neuroleptics, and anti-epileptics. European Journal of Epidemiology, 18, 769–771.

Mynors-Wallis, L., Gath, D., Lloyd-Thomas, A., and Tomlinson, D. (1995). Randomized controlled trial comparing problem solving treatment with amitriptyline and placebo for major depression in primary care. *British Medical Journal, 310*, 441–445.

Mynors-Wallis, L., Gath, D., Day, A., and Baker, F. (2000). Randomized controlled trial of problem solving treatment, antidepressant medication, and combined treatment for major depression in primary care. *British Medical Journal, 320*, 26–30.

Nadeem, E., Lange, J.M., Edge, D., Fongwa, M., Belin, T., and Miranda, J. (2007). Does stigma keep poor young immigrant and U.S.-born black and Latina women from seeking mental health care? *Psychiatric Services, 58*, 1547–1554.

National Committee on Quality Assurance. (2005). *NCQA Report Shows Health Care Quality Up, But Enrollment Down in Plans that Report on Performance.* News Release, National Committee on Quality Assurance, October 3. Available: http://www.ncqa.org/tabid/257/Default.aspx [accessed March 9, 2009].

National Committee on Quality Assurance. (2008). Antidepressant medication management. In *The State of Health Care Quality 2008* (pp. 23–25). Washington, DC: Author. Available: http://www.ncqa.org/Portals/0/Newsroom/SOHC/SOHC_08.pdf [accessed March 9, 2009].

Navaie-Waliser, M., Martin, S.L., Tessaro, I., Campbell, M., and Cross, A. (2000). Social support and psychological functioning among high-risk mothers: The impact of the Baby Love Maternal Outreach Worker Program. *Public Health Nursing, 17*, 280–291.

Nolan, P., and Badger, F. (2005). Aspects of the relationship between doctors and depressed patients that enhance satisfaction with primary care. *Journal of Psychiatric and Mental Health Nursing, 12*, 146–153.

Nulman, I., Rovet, J., Stewart, D.E., Wolpin, J., Pace-Asciak, P., Shuhaiber, S., and Koren, G. (2002). Child development following exposure to tricyclic antidepressants or fluoxetine throughout fetal life: A prospective, controlled study. *American Journal of Psychiatry, 159*, 1889–1895.

Nunes, E.V., and Levin, F.R. (2004). Treatment of depression in patients with alcohol or other drug dependence: A meta-analysis. *Journal of the American Medical Association, 291*, 1887–1896.

Oberlander, T.F., Reebye, P., Misri, S., Papsdorf, M., Kim, J., and Grunau, R.E. (2007). Externalizing and attention behaviors in children of depressed mothers treated with selective serotonin reuptake inhibitor antidepressants during pregnancy. *Archives of Pediatric and Adolescent Medicine, 161*, 22–29.

Oberlander, T.F., Warburton, W., Misri S., Aghajanian, J., and Hertzman, C. (2006). Neonatal outcomes after prenatal exposure to selective serotonin reuptake inhibitor antidepressants and maternal depression using population-based linked health data. *Archives of General Psychiatry, 63*, 898–906.

Oren, D.A., Wisner, K.L., Spinelli, M., Epperson, N., Peindl, K.S., Terman, J.S., and Terman, M. (2002). An open trial of morning light therapy for treatment of antepartum depression. *American Journal of Psychiatry, 159*, 666–669.

Oxman, T.E., Dietrich, A.J., Williams, J.W., and Kroenke, K. (2002). A three-component model for reengineering systems for the treatment of depression in primary care. *Psychosomatics, 43*, 441–450.

Padgett, D.K., Patrick, C., Burns, B.J., and Schlesinger, H.J. (1994). Ethnicity and the use of outpatient mental health services in a national insured population. *American Journal of Public Health, 84*, 222–226.

Park, S.Y., and Bernstein, K.S. (2008). Depression and Korean American immigrants. *Archives of Psychiatric Nursing, 22*, 12–19.

Parker, G., Parker, I., Brotchie, H., and Stuart, S. (2006). Interpersonal psychotherapy for depression? The need to define its ecological niche. *Journal of Affective Disorders, 95*, 1–11.

Pescosolido, B.A. (1996). Bringing the "community" into utilization models: How social networks link individuals to changing systems of care. *Research in the Sociology of Health Care, 13A*, 171–197.

Pickett-Schenk, S.A., Cook, J.A., Steigman, P., Lippincott, R., Bennett, C., and Grey, D.D. (2006). Psychological well-being and relationship outcomes in a randomized study of family-led education. *Archives of General Psychiatry, 63*, 1043–1050.

Pilkington, K., Kirkwood, G., Rampes, H., and Richardson, J. (2005). Yoga for depression: The research evidence. *Journal of Affective Disorders, 89*, 13–24.

Pilkington, K., Rampes, H., and Richardson, J. (2006). Complementary medicine for depression. *Expert Review of Neurotherapeutics, 6*, 1741–1751.

Pilowsky, D.J., Wickramaratne, P.J., Rush, A.J., Hughes, C.W., Garber, J., Malloy, E., King, C.A., Cerda, G., Sood, A.B., Alpert, J.E., Wisiewski, S.R., Trivedi, M.H., Talati, A., Carlson, M.M., Liu, H.H., Fava, M., and Weissman, M.M. (2006). Children of currently depressed mothers: A STAR*D ancillary report. *Journal of Clinical Psychiatry, 67*, 126–136.

Quello, S.B., Brady, K.T., and Sonne, S.C. (2005). Mood disorders and substance abuse disorders: A complex comorbidity. *Science Practice Perspectives, 3*, 13–21.

Rahimi, R., Nikfar, S., and Abdollahi, M. (2009). Efficacy and tolerability of hypericum perforatum in major depressive disorder in comparison with selective serotonin reuptake inhibitors: A meta-analysis. *Progress in Neuropsychopharmacology and Biological Psychiatry, 33*, 118–127.

Regier, D.A., Farmer, M.E., Rae, D.S., Locke, B.Z., Keith, S.J., Judd, L.L., and Goodwin, F.K. (1990). Comorbidity of mental disorders with alcohol and other drug abuse. Results from the Epidemiologic Catchment Area (ECA) Study. *Journal of the American Medical Association, 264*, 2511–2518.

Revicki, D.A., Siddique, J., Frank, L., Chung, J.Y., Green, B.L., Krupnick, J., Prasad, M., and Miranda, J. (2005). Cost-effectiveness of evidence-based pharmacotherapy or cognitive behavior therapy compared with community referral for major depression in predominantly low-income minority women. *Archives of General Psychiatry, 62*, 868–875.

Ro, L.J., Treadwell, H.M., and Northridge, M. (2003). *Community Health Workers and Community Voices. Promoting Good Health. A Community Voices Publication.* National Center for Primary Care, Morehouse School of Medicine. Available: http://www.community voices.org/Uploads/CHW_FINAL_00108_00042.pdf [accessed March 30, 2009].

Rojas, G., Fritsch, R., Solis, J., Jadresic, E., Castillo, C., Gonzalez, M., Guojardo, V., Lewis, G., Peters, T.J., and Araya, R. (2007). Treatment of postnatal depression in low-income mothers in primary-care clinics in Santiago, Chile: A randomized controlled trial. *Lancet, 370*, 1629–1637.

Rost, K., Nutting, P., Smith, J., Werner, J., and Duan, N. (2001). Improving depression outcomes in community primary care practice. *Journal of General Internal Medicine, 16*, 143–149.

Rost, K., Smith, J.L., and Dickinson, M. (2004). The effect of improving primary care depression management on employee absenteeism and productivity: A randomized trial. *Medical Care, 42*, 1202–1210.

Rounsaville, B.J., Anton, S.F., Carroll, K., Budde, D., Prusoff, B.A., and Gawin, F. (1991). Psychiatric diagnoses of treatment seeking cocaine abusers. *Archives of General Psychiatry, 48*, 43–51.

Sadavoy, J., Meier, R., and Ong, A.Y.M. (2004). Barriers to access to mental health services for ethnic seniors: The Toronto study. *Canadian Journal of Psychiatry, 49*, 192–199.

Sanchez, F., and Gaw, A. (2007). Mental health care of Filipino Americans. *Psychiatric Services, 58*, 810–815.

Scuglik, D.L., Alarcon, R.D., Lapeyre, A.L., III, Williams, M.D., and Logan, K.M. (2007). When the poetry no longer rhymes: Mental health issues among Somali immigrants in the USA. *Transcultural Psychiatry, 44*, 581–595.

Segal, Z.V., Williams, J.M.G., and Teasdale, J.D. (2002). *Mindfulness-Based Cognitive Therapy for Depression: A New Approach for Preventing Relapse.* New York: Guilford Press.

Seligman, M.E.P., Schulman, P., DeRubeis, R.J., and Hollon, S.D. (1999). The prevention of depression and anxiety. *Prevention and Treatment, 2*(1).

Shin, J.K. (2002). Help-seeking behaviors by Korean immigrants for depression. *Issues in Mental Health Nursing, 23*, 461–476.

Simon, G.E. (1998). Can depression be managed appropriately in primary care? *Journal of Clinical Psychiatry, 59*, 3–8.

Simon, G.E., Fleck, M., Lucas, R., Bushnell, D.M., and the LIDO Group. (2004). Prevalence and predictors of depression treatment in an international primary care study. *American Journal of Psychiatry, 161*, 1626–1634.

Simon, G.E., Katon, W.J., Lin, E.H., Rutter, C., Manning, W.G., Von Korff, M., Ciechanowski, P., Ludman, E.J., and Young, B.A. (2007). Cost-effectiveness of systematic depression treatment among people with diabetes mellitus. *Archives of General Psychiatry, 64*, 65–72.

Sleath, B., and Rubin, R.H. (2002). Gender, ethnicity, and physician-patient communication about depression and anxiety in primary care. *Patient Education and Counseling, 48*, 243–252.

Sleath, B., West, S., Tudor, G., Perreira, K., King, V., and Morrissey, J. (2005). Ethnicity and depression treatment preferences of pregnant women. *Journal of Psychosomatic Obstetrics and Gynecology, 26*, 135–140.

Smith, C.A., and Hay, P.P. (2005). Acupuncture for depression. *Cochrane Database of Systematic Reviews*, (2), CD004046.

Spek, V., Cuijpers, P., Nykicek, I., Riper, H., Keyzer, J., and Pop, V. (2007). Internet-based cognitive behaviour therapy for symptoms of depression and anxiety: A meta-analysis. *Psychological Medicine, 37*, 319–328.

Spinelli, M.G., and Endicott, J. (2003). Controlled clinical trial of interpersonal psychotherapy versus parenting education program for depressed pregnant women. *American Journal of Psychiatry, 160*, 555–562.

Stathopoulou, G., Powers, M.B., Berry, A.C., Smits, J.A.J., and Otto, M.W. (2006). Exercise interventions for mental health: A quantitative and qualitative review. *Clinical Psychology: Science and Practice, 13*, 179–193.

Stewart, W.F., Ricci, J.A., Chee, E., Hahn, S.R., and Morganstein, D. (2003). Cost of lost productive work time among U.S. workers with depression. *Journal of the American Medical Association, 289*, 3135–3144.

Su, K.P., Huang, S.Y., Chiu, T.H., Huang, K.C., Huang, C.L., Chang, H.C., and Pariante, C.M. (2008). Omega-3 fatty acids for major depression during pregnancy: Results from a randomized, double-blind, placebo-controlled trial. *Journal of Clinical Psychiatry, 69*, 644–651.

Suri, R., Altshuler, L., Helleman, G., Burt, V.K., Aquino, A., and Mintz, J. (2007). Effects of antenatal depression and antidepressant treatment on gestational age at birth and risk of preterm birth. *American Journal of Psychiatry, 64*, 1206–1213.

Swartz, H.A., Shear, M.K., Frank, E., Cherry, C.R., Scholle, S.H., and Kupfer, D.J. (2002). A pilot study of community mental health care for depression in a supermarket setting. *Psychiatric Services, 53*, 1132–1137.

Takeuchi, D.T., Zane, N., Hong, S., Chae, D.H., Gong, F., Gee, G.C., Walton, E., Sue, S., and Alegría, M. (2007). Immigration-related factors and mental disorders among Asian Americans. *American Journal of Public Health, 97*, 84–90.

Tam, W.H., Lee, D.T.S., Chin, H.F.K., Ma, K.C., Lee, A., and Chung, T.K.H. (2003). A randomized controlled trial of educational counselling on the management of women who have suffered suboptimal outcomes in pregnancy. *British Journal of Obstetrics and Gynecology, 110*, 853–859.

Tandon, S.D., Parillo, K.M., Jenkins, C., and Duggan A.K. (2005). Formative evaluation of home visitor's role in addressing poor mental health, domestic violence and substance abuse among low-income pregnant and parenting women. *Maternal and Child Health Journal, 9*, 273–283.

Thase, M.E., Entsuah, A.R., and Rudolph, R.L. (2001). Remission rates during treatment with venlafaxine or selective serotonin reuptake inhibitors. *British Journal of Psychiatry, 178*, 234–241.

Thompson, C., Kinmonth, A.L., Stevens, L., Peveler, R.C., Stevens, A., Ostler, K.J., Pickering, R.M., Baker, N.G., Henson, A., Preece, J., Cooper, D., and Campbell, M.J. (2000). Effects of a clinical practice guideline and practice-based education on detection and outcome of depression in primary care: Hampshire Depression Project randomized controlled trial. *Lancet, 355*, 185–191.

Thompson, V.L.S., Bazile, A., and Akbar, M. (2004). African Americans' perceptions of psychotherapy and psychotherapists. *Professional Psychology: Research and Practice, 35*, 19–26.

Tiet, Q.Q., and Mausbach, B. (2007). Treatments for patients with dual diagnosis: A review. *Alcoholism: Clinical and Experimental Research, 31*, 513–635.

Trivedi, M.H., Rush, A.J., Crismon, M.L., Kashner, T.M., Toprac, M.G., Carmody, T.J., Key, T., Biggs, M.M., Shores-Wilson, K., Witte, B., Suppes, T., Miller, A.L., Altshuler, K.Z., and Shon, S.P. (2004). Clinical results for patients with major depressive disorder in the Texas Medication Algorithm Project. *Archives of General Psychiatry, 61*, 669–680.

Trivedi, M.H., Rush, A.J., Wisniewski, S.R., Nierenberg, A.A., Warden, D., Ritz, L., Noquist, G., Howland, R.H., Lebowitz, B., McGrath, P.J., Shores-Wilson, K., Biggs, M.M., Balasubramani, G.K., Fava, M., and the Star Study Team. (2006). Evaluation of outcomes with citalopram for depression using measurement-based care for STAR*D: Implications for clinical practice. *American Journal of Psychiatry, 163*, 28–40.

Trostel, P., Walker, I., and Woolley, P. (2002). Estimates of the economic return to schooling for 28 countries. *Labour Economics, 9*, 1–16.

Tuunainen, A., Kripke, D.F., and Endo, T. (2004). Light therapy for non-seasonal depression. *Cochrane Database of Systematic Reviews*, (2), CD004050.

U.S. Department of Health and Human Services. (2001). *Mental Health: Culture, Race, and Ethnicity—A Supplement to Mental Health: A Report of the Surgeon General*. Rockville, MD: Author, Substance Abuse and Mental Health Services Administration, Center for Mental Health Services.

U.S. Food and Drug Administration. 2004. *Effexor and Effexor XR*. Available: http://www.fda.gov/medwatch/safety/2004/safety04.htm#effexor [accessed March 9, 2009].

U.S. Surgeon General. (1999). *Mental Health: A Report of the Surgeon General*. Washington, DC: U.S. Department of Health and Human Services.

Vallejo, Z., and Amaro, H. (in press). Adaptation of mindfulness-based stress reduction program for addiction relapse prevention. *Humanistic Psychology*.

van Os, T.W.D.P., van den Brink, R.H.S., Tiemens, B.G., Jenner, J.A., van der Meer, K., and Ormel, J. (2005). Communicative skills of general practitioners augment the effectiveness of guideline-based depression treatment. *Journal of Affective Disorders, 84*, 43–51.

van Straten, A., Cuijpers, P., and Smits, N. (2008). Effectiveness of a web-based self-help intervention for symptoms of depression, anxiety, and stress: Randomized controlled trial. *Journal of Medical Internet Research, 10*, e7.

Van Voorhees, B.W., Walters, A.E., Prochaska, M., and Quinn, M.T. (2007). Reducing health disparities in depressive disorders outcomes between non-Hispanic whites and ethnic minorities: A call for pragmatic strategies over the life course. *Medical Care Research and Review, 64,* 157S–194S.

Vega, W.A., Kolody, B., Aguilar-Gaxiola, S., Alderete, E., Catalano, R., and Caraveo-Anduaga, J. (1998). Lifetime prevalence of DSM-III-R psychiatric disorders among urban and rural Mexican Americans in California. *Archives of General Psychiatry, 55,* 771–778.

Wagner, E., Austin, B., and VonKorff, M. (1996). Organizing care for patients with chronic illness. *Millbank Quarterly, 74,* 511–544.

Wang, P.S., Patrick, A., Avorn, J., Azocar, F., Ludman, E., McCulloch, J., Simon, G., and Kessler, R. (2006). The costs and benefits of enhanced depression care to employers. *Archives of General Psychiatry, 63,* 1345–1353.

Wang, P.S., Simon, G.E., Avorn, J., Azocar, F., Ludman, E.J., McCulloch, J., Petukhova, M.Z., and Kessler, R.C. (2007). Telephone screening, outreach, and care management for depressed workers and impact on clinical and work productivity outcomes: A randomized controlled trial. *Journal of the American Medical Association, 298,* 1401–1411.

Ward, E.C. (2007). Examining differential treatment effects for depression in racial and ethnic minority women: A qualitative systematic review. *Journal of the National Medical Association, 99,* 265–274.

Weier, K.M., and Beal, M.W. (2004). Complementary therapies as adjuncts in the treatment of postpartum depression. *Journal of Midwifery and Women's Health, 49,* 96–104.

Weiss, R.D., Griffin, M.L., Greenfield, S.F., Najavits, L.M., Wyner, D., Soto, J.A., and Hennen, J.A. (2000). Group therapy for patients with bipolar disorder and substance dependence: Results of a pilot study. *Journal of Clinical Psychiatry, 61,* 361–367.

Weissman, M.M. (2007). Cognitive therapy and interpersonal psychotherapy: 30 years later. *American Journal of Psychiatry, 164,* 693–696.

Weissman, M.M., Wickramaratne, P., Nomura, Y., Warner, V., Pilowsky, D., and Verdeli, H. (2006). Offspring of depressed parents: 20 years later. *American Journal of Psychiatry, 163,* 1001–1008.

Wells, K.B., Sherbourne, C., Schoenbaum, M., Duan, N., Meredity, L., Unutzer, J., Miranda, J., Carney, M.F., and Rubenstein, L.V. (2000). Impact of disseminating quality improvement programs for depression in managed primary care. *Journal of the American Medical Association, 283,* 212–220.

Whaley, A.L. (2004). Ethnicity/race, paranoia, and hospitalization for mental health problems among men. *American Journal of Public Health, 94,* 78–81.

Whitby, D.H., and Smith, K.M. (2005). The use of tricyclic antidepressants and selective serotonin reuptake inhibitors in women who are breastfeeding. *Pharmacotherapy, 25,* 411–425.

Whooley, M.A., and Simon, G.E. (2000). Managing depression in medical outpatients. *New England Journal of Medicine, 343,* 1942–1950.

Wisner, K.L., Hanusa, B.H., Perel, J.M., Peindl, K.S., Piontek, C.M., Sit, D.K.Y., Findling, R.L., and Moses-Kolko, E.L. (2006). Postpartum depression: A randomized trial of sertraline versus nortriptyline. *Journal of Clinical Psychopharmacology, 26,* 353–360.

Wisner, K.L., Perel, J.M., Peindl, K.S., Hanusa, B.H., Findling, R.L., and Rapport, D. (2001). Prevention of recurrent postpartum depression: A randomized clinical trial. *Journal of Clinical Psychiatry, 62,* 82–86.

Wisner, K.L., Perel, J.M., Peindl, K.S., Hanusa, B.H., Piontek, C.M., and Findling, R.L. (2004). Prevention of postpartum depression: A pilot randomized clinical trial. *American Journal of Psychiatry, 161,* 1290–1292.

Witkiewitz, K., and Marlatt, G.A. (2004). Relapse prevention for alcohol and drug problems: That was Zen, this is Tao. *American Psychology, 59,* 340–341.

Wong, E.C., Marshall, G.N., Schell, T.L., Elliott, M.N., Hambarsoomians, K., Chun, C.A., and Berthold, S.M. (2006). Barriers to mental health care utilization for U.S. Cambodian refugees. *Journal of Consulting and Clinical Psychology, 74,* 1116–1120.

World Health Organization. (2008). *Integrating Mental Health Into Primary Care: A Global Perspective.* Available: http://www.who.int/mental_health/resources/mentalhealth_PHC_2008.pdf [accessed January 17, 2009].

Wright, J.H., Wright, A.S., Albano, A.M., Basco, M.R., Goldsmith, L.J., Raffield, T., and Otto, M.W. (2005). Computer-assisted cognitive therapy for depression: Maintaining efficacy while reducing therapist time. *American Journal of Psychiatry, 162,* 1158–1164.

Wyeth Pharmaceuticals. (2008). *Effexor XR® (venlafaxine hydrochloride) Extended-Release Capsules.* Available: http://www.wyeth.com/content/showlabeling.asp?id=100 [accessed March 9, 2009].

Yawn, B.P. (2008). *Parental Depression in Family Medicine and Rural Medicine.* Workshop on Depression and Parenting, Committee on Depression, Parenting Practices, and the Healthy Development of Children, Irvine, CA.

Young, M.A., Fogg, L.F., Scheftner, W.A., and Fawcett, J.A. (1994). Interactions of risk factors in predicting suicide. *American Journal of Psychiatry, 151,* 434–435.

7

Prevention of Adverse Effects

SUMMARY

Prevention Interventions That Specifically Target Families with Depressed Parents

• Studies of interventions that target families with depressed parents have shown the potential to prevent adverse outcomes in children across all developmental stages. These include interventions that prevent or treat depression in the parent, those that target the vulnerabilities of the children, and those that improve parent-child relationships and parenting practices. However, the evaluation of these interventions has rarely included large-scale trials or widespread implementation or dissemination.

Broadly Focused Prevention Interventions in Families with Depressed Parents

• Some evidence suggests that prevention strategies that focus more broadly on parenting and child development can be effective even when there is a high rate of depression among parents. However, most evidence-based prevention strategies have not been evaluated for their relative effectiveness in families with depressed parents. Enhancements of these strategies with components targeted specifically to families with depressed parents have also rarely been evaluated.

- Existing service programs for families, such as early childhood education and home visitation, often provide preventive services that focus more broadly on parenting and child development. These service programs often serve a large number of depressed parents. Although these programs offer opportunities to identify depression in parents and to integrate treatment and prevention services, few programs routinely do so.

Prevention for Vulnerable Families

- Some prevention programs targeted to families with depression have been shown to be effective in low-income families and in families from varied cultural and linguistic backgrounds. There is less evidence on the effectiveness of these programs in families with co-occurring conditions such as exposure to trauma and co-existing mental and substance abuse disorders.
- A variety of existing service programs serve vulnerable families, such as social welfare programs and substance abuse services. Although these programs offer opportunities to identify depression in parents and to integrate treatment and prevention services, few programs routinely do so.

As described in this report, major depression is a highly prevalent disorder among adults of parenting age, and, as a consequence, millions of children in the United States are exposed every year to the risk associated with depression in a parent. Even more children are exposed to heightened levels of depressive symptoms in parents who do not meet diagnostic criteria; these children have also been demonstrated to be at increased risk. So far we have focused on identifying and treating depression in parents. This chapter focuses on efforts to prevent the effects that depression in parents can have on their families, as described in Chapter 4. The importance of preventive efforts is underscored by the scope of the problem and by the high percentage of adult depression, including parents, that goes untreated. Treating parental depression, attending to children's needs, and assisting parenting are all necessary components to foster resilience, promote health, and prevent disorder in families in which parents are depressed.

An important framework exists for understanding the available literature. The National Academies recently published a report on the prevention of mental, emotional, and behavioral disorders among young people (National Research Council and Institute of Medicine, 2009). The committee strongly supports the overall perspective on prevention presented in

Preventing Mental, Emotional, and Behavioral Disorders Among Young People: Progress and Possibilities. The report emphasizes several general points about prevention that apply to the prevention of depression in families: (1) prevention requires a shift to a public health focus from the traditional disease model, in which one waits for the occurrence of disease before action; (2) not only are the immediate needs of the child and family important but also their longer term needs; (3) mental health and physical health are inseparable and should be viewed as different aspects of the same underlying developmental processes; (4) mental, emotional, and behavioral disorders and their prevention are inherently developmental, and coordinated systems-level interventions are needed to address them. The prevention report emphasizes the need for a developmental perspective—just as this report does in considering the prevention of adverse outcomes of parental depression. The needs of children are quite different at ages 4, 8, or 12, so different interventions need to be tailored for children and their parents at different developmental stages.

Studies of parental depression can involve different types of focus. In some studies, severely ill parents with depression are identified, and the interventions focus primarily on depression. In others, depression in parents often serves as the identifier of a constellation of adversities that may include poverty, minority status, living in low-resource, difficult neighborhoods, social isolation, and exposure to violence. Although parental depression is an important condition to be addressed, comprehensive prevention efforts must also address these other factors. Additional risk factors that often need to be addressed systematically include comorbidity, divorce, and diminished social status.

The committee reviewed the relevant literature in order to identify examples of interventions or programs that target families with a depressed parent or that illustrate important conceptual principles for addressing the needs of these families, as well as to identify areas in which relatively little intervention research has been conducted. The committee did not seek to systematically identify all existing interventions and program evaluations. We drew on existing meta-analyses and systematic reviews whenever possible and supplemented with additional literature searches to identify relevant evidence-based programs. Whenever possible, we limited our review to interventions that have been evaluated in at least one randomized trial. In some cases, nonrandomized studies are discussed if that was the best available evidence for an approach to families with a depressed parent. The chapter text focuses on concepts and major outcomes. A table at the end of the chapter summarizes methodological details, study population demographics, and outcome measures for interventions that target families with a depressed parent.

The chapter begins with the available evidence on prevention of depression in parents, which is a first-line approach to preventing the adverse effects on children. The main focus of the chapter, however, is on approaches to reduce adverse outcomes in children, with a special emphasis whenever possible on interventions that take a two-generation approach to addressing the parent's depression, parenting, and child outcomes.

The committee's review revealed promising programs and important conceptual frameworks related to preventing the effects that depression in parents can have on families. These studies themselves and the broader context of prevention research indicate that there is a considerable promise to the approach and that current lines of investigation need expansion. However, despite the immense costs of parental depression in many different areas of life, as yet there are no large-scale, widely implemented prevention programs within systems in the United States to address parental depression. There is, therefore, a need to develop large-scale programs based on the existing knowledge base and on promising programs and, at the same time, to refine and evaluate these programs at various levels in order to determine the most effective and cost-effective preventive interventions.

A FRAMEWORK FOR PREVENTIVE INTERVENTIONS

Significant interest and a substantial knowledge base in the area of prevention have accumulated over the past 15 years. A broad framework for preventive interventions has been presented by the Institute of Medicine (IOM) report *Reducing Risks for Mental Disorders* (1994) and the previously mentioned report *Preventing Mental, Emotional, and Behavioral Disorders Among Young People* (National Research Council and Institute of Medicine, 2009). As outlined in the these reports, the usual sequence leading to the eventual widespread dissemination of preventive interventions is, first, the identification of risk factors and protective mechanisms, then the development of promising approaches and efficacy studies of preventive interventions, followed by large-scale effectiveness and dissemination studies, and finally the implementation of prevention programs. Chapter 4 described evidence related to the first step in prevention research, reviewing a number of identified mechanisms that mediate the association between depression in parents and adverse outcomes in children, including biological, psychological, and interpersonal processes. This chapter considers preventive interventions, with a focus on those that have been designed to directly address the source of risk for children by reducing parental depression through prevention or treatment and by targeting possible mechanisms of risk, including psychological vulnerabilities in children of depressed parents (e.g., Clarke et al., 2001), family relationships (e.g., Beardslee et al., 2007), and parenting and children's ways of coping (e.g., Compas, Forehand, and Keller, 2009).

The IOM framework defines prevention as intervening before the onset of a disorder in order to prevent or reduce risk for the disorder. This is distinct from treatment, which is targeted to individuals with a diagnosable disorder and is intended to cure the disorder or reduce its symptoms or negative effects on that individual. The framework also distinguishes between preventive interventions delivered to the general population (called *universal* prevention), to individuals exposed to known risk factors (*selective* prevention), and to individuals exhibiting signs or symptoms of a disorder (*indicated* prevention). By definition, interventions that target the children of parents with current or past depression are either selective or indicated: the target populations are identified by exposure to the risk of parental depression (selective prevention) and, in some cases, by the onset in the children and adolescents of symptoms of related adverse outcomes (indicated prevention). Preventive interventions have been delivered in a variety of contexts, including health care settings, early childhood settings, schools, and communities. Evaluating the effects of prevention programs is complex, as effects may not manifest for months or years after delivery of the intervention, and lasting preventive effects must be documented over long periods of time.

PREVENTION OF DEPRESSION IN PARENTS

Adults and Adolescents of Parenting Age

A first-line approach to preventing the effects of depression in parents is prevention of depression in adults and adolescents of parenting age. This is an important aspect, along with treatment, of reducing the burden of disease and its effects on parenting and child development. A recent meta-analysis reviewed 19 studies that used a randomized design to examine whether prevention programs are capable of reducing the incidence of depression (Cuijpers et al., 2008). This review was not designed to examine depression in parents but did include some studies of parents or adults of parenting age. Of these 19 studies, 11 included interventions with adults and 7 involved adolescents. Of the 11 studies with adults, 4 involved interventions delivered to pregnant women, 3 with women during the postpartum period, 1 with older adults, and 3 with adults in the typical parenting age range (ages 18–50). Interventions were delivered in a variety of settings using universal, selective, and indicated approaches. The mean incidence rate ratio was 0.78, indicating a reduction in incidence of depression by 22 percent, although the limited duration of follow-up in most studies makes it difficult to distinguish whether this reflects a true reduction in incidence or a delay in onset.

Thus, as reflected in this meta-analysis, there is promising evidence that it is feasible to reduce depression in adults and adolescents through preventive interventions, and these approaches could potentially be used to target parents of children at all developmental stages, starting with preconception. Although some of the existing interventions that have been rigorously tested were delivered to adults of parenting age, with the exception of strategies specifically targeting pregnant or postpartum women (see the next section), they were not designed specifically to prevent depression in parents, nor did they assess whether the subjects were parents or analyze outcomes for parents as a distinct subgroup. Indeed, just as there is a limited number of treatment studies analyzing outcomes in parents, there is a lack of evidence on effective prevention strategies targeted to parents and on the relative effectiveness in parents of current prevention strategies devised for adults in general. Further evaluation of current preventive interventions is needed in which the parenting status of the participants is tracked and outcomes for parents are analyzed. In addition, evaluations are needed of new interventions or adaptations of existing interventions that incorporate approaches specifically targeted to adults or adolescents who are parents, including, for example, multigenerational approaches such as those described in this chapter.

Pregnant and Postpartum Women

Although broad intervention approaches to prevent depression in adults are generally not targeted to parents, there are prevention strategies specifically focusing on pregnancy and the postpartum period. A variety of approaches have been used in interventions designed to prevent depression in the postpartum period. These include psychotherapeutic approaches based on the same principles as approaches for the treatment of postpartum depression, including cognitive-behavioral therapy (CBT) and interpersonal psychotherapy (IPT), along with psychoeducation, social support, and other supportive services. Evidence from rigorous evaluations of prevention models is limited, and the results are mixed. Although a few programs have been shown to be promising, others fail to demonstrate significant effects on measures of depressive symptoms or a diagnosis of depression (Battle and Zlotnick, 2005; Dennis, 2005; Dennis and Creedy, 2004). A few examples of programs that have shown promise in at least one randomized trial are described below. In addition, most evaluations of interventions to prevent postpartum depression do not include measures of child outcomes, so the impact of these interventions on reducing adverse outcomes for children is not known. Further evaluation of these approaches in diverse populations of mothers and delivered in diverse settings is needed to determine if more widespread implementation would be warranted.

The ROSE Program: Zlotnick conducted two randomized clinical trials of an interpersonal psychotherapy-based group intervention to prevent depression in pregnant women receiving public assistance who were at high risk for depression (Zlotnick et al., 2001, 2006). Known as the ROSE Program (Reach Out, Stand Strong, Essentials for New Mothers), the intervention is designed to help an ethnically diverse group of mothers-to-be on public assistance improve close interpersonal relationships, build social support networks, and master their transition to motherhood. At 3 months' postpartum, mothers in the intervention group were significantly less likely to have a diagnosis of postpartum depression.

Telephone Peer Support: Using a different approach, Dennis et al. (2009) reported a large, randomized trial of an individualized, telephone-based peer support intervention. The participants were women receiving postpartum care in seven health regions in Canada who were identified as high risk for depression owing to elevated depressive symptoms. They were matched with trained peer volunteers who had recovered from postpartum depression and received a minimum of four peer-support phone sessions starting at 2 weeks' postpartum. At 12 weeks' postpartum, a significantly fewer number of the mothers in the intervention group had scores on the Edinburgh Postnatal Depression Scale (EPDS) consistent with postpartum depression.

Other interventions designed to prevent depression in the postpartum period through psychotherapeutic, psychoeducational, and social support approaches have been evaluated in randomized trials but have not demonstrated an effect. For example, some approaches that have not demonstrated similar success have included a six-session group cognitive-behavioral therapy–based program targeted at mothers of very preterm infants (Hagan, Evans, and Pope, 2004); a single, individual critical incident stress debriefing session after childbirth (Priest et al., 2003); and a series of six weekly prenatal and one postnatal group classes focused on cognitive and problem-solving approaches and enhancing social support (Brugha et al., 2000).

This difference in outcomes may result from methodological differences and intervention design, but it may also be explained by the level of risk in the study population. The ROSE Program is distinct from these other trials because it targeted a high-risk population in terms of both demographics and depressive symptoms. The peer telephone support intervention was evaluated in a more general demographic population but was also targeted to women at high risk based on symptoms. Thus, there appears to be promise for indicated prevention approaches to address postpartum depression in women at high risk, but universal approaches have not been as successful. Universal prevention is discussed later in this chapter.

Infant Sleep: Maternal depression has been associated with infant sleep problems (Bayer et al., 2007), and a recent randomized trial tested the effects of an infant sleep intervention on depression in mothers. A behavior modification program designed to improve infant sleep was delivered by well-child nurses to 8-month-old infants in well-child care centers in Australia with mothers reporting a problem with their infants' sleep (Hiscock et al., 2007, 2008). Infant sleep problems were significantly reduced at 10 and 12 months compared with the control group, maternal depressive symptoms were also significantly reduced for the sleep intervention group, and the EPDS scores of the intervention group improved consistent with a reduction in postpartum depression. Parenting practices were also assessed using the Parent Behavior Checklist, as was child mental health using the Child Behavior Checklist. Neither measure differed markedly between the intervention and control groups (Hiscock et al., 2008). This trial was conducted in a more generalized population of mothers and suggests that targeting infant sleep problems may be an additional promising approach to preventing postpartum depression.

PREVENTION OF ADVERSE OUTCOMES IN CHILDREN

There are at least six potential models preventive interventions for children of depressed parents: (1) treatment of depression in adults (including parents), (2) early childhood interventions, (3) teaching parenting skills, (4) cognitive-behavioral interventions to address the children's risk factors, (5) interventions to strengthen family functioning, and (6) family cognitive-behavioral interventions to teach both parenting skills to depressed parents and coping skills to their children. Research on these approaches is at various stages of maturity.

Treatment of Parents' Depression

Arguably the most direct method of prevention of adverse outcomes in children of depressed parents would involve the treatment of parents' depression to remission and prevention of relapse. However, only a few investigations have examined the influence of antidepressants or psychotherapy on parenting or child outcomes. Therefore, key questions remain about the effects of treatment on families and the role of treatment in the prevention of adverse outcomes for children of depressed parents.

Gunlicks and Weissman (2008) reviewed the findings of 10 studies that examined the association between improvement in parents' depression and their children's psychopathology. They conclude that, although there is some evidence that successful treatment of parents' depression has been associated with improvement in children's symptoms and functioning, treatment may not be sufficient for improving cognitive and other aspects of child development. However, they note that research on the effects of treating parents' depression as a means of preventing adverse outcomes in children is in its early stages and that further study is needed. This review was not limited to interventions evaluated in randomized trials. It includes some randomized trials of interventions focused specifically on treatment for the parent (included in the examples described immediately below) as well as interventions that included components targeting parent-child interaction (described in the later section on parenting interventions).

Findings from the child component of the Sequence Treatment Alternatives to Relieve Depression (STAR*D) trial are illustrative of the status of research on the effects of treatment of parents' depression on children's mental health (Weissman et al., 2006). The study found that successful pharmacological treatment of mothers' depression to remission over 3 months was associated with significant reductions in mental health problems in their children compared with baseline. During the year following initiation of treatment for maternal major depressive disorder, decreases in the children's psychiatric symptoms were significantly associated with decreases in maternal depression severity (Pilowsky et al., 2008). An additional analysis of the STAR*D trial examined the fates of single mothers: investigators found that this population was much less likely to complete treatment and less likely to remit if they remained in treatment (Talati et al., 2007). The impact of the single mother's remission on her children was less dramatic than that found with two-parent households, but these results failed to achieve statistical significance.

Two other studies examined the familial impact of successfully treating dysthymia, a persistent form of low-grade depressive illness (Browne et al., 2002; Byrne et al., 2006). The authors reported a decrease in emotional and behavioral symptoms for children whose parents had successfully responded to pharmacotherapy (sertraline), interpersonal psychotherapy, or a combination thereof.

Other studies have focused specifically on treatment of postpartum depression. A study reported by Murray et al. (2003) and Cooper et al. (2003) investigated the effects of three different psychological treatments delivered by home visits for depressed postnatal women on maternal and childhood outcomes. They measured immediate and long-term maternal mood and depression as well as child and parenting outcomes. Although there were initial benefits at 4.5 months postpartum, the effects on maternal depression did not persist after 9 months, and they found no persistent impact of parental treatment on behavioral management, childhood attachment, or cognitive outcomes (Cooper et al., 2003; Murray et al., 2003).

Another study investigated the impact of interpersonal psychotherapy for maternal postpartum depression on child and parent outcomes. Although treatment improved maternal depression, it did not have a significant impact on parenting or child outcomes, even when mothers who responded successfully to treatment were analyzed separately (Forman et al., 2007; O'Hara et al., 2000).

Based on the available data, treatment to remission seems promising for reduction of child psychopathology in older children. However, these studies have not measured possible changes in parenting behaviors as a function of mothers' depression status, leaving unanswered at present the question of the role of possible improvements in parenting that are sufficient to improve child outcomes. In addition, treatment interventions have not shown sustained success in infant children of depressed mothers or in improving parenting skills, parent-child relationships, or child developmental outcomes other than psychopathology. In addition, it remains unclear whether treatment that improves symptoms but does not lead to remission can have any benefits for child outcomes or whether any beneficial effects of parental treatment to remission are lost if the depression recurs. Gunlicks and Weissman (2008) call for more careful documentation of the relation between parental and child symptoms, the differential effect of parents' treatment with psychological versus pharmacological treatment, and possible mediators and moderators of the relation between parental improvement and child psychopathology. In addition to measures of children's symptoms and diagnoses related to psychopathology, it is important to more fully understand the effects of parents' treatment on other functional developmental outcomes for children, such as social, emotional, and academic competence, as well as on quality of parenting.

Interventions for Children of Depressed Parents in Early Childhood

There is good evidence that intensive intervention early in life for high-risk children and their parents can have significant long-term effects on children's outcomes (National Research Council and Institute of Medicine, 2009). These interventions target those at risk because of multiple factors, including in some cases parental depression; when reported, parental depression is found to be highly prevalent in some studies of early childhood interventions, such as Early Head Start (Administration for Children and Families, 2002). Early childhood interventions take place in a variety of settings, and many target multiple domains, such as health, mental health, social and emotional development, relationships, and parenting.

The effectiveness of these interventions for children of parents with depression has not been specifically examined in most studies. In addition, there are few examples of programs that deliver interventions designed to target changes in both children's outcomes and parents' depression, either when parental depression is the primary concern or when depression serves as the identifier of a constellation of risk factors. Examples of approaches or programs with promise or informative evidence for future interventions are described below.

Home Visitation

A wide range of home visitation services exist that are intended to improve maternal well-being and to promote optimal child development, but only a few have been rigorously evaluated. A recent meta-analysis showed that home visiting programs do have significant cognitive and social-emotional development gains for children (Sweet and Appelbaum, 2004). Two national models, the Nurse-Family Partnership (NFP) and Healthy Families America (HFA), have each been subjected to at least three randomized controlled trials. Significant outcomes replicated across two or more trials include (1) improved prenatal health, (2) fewer childhood injuries, (3) increased maternal employment, and (4) improved school readiness. Evidence for the prevention of child maltreatment—a major community justification for funding these programs—has proven harder to document, although several recent evaluations point to reductions in maternally reported maltreatment and harsh parenting.

Home visiting programs offer an opportunity for access to depressed mothers and their children, and home visiting has been evaluated as a setting for treatment of postpartum depression (see Chapter 6). However, there have not been many rigorous, randomized evaluations of home visiting programs or program enhancements designed specifically for mothers with depression and their children, nor have there been many studies specifically assessing the links between child outcomes and maternal depression in home visiting programs. There have been some small trials of interventions delivered through home visiting that have evaluated both maternal and child outcomes. These include the treatment intervention described earlier, which showed some short-term benefit for maternal depression but had no effect on parenting or child outcomes (Cooper et al., 2003; Murray et al., 2003) as well two mother-child interventions described later in this chapter, which showed some promising effects on parent-child interaction and child development but no effect on maternal depressive symptoms (Horowitz et al., 2001; van Doesum et al., 2008).

There is also some limited evidence on the effects of maternal depression on the effectiveness of more broadly targeted home visiting programs. Program developers and researchers have identified three major impediments to effectiveness that transcended the different home visiting service models: domestic violence, substance abuse, and maternal depression

(National Research Council and Institute of Medicine, 1999). These are widely recognized as seriously undermining maternal engagement, motivation, and the utilization of skills and opportunities offered by home visitation services, and a 1999 National Academies workshop report observed that "depression, for example, interferes with engagement and motivation to follow up on visits, which makes it more likely that a family will not fully experience the program" (National Research Council and Institute of Medicine, 1999, p. 11). An evaluation of Healthy Families Massachusetts (Jacobs et al., 2005) found that symptoms of depression interfered with parenting beliefs, knowledge, and confidence and was negatively correlated with peer social support. Maternal depression was also a significant predictor of decreased emotional availability of the child.

Given that maternal depression can interfere with the effectiveness of home visiting programs, and home visiting offers an opportunity to deliver interventions to address maternal depression, one promising approach may be to both embed ways to recognize parental depression in existing programs and enrich these programs with interventions specifically for depressed parents when needed.

Early Childhood Education

Early education programs that combine early education with comprehensive health and social services have been shown to have a lasting impact on children's cognitive scores, behavioral development, school retention, and adult productivity (Nelson, Westhues, and MacLeod, 2003). Although there are several different effective programs, few examples of interventions in this setting specifically address depression in parents.

Early Head Start has been evaluated in a large-scale random assignment study (Administration for Children and Families, 2002). Designed for children from birth to age 3, Early Head Start includes early education, parenting education, health and mental health services, and family support. The data suggest that Early Head Start strengthens parenting and has significant but somewhat modest effects on child development. The strongest findings were in programs that had both home visiting and center-based services and programs that were well implemented—that is, the most comprehensive programs had the largest effect. However, the program did not have a favorable impact for families with three or more demographic risk factors (single parent, receiving public assistance, unemployed parent, teenage parent, parent lacking high school diploma or GED).

Although not designed to target parental depression, in a subsample of programs that measured depression, about half of mothers in the project were depressed. Greater positive effects of Early Head Start on some parenting and child outcomes were seen in families in which the mother was at risk for depression compared with children whose mothers were not at risk (Administration for Children and Families, 2002). Early Head Start had no effect on maternal depression 1 year after enrollment, but, after 3–5 years, depressive symptoms were reduced. The earlier impacts on child outcomes mediated this effect on maternal depression (Chazan-Cohen et al., 2007).

Given the high prevalence of maternal depression in early childhood programs such as Early Head Start, these programs offer an opportunity to deliver interventions to address maternal depression. Therefore, as with home visitation programs, one promising approach may be to embed ways to recognize parental depression in existing early childhood programs and to enrich these programs with parenting interventions specifically for depressed parents and referral for mental health services. In addition, because the combination of multiple risk factors was associated with worse outcomes, program enhancements to address other family needs, for example, income and educational needs, may also be warranted in order to maximize program outcomes.

Interventions for Children of Depressed Parents in Childhood and Adolescence

Clarke and colleagues have developed a cognitive-behavioral preventive intervention for youth at high risk of depression and have evaluated it specifically in children of depressed parents (Clarke et al., 1995, 2001). Adolescent youth with subdiagnostic depressive symptoms whose parents were being treated for depression received 15 1-hour group sessions or usual care (Clarke et al., 2001). Adolescents in the intervention reported significantly fewer symptoms of depression at postintervention and 12-month follow-up and a significantly lower rate of newly diagnosed major depressive episodes at 12-month follow-up. This trial has recently been replicated in a larger, four-site randomized trial (Garber et al., 2007, 2009). In this case, the participants had current depressive symptoms or a history of depression or both and also had a parent with a current or past episode of major depression. At 8 months after enrollment, a significant preventive effect was found, but this was moderated by parental depression at enrollment. For adolescents with parents with a history of depression but not currently depressed at baseline, the intervention led to reduced onset of depression. However, when the adolescents in the intervention group had a parent with current depression at enrollment, the rates of new depression posttreatment were not significantly different.

Depression is one of the major adverse outcomes for children of depressed parents, and this intervention demonstrates that it is possible to prevent episodes of major depression in these children. However, the importance of the current status of the parent's depression in the expanded replication trial highlights the concept that preventive interventions targeting the children of depressed parents may not be sufficient unless the depressed parent is also adequately treated.

Interventions Targeting Parent-Child Relationships and Parenting Skills

As described in Chapter 4, parenting skills and practices are disrupted and impaired in parents with depression. Therefore, a third approach to preventive intervention for their children is to address parenting as a mediator of the effects of the depression. Many parent training approaches have demonstrated effectiveness on a range of child and parent outcomes (Kaminski et al., 2008; National Research Council and Institute of Medicine, 2009). However, only a few parenting interventions have been specifically designed to improve the quality of parenting by depressed parents or have been evaluated specifically in a population of depressed parents.

There is some evidence, however, on the relative effectiveness of parenting interventions for parents with depression in evaluations of more broadly targeted parenting interventions. On one hand, some parenting interventions have been shown not only to improve outcomes for children of depressed parents but also to reduce depressive symptoms in parents. On the other hand, elevated symptoms of depression have been found in some studies to limit the effectiveness of parenting interventions. Thus, although parents who are struggling with depressive symptoms may be less likely to benefit from efforts to improve their parenting skills, participation in parenting interventions can contribute to a reduction in parents' depressive symptoms and improve child outcomes.

Parent-Child Interactions in Infancy and Early Childhood

Many of the treatment and preventive interventions described earlier in this chapter and in Chapter 6 that target depression in postpartum women have not assessed outcomes for children or focused on the parenting relationship. However, there is a robust literature on approaches in early childhood that foster interactions between mothers and infants or toddlers, and some of these approaches have been evaluated in mothers with depression or depressive symptoms. In these evaluations, these interventions have shown positive effects on parent-child interactions, indicating that these interventions can be effective even in the presence of maternal depression and in both low-income mothers and more generalized populations. Some have also been shown to treat maternal depression.

Horowitz et al. (2001) evaluated interaction coaching in the setting of home visits for depressed mothers with the goal of improving maternal responsiveness or the mother's ability to accommodate to an infant's behavior through regulation of her own behavioral responses. Interaction coaching took place during three home visits when the infants were ages 4–18 weeks. The researchers found significant improvements in maternal-infant responsiveness but did not find an effect on depressive symptoms.

In another recent example, an individually tailored mother-baby intervention was delivered through home visits in the Netherlands to depressed mothers with infants ages 1–12 months (van Doesum et al., 2008). The mothers met diagnostic criteria for a major depressive episode or dysthymia and were under concurrent outpatient treatment that was not part of the intervention. The major components of the intervention were modeling of parenting, cognitive restructuring, practical pedagogical support, and infant massage. At 6-month follow-up, the intervention group showed significant improvements in infant attachment security, mother-child interaction, and child socioemotional competence. Child externalizing, internalizing, and dysregulation measures were not significant. The improvement in maternal-infant interaction for the intervention group was not attributable to decreased maternal depressive symptoms, which decreased equally in both groups.

In another approach to improving mother-infant interaction, depressed lower-income mothers were trained to assess their newborn infants' behavior using an instrument called Mother's Assessment of the Behavior of Her Infant (Hart, Field, and Nearing, 1998). Mothers then carried out this assessment weekly for 1 month. This intervention led to significant improvements compared with control mother-infant pairs on measures of the Neonatal Behavioral Assessment Scale. The intervention did not have any effect on maternal depression.

Field et al. (2000) evaluated a more comprehensive intervention for low-income adolescent mothers with depressive symptoms and their infants. This multicomponent intervention was delivered in a public vocational school and consisted of free day care for the infants; social, educational, and vocational programs for the mothers; several mood induction interventions for the mothers, including relaxation therapy and music mood induction; and infant massage therapy and mother-infant interaction coaching, which have previously been shown to improve child outcomes and parenting interactions for mothers with depression (Field et al., 1996; Malphurs et al., 1996; Pelaez-Nogueras et al., 1996). At 12 months postpartum, the mothers who received the intervention had significantly reduced depressive symptoms compared to depressed mothers who did not receive the intervention, although they were not reduced to the level of nondepressed control mothers. Their parent-child interactions also significantly improved, and their infants scored significantly better on measures of infant development.

Another approach in early childhood that targets both the parent and the child and has been evaluated in mothers with depression is toddler-parent psychotherapy (TPP) (Lieberman, Weston, and Pawl, 1991). In TPP, mothers and their toddlers are seen in joint sessions with a therapist with the aim of improving the mother-child interaction and maternal responsivity. TPP has been shown to increase attachment security and foster cognitive development in children of depressed mothers (Cicchetti, Rogosch, and Toth, 2000; Cicchetti, Toth, and Rogosch 1999). In more recently published evaluation results, Cicchetti and colleagues (Cicchetti, Toth, and Rogosch, 2004; Toth et al., 2006) again demonstrated the efficacy of TPP in fostering secure attachment in mothers with depression. There were no effects on the mothers' depression.

Parent Training Interventions

In a review of the effects of group-based parenting programs on maternal psychological health, Barlow, Coren, and Stewart-Brown (2008) identified 11 programs that measured depression or depressive symptoms using a range of standardized instruments. A meta-analysis of these programs showed a small but significant improvement in the intervention groups. Of the 11 studies, 7 showed no difference or only a nonsignificant difference favoring the parents who received the intervention (Cunningham, Bremner, and Boyle, 1995; Greaves, 1997; Gross, Fogg, and Tucker, 1995; Irvine et al., 1999; McGillicuddy et al., 2001; Nixon and Singer, 1993; Patterson et al., 2002), and 4 of the individual studies showed significant effects (Pisterman et al., 1992; Scott and Stradling, 1987; Sheeber and Johnson, 1994; Taylor et al., 1998). Although depression was measured as an outcome for parents, none of these four trials was specifically targeted to parents with depression.

Scott and Stradling (1987) demonstrated significant improvement in depression levels on the Irritability, Depression, and Anxiety Scale for mothers of children with parent-reported behavior problems after a seven-session series of behavioral parenting sessions. Sheeber and Johnson (1994) studied a series of nine weekly sessions of a program focused on behavioral strategies for parents of children with "difficult temperaments." They found a significant reduction in levels of depression on the depression subscale of the Parenting Stress Index. In an evaluation of the Parent and Child Series (PACS) Program, Taylor et al. (1998) found significant improvements in depression as measured by the Beck Depression Inventory (BDI). This intervention used videotape modeling for parents of children with a diagnosis of conduct disorder. In contrast, two other studies evaluating the PACS Program (Gross, Fogg, and Tucker, 1995; Patterson et al., 2002) did not find significant effects. Pisterman et al. (1992) found significant improvement on the depression subscale of the Parenting Stress Index for parents of children with attention deficit disorder with hyperactivity who participated in 12 weekly parent training sessions focused on improving parent-child interaction and child compliance.

In another, more recent, example of a parenting program with a demonstrated effect on depression in parents, DeGarmo, Patterson, and Forgatch (2004) found that changes in parenting by single or separated mothers led to subsequent reductions in their sons' (mean age 8 years at baseline) externalizing and internalizing behavior problems. Changes in the sons' behavior problems in turn led to reductions in mothers' depressive symptoms over a period of 2.5 years. Thus, in this intervention, the effects of teaching parenting skills on maternal depressive symptoms were mediated by the decrease in children's behavior problems. Tonge et al. (2006) also found that a parent education and behavior management intervention led to improvements in parents' depression. This intervention for parents of children with autism led to a reduction on the depression measure of the General Health Questionnaire for parents who began the trial with high levels of depressive symptoms. Effects on child outcomes were not reported.

These studies provide evidence that teaching parenting skills—such as responsive and nurturing behavior, effective use of positive reinforcement, consistency in responding to child behavior, positive interactions with the child, promoting social skills—not only can improve outcomes for children but also can contribute to reductions in parents' depressive symptoms, similar to interventions to improve parent-child interactions in infancy and early childhood. Kaminski et al. (2008) note that an increased sense of self-efficacy that results from improvement in parenting skills and reductions in children's behavior problems may contribute directly to reductions in parents' depressive symptoms. However, it is also possible that parenting interventions help to mobilize parents to seek additional mental health services that are responsible for reducing their depressive symptoms. Most of these parent training programs evaluating effects on depression in parents have not been targeted to parents with depression. Rather, they have been targeted to parents of children with behavioral problems or clinical diagnoses or parents experiencing additional stressors, such as separation. It is therefore not clear how well these results can be generalized to a broader population of families.

There is also some evidence that parental depression can reduce the effectiveness of some parenting programs, as was seen with the home visiting and early childhood programs described above. The Incredible Years, for example, is a training program that includes components for parents, teachers, and children designed to promote social, emotional, and academic competence, to reduce children's aggression and behavioral problems, and to prevent them from developing conduct problems. Two randomized trials in Head Start have shown that the Incredible Years Parenting Training Program resulted in significant improvement in parent-child interactions and child behaviors (Webster-Stratton, 1998; Webster-Stratton, Reid, and Hammond, 2001). In an evaluation of the role of mental health factors and parental engagement, researchers found that parental depression had a small negative effect on program engagement, a factor that was associated with program benefits in a dose-response fashion. The estimates of program effectiveness were also slightly lower for parents with elevated levels of depressive symptoms. However, these differences were small, and families with a depressed parent nonetheless significantly benefited from the program (Baydar, Reid, and Webster-Stratton, 2003). This suggests that parents with depression can benefit from parenting programs and from enhancements to increase their engagement and link them to treatment. The Triple P Program, for example, is a parenting intervention with multiple levels of interventions, including an enhanced component that provides skills and support to deal with parental depression, marital discord, or other family challenges (Sanders, 1999).

Combining Parent Training and Treatment of Depression

Two randomized controlled trials have combined interventions to teach parenting skills with treatment for parents' depression and assessed the effects of the interventions on maternal depression and childhood behavioral problems (Sanders and McFarland, 2000; Verduyn et al., 2003). Sanders and McFarland (2000) randomized a small number of families with depressed mothers of young children with behavior problems to either a behavioral family intervention or a family intervention integrating CBT strategies for treatment of depression with the teaching of parenting skills. Both treatments were equally effective in reducing depressive symptoms in the mothers and behavior problems in the children immediately post-intervention. However, at 6 months, more families that received the CBT family intervention maintained the reductions in both depressive symptoms and had concurrent changes in depressive symptoms and child behavior problems than the families receiving behavioral therapy. Verduyn et al. (2003) also examined CBT for depression with parenting skills enhancement for depressed mothers of young children in a randomized trial with a mothers' support group and no intervention as comparison groups. Although within-group analyses revealed improvement of child behavior problems and maternal depression in the CBT group pretest to posttest at 6 and 12 months, there was no difference among the three randomized comparison groups.

Two-Generation Preventive Interventions

Based on the evidence for the effects of depression on parenting quality and child outcomes, there is a strong theoretical basis to suggest that the most effective prevention interventions will incorporate multiple approaches and target both generations by including active components for both parents and children. There is therefore a need to design and evaluate comprehensive, two-generation interventions that focus on parenting and take preventive approaches to address the needs of children and their depressed parents.

Family Talk Intervention

Beardslee and colleagues have developed and evaluated a preventive intervention for children at risk for depression owing to their parents' depression. This intervention was designed so that it could be used with all families facing parental depression. Its aim is to increase protective processes in the family—for example, better communication, increased understanding of one another and of the illness, and support for resilience-enhancing activities in children, such as accomplishing age-appropriate developmental tasks or experiencing good peer relationships (Beardslee and Podorefsky, 1988).

This intervention has been evaluated in three randomized trials comparing two active forms of intervention, one a two-session lecture for parents in a group format and the other a clinician-facilitated intervention of a series of sessions with both family meetings and separate meetings with parents and children. In both the first pilot study and a second larger trial, sustained changes were found in behaviors and attitudes toward the illness as well as reported increases in family communication and attention to the children's experience in both groups, with a significantly greater change in the clinician-facilitated group (Beardslee et al., 1997, 2003). Analysis of the combined sample from the first two trials at 2.5 and 4.5 years after enrollment showed a sustained increase for both sets of intervention groups in the two main targets of intervention (behavior and attitudes toward the illness in the parents and understanding of parental illness in the children), with a significantly greater effect in the clinician-facilitated group. Parents who changed the most in behavior and attitude had children who increased the most in understanding (Beardslee et al., 2003, 2007). In addition, in both groups, there was a gradual increase in both parents' and children's Family Relationship Inventory scores and a decline in scores on the Youth Self-Report Depression Subscale, but there were no significant differences between the clinician-facilitated group and the lecture comparison group. Recognition and treatment of depression when it occurred was also increased in both intervention groups compared with the recognition of depression prior to enrollment (Beardslee et al., 2007). Similar effects were found in a third, small, randomized trial to evaluate an adaptation for use with single mothers who were members of minority groups (Podorefsky, McDonald-Dowdell, and Beardslee, 2001).

The principles in this approach and the specific Family Talk Intervention have been used in a number of large-scale efforts to address children of the mentally ill and specifically children of parents with depression. For example, the lecture sessions were adapted for use in the state of Delaware by the Delaware Mental Health Association. The Family Talk Intervention has also been selected for use in several large-scale programs for children of the mentally ill in Holland and Finland (Beardslee et al., in press; Solantaus and Toikka, 2006). This large-scale implementation effort is discussed in more detail in Chapter 8.

Family Cognitive-Behavioral and Parenting Skills Intervention

Building on the work of Clarke and Beardslee, Compas and colleagues have developed and evaluated a preventive intervention for depressed parents and their children with two active components—teaching parenting skills to parents and teaching children skills to cope with their parents' depression (Compas, Forehand, and Keller, 2009; Compas, Keller, and Forehand, in press). This intervention model is based on evidence that parents' depression is associated with increased levels of withdrawn and irritable or intrusive parenting and that these patterns of parenting are associated with increased levels of children's internalizing and externalizing problems (Jaser et al., 2005; Langrock et al., 2002). Conversely, children's use of secondary control coping (acceptance, cognitive reappraisal, distraction) to cope with these stressful interactions with their parents is associated with lower internalizing and externalizing problems (Langrock et al., 2002; Jaser et al., 2005, in press).

An open-trial pilot study established the feasibility, acceptability, and initial effects of an earlier version of this family intervention (Compas, Keller, and Forehand, in press). A total of 34 families participated. Each family had a parent who had experienced at least one episode of depression during the lifetime of his or her children; half of the sample had a parent who met criteria for a current depressive episode at the time of assessment. After 10 small-group interventions, parents' reports of their children's problems showed significant decreases in aggressive behavior problems, withdrawn behavior, total internalizing problems, and total externalizing problems. Significant effects were also found on self-reports of depression in the parents on the BDI-II.

Initial findings from an ongoing, randomized clinical trial in a sample of 111 families further suggest that this is a promising approach to the prevention of adverse outcomes in children of depressed parents (Compas, Forehand, and Keller, 2009). Compared with a psychoeducational information comparison condition, significant effects have been found favoring the intervention group on adolescents' self-reports of their depressive symptoms and other internalizing and externalizing problems, as well as on parents' reports of adolescents' externalizing symptoms over the first 12 months after the intervention. Furthermore, significantly greater reductions have been found in the group intervention on parents' depressive symptoms on the BDI-II at 2 months after enrollment; however, effects on parents' depressive symptoms were not sustained at 6- or 12-month follow-ups.

These interventions demonstrate that a focus on parenting in combination with several prevention approaches that address the needs of the children as well as the needs of parents with depression has great promise for addressing the adverse effects of depression on families. A comprehensive, two-generation approach to intervention design is directly related to the impairments in parenting described in Chapter 4, underscoring a strong theoretical basis. The examples described above offer a preliminary base of evidence in practice; however, further replication and larger scale studies are needed to evaluate the feasibility and effectiveness of implementing these kinds of programs in real-world settings in which parents can be reached.

UNIVERSAL AND PUBLIC HEALTH APPROACHES

Although not the focus of this chapter, it is worth noting that a potentially important part of any comprehensive approach to supporting families dealing with depression is a broad awareness of the need for universal public health strategies. Such efforts focus on wellness and mental health promotion as a way to reduce the incidence of depression for adults and adolescents, including those who are or may become parents. These efforts may include a focus on diet and nutrition, exercise, sleep, stress reduction, social support, and education. For pregnant women, these approaches also include quality prenatal care, adequate nutrition, and avoidance of harmful substances, all of which can improve health outcomes for both mothers and children (Bodnar and Wisner, 2005; Clapp, 2002; Honikman, 2002).

Universal prevention and public health approaches are challenging to design. It can be very difficult to evaluate the extent to which they can lead to prevention of depression in parents and of adverse outcomes in children of depressed parents. There is a very limited evidence base for effects of universal prevention and public health approaches on depression in families, and very few programs have had rigorous evaluations.

The work that has been done has centered around pregnancy and the postpartum period. Social support and education have commonly emerged as possible avenues to reduce stress and other risks for depression and to increase awareness about depressive symptoms. One approach has been broad public awareness campaigns and strategies to institute universal education for expectant families about postpartum depression. These are discussed in more detail in Chapter 8. Elements of social support and education are also evident in interventions for pregnant and postpartum women that are both universally and selectively targeted, such as the preventive interventions described earlier in this chapter for which there was greater success in programs targeted to high-risk mothers. This is consistent with a systematic review of randomized trials of postpartum support and education. Shaw et al. (2006) found that universal interventions delivered to unselected women did not result in statistically significant improvements in any outcomes related to maternal mental health, parenting, quality of life, or physical health. A more recent large multicommunity universal intervention effort in Australia called PRISM (Program of Resources, Information, and Support for Mothers) incorporated not only community-based education and supportive services for mothers but also training for health care providers with the aim of improving their recognition of maternal depression and their capacity to address it (Lumley et al., 2006). However, in a cluster randomized trial, the intervention was not effective in reducing depression at 6 months postpartum, a result that the authors attributed in part to the smaller than expected impact of education and training of the primary caregivers.

Although there is a lack of strong direct evidence for effects on maternal depression, universal approaches focused on prenatal and postpartum support are an area of public health program design and implementation. Thus, like the areas of home visiting, early childhood, and parenting programs described earlier, research is warranted to explore these programs as opportunities to rigorously evaluate embedded strategies to recognize parental depression and to enrich them with interventions specifically for depressed parents and referral for mental health services.

For example, one emerging approach to universal supportive care in pregnancy is the group care model. The Centering Healthcare Institute offers two group care models, one for pregnant mothers (Centering Pregnancy) and one for new mothers (Centering Parenting) (Agency for Healthcare Research and Quality, 2008). Centering Pregnancy brings together groups of 8 to 12 pregnant women who are at a similar stage in their pregnancy. The groups meet in 10 2-hour sessions in which participants receive physical assessment, education and skills building, and support through facilitated group discussion. This group care model has been shown in a randomized controlled trial to produce improved pregnancy and birth outcomes (Ickovics et al., 2007). Centering Parenting brings together 5 or 6 mother-baby pairs and follows a schedule according to well-baby visits. A notable benefit of this approach is that the care is billable and sustainable (as a part of prenatal care and well-baby care). Although results have not been published on the effects of this model of care on antepartum or postpartum depression, the program is currently being evaluated for its impact on psychosocial outcomes, including stress and depression (Ickovics, 2008, personal communication).

PREVENTION FOR VULNERABLE FAMILIES

Many factors contribute to a heightened risk for depression in families, including poverty, housing and employment insecurity, and distressed neighborhoods; minority and immigrant status; co-occurring conditions, such as substance abuse, trauma, child abuse, and domestic violence; and family stressors. Some prevention intervention evaluations have examined the moderating effects of these risk factors. There are also interventions that directly address some of these risk factors in families, but there is limited evidence for the effects of these interventions on depression in families or for their relative effectiveness in families with depression. Examples of interventions with some specific evidence or highly applicable principles are reviewed here.

A recurring theme is that interventions for high-risk families can operate in many ways. In some cases, interventions targeted at risk factors reduce depression in parents as well as improve parenting and child outcomes. In other cases, the presence of depression in a family can alter the effectiveness of the interventions. Depression can sometimes decrease the effectiveness of the program, presumably by interfering with the quality of the family's participation. In other examples, programs are more effective for families with depression, presumably because the higher level of risk in these families at the outset makes them most amenable to improvement as a result of the intervention.

Poverty and Related Risk Factors

There is increasing awareness of the inseparability of poverty and both risk for depression and child developmental outcomes. The 2009 National Research Council and Institute of Medicine prevention report highlighted the risk that poverty can confer and emphasized that "the future mental health of the nation depends crucially on how, collectively, the costly legacy of poverty is dealt with" (National Research Council and Institute of Medicine, 2009, p. xv). Previous chapters of this report have emphasized how the study of parental depression strongly reinforces the need to address poverty and health disparities.

As described earlier in this chapter, early childhood intervention programs, including Early Head Start and some home visitation programs, were targeted to low-income families, and the rates of depression were found to be very high. This has also been seen in other emerging approaches to improving outcomes for low-income mothers. For example, a pilot project in Chicago found high rates of depression in the participants in a program evaluating the use of a community-based doula (a new mother's aid) for young mothers in low-income communities, which is now being implemented more broadly and is undergoing a randomized controlled, longitudinal study (Altfeld, 2003; Robert Wood Johnson Foundation, 2008).

Although, in most programs, evaluation is needed of the relative effectiveness of these early childhood programs when a parent is depressed, the available evidence does indicate that interventions to prevent adverse effects of depression in parents can be effective in low-income families. For example, many of the effective interventions for families with depression described earlier in this chapter, especially in pregnancy, postpartum, and early childhood, were targeted to low-income families (e.g., ROSE and some parent-child interaction interventions).

For interventions that focus on parent training, a recent meta-analysis of parent training interventions similarly found consistent evidence for positive outcomes for families in poverty (Reyno and McGrath, 2006). However, depressive symptoms in the parent were a significant threat to the success of many of these interventions, with the interpretation that depressive symptoms work against parents' motivation to attend and to consistently apply what is taught. As described earlier, however, depressive symptoms in parents can also correlate with greater improvement in response to an intervention. In an evaluation of the Incredible Years in low-income Head Start children, for example, increased parenting capability reduced child behavior problems at home and in the classroom, and the level and duration of maternal participation were associated with positive child outcomes (Baydar, Reid, and Webster-Stratton, 2003; Reid, Webster-Stratton, and Baydar, 2004). Depressive symptoms did reduce maternal engagement. Despite this, symptomatic mothers benefited from the intervention as much as, or more than, nonsymptomatic mothers, which was attributed to their poorer initial parenting skills (Baydar, Reid, and Webster-Stratton, 2003).

Given the high prevalence of maternal depression in prevention programs targeted to low-income families and the potential for depression to interfere with the effectiveness of programs in this vulnerable population, in order to maximize outcomes in these programs there is once again cause to consider developing and evaluating approaches to embed recognition of parental depression and referral for mental health services along with programmatic enrichment for the subpopulation of depressed parents.

Employment and Income Assistance Programs

As just described, prevention interventions designed to improve outcomes for children and families can be effective in low-income families. In addition, programs that address poverty by increasing employment and income can have positive effects on parenting and on child outcomes (Morris, Duncan, and Clark-Kauffman, 2005). However, based on available evidence, it is not clear whether programs designed to address employment, poverty, and housing can also affect depression in parents or improve child outcomes specifically in families with depression, because few studies have directly addressed this question. A few examples of projects using randomized designs that have included some evaluation of depression in parents, parenting, or child developmental outcomes are described below.

New Hope Project: The New Hope project in Milwaukee, Wisconsin, provided income supplementation, job search assistance, and subsidized health insurance and child care in families that were primarily African American and Hispanic (Epps and Huston, 2007; Huston et al., 2005; Miller et al., 2008). The program increased parental employment and family income while the benefits were in place. There were significant improvements in children's academic performance and positive social behavior as well as a decrease in problem behavior. There was little impact on parenting practices and parent-child relations or psychological well-being in parents.

Minnesota Family Investment Program: The Minnesota Family Investment Program (MFIP) provided financial incentives to encourage work as well as employment-focused activities and services to predominantly non-Hispanic European Americans and African Americans in urban counties in Minnesota (Gennetian and Miller, 2002). MFIP increased employment, earnings, and income in families through 3 years after entry into the study. Children in families receiving the program were less likely to exhibit problem behaviors and more likely to perform better and be more engaged at school. The program reduced the incidence of mothers at high risk for depression (Center for Epidemiologic Studies Depression Scale [CESD] score of 24 or above) but did not have effects on the home environment and parenting, except for a significant increase in parental supervision of children.

New Chance Project: The New Chance demonstration project, which took place in 10 states, focused on young women who bore children as teenagers and were high school dropouts. The project provided adult education, occupational skills training, job assistance, health and family planning classes and services, group and individual counseling to address problems in the mothers' lives, parenting classes, and classes on life skills, such as communication and decision making (Quint, Bos, and Polit, 1997). Over half of the overall sample at the outset of the study were at risk of clinically significant depression based on CESD scores. The percentage at risk for depression decreased in both the experimental and control groups, but the intervention did not have a significant effect on depression relative to the control group. CESD scores improved more for mothers in the control group than for mothers in the New Chance group, and, at 42-month follow-up, the mothers in the program group were at higher risk of depression than those in the control group. This was hypothesized to result from the greater instability in living arrangements in the program group as well as from raised expectations for improvement that remained unmet. The program group also reported higher levels of parental stress and rated their children as having more behavior problems, an effect that was concentrated among those mothers who were at risk of depression at baseline.

At the 18-month follow-up, children in the New Chance group did have more favorable home environments than the control group based on the Home Observation for Measurement of the Environment (HOME) scale, which evaluates aspects of the home environment, such as cognitive stimulation, safety, emotional support in mother-child interactions, and harshness of discipline. By the 42-month follow-up, however, this effect persisted only for the subset of mothers who were not at initial risk of depression. An in-depth examination of parenting behavior and child development in a subset of families, using coded videotaped observations of interactive tasks for the mother and child, showed that, at an average of 21 months after enrollment, the program had positive effects on parenting, but these were not accompanied by a difference in child developmental outcomes measures (Zaslow and Eldred, 1998).

Moving to Opportunity: In a randomized housing mobility experiment as part of a demonstration project called Moving to Opportunity, families living in high-poverty public housing projects in five U.S. cities were given vouchers and counseling to help them move to private housing in neighborhoods with lower levels of poverty. The study population was comprised predominantly of African American or Hispanic female heads of household with children. The families were offered housing vouchers, allowing them to move to neighborhoods that were safer and had significantly lower poverty rates than those of control families who were not offered vouchers. There were significant reductions in psychological distress and in the probability of a diagnosis of a major depressive episode, with systematically larger effect sizes for the group experiencing larger changes in neighborhood poverty rates (Kling et al., 2004; Kling, Liebman, and Katz, 2007).

Taken together, these findings support the principle that policies and programs that target poverty and related risk factors, such as employment, income, and housing, have some potential for beneficial effects on child outcomes, parenting, and depression in families. However, the evidence in this area is mixed, and in some cases outcomes appear to be worse for families with depression or parents at high risk for depression. Therefore, further evaluation is needed, both of the effects of these programs on the subset of participating families with depression and, as noted in previous discussions, of enhancing the intervention to maximize the benefits for these high-risk families, such as incorporating access to mental health services and providing more intensive outreach, engagement, and support services to both parents and children in families with depression. Subsequent intervention research of this kind can be further informed by studies that have identified compensatory actions that parents can take to reduce the adverse effects of poverty and other social risk factors on children (e.g., Jarrett and Burton, 1999).

The data on the effects of employment, income, and housing interventions in families with depression, although limited, are also sufficient to suggest that a complementary approach is also worth considering. Comprehensive early childhood and parenting programs that are targeted to or serve low-income families with depression may benefit from designing and evaluating enhancements that offer income, employment, and housing support as a possible means to increase their effectiveness in this vulnerable population.

Families with Co-occurring Conditions

As described in this report, families with depression are more vulnerable to potential adverse outcomes when there is a co-occurrence of such conditions as substance abuse, trauma, child abuse, family conflict, and domestic violence. Although these coexisting risk factors are likely to play a role in the effectiveness of many of the interventions discussed in this chapter, there is very limited rigorous evidence to examine how these factors interact with parental depression in approaches to preventing adverse outcomes in children.

In the area of substance abuse, for example, there are programs that take a family-based approach to prevention of substance abuse in children and adolescents, such as the Strengthening Families Program (Spoth et al., 2002; Spoth, Redmond, and Shin, 2001). This is a highly regarded, evidence-based, family skills training program, but it is not targeted at families with parents with substance abuse or co-occurring depression. In addition, the relative effectiveness for such families is not known, although there is some indication that the intervention works equally well in high-risk and low-risk families, based on a broad measure of risk that includes internalizing symptoms in parents (Guyll et al., 2004; Spoth et al., 2006). Several substance abuse prevention programs are specifically targeted to children growing up in homes in which caregivers have substance use disorders. For example, Alateen is a program for children of alcoholics based on the Alcoholics Anonymous 12-Step Program of Recovery, which has been widely adopted. However, at the present time, very few evaluation data on the effectiveness of Alateen are available. In general, a review of the prevention and intervention programs targeted to children of caregivers with alcohol or substance use disorders showed that they have not received enough rigorous evaluation to demonstrate prevention or reduction in alcohol or drug use consumption (Emshoff and Price, 1999), and there are no data on the relative effectiveness for families also coping with depression in the parents.

As described in Chapter 6, residential substance abuse programs for women and their children, such as those that are part of the Boston Public Health Commission and PROTOTYPES, take comprehensive, innovative approaches with potential for addressing the overlapping challenges of substance abuse, depression, and trauma (see Box 6-2). Although rigorous data for child outcomes are not available, the two-generation approach that includes treatment interventions for the parent, parenting training, and preventive interventions for the children is a formula that warrants attention for further evaluation and as an informative model for the design of other intervention programs.

Cultural and Linguistic Competence and Adaptation in Design and Implementation of Prevention Interventions

The availability of culturally and linguistically appropriate interventions is an important element in addressing disparities in attention to depression in vulnerable populations. The discussion of issues of engagement and barriers to care in Chapter 6 applies as well to preventive interventions as it does for treatment.

A crucial component in the effective implementation of programs to prevent the adverse outcomes of depression in vulnerable families is the cultural and linguistic appropriateness of the design and delivery of interventions to serve diverse populations. Van Vorhees and colleagues conducted a systematic review of the literature to identify modifiable mechanisms and effective interventions for the prevention of depression in the health care setting at the system, community, provider, and individual patient level (Van Voorhees et al., 2007; see also Chapter 6). From their review of the limited number of studies that examined potential effects of preventive interventions for adult depression on disparities, Van Vorhees and colleagues concluded that adapting standard preventive interventions to enhance cultural relevance to Hispanics (Muñoz et al., 1995), African Americans (Napholz, 2005; Phillips, 2000), and American Indians (Manson and Brenneman, 1995) showed promising results. Similarly, many of the interventions described in this chapter, particularly those targeted to early childhood, were evaluated primarily in minority populations, and thus have demonstrated effectiveness in these groups.

In other cases, such as the Family Talk Intervention, trials subsequent to the pilot study have focused on culturally specific adaptations for new populations. As described earlier, the Family Talk Intervention was adapted for use with inner-city, single-parent, minority families with positive results (Podorefsky, McDonald-Dowdell, and Beardslee, 2001). The intervention approach has also been recently adapted for use with Hispanic clients, and a manual for the conduct of the intervention in Spanish has been developed. The modifications include delivering the intervention both in English and Spanish, a focus on acculturation stress and the immigration experience as well as depression, flexibility in delivering the sessions, and careful attention to treating the families with respect. An open trial involving nine families with pre- and postassessment receiving the clinician-centered intervention has shown that it is safe and feasible and led to significant changes in behaviors and attitudes toward the illness. The families also had high scores on a standard self-report rating of the parents' therapeutic alliance with the therapist providing the intervention (D'Angelo et al., 2009).

Future work on interventions to serve families with depression can also draw on the example of successfully adapted interventions in related domains. For example, Beeber, Perreira, and Schwartz (2008) have adapted an intervention to increase social support for low-income mothers, including recently immigrated Latina women. The Incredible Years, a parenting program described earlier in this chapter, can also serve as an informative model for successful wide adaptation of a parenting intervention.

PREVENTION APPROACHES IN COMMUNITY SETTINGS

Community and faith-based organizations may offer an important setting for education and other prevention programs for families with depression, especially in some minority communities. In many rural and low-income communities, churches are the primary institutions of social support, and community settings may offer the most promise for access to needed interventions. However, there are important questions about capacity and whether organizations in these settings have the knowledge, education, and skilled staff necessary to implement programs.

Schools have been a more common setting for preventive interventions for children, including some parenting and family-focused interventions (National Research Council and Institute of Medicine, 2009). However, with the exception of the parenting interventions described above, few programs have been evaluated in school settings that target children of depressed parents in their program design or program evaluation.

The Internet offers an emerging opportunity to deliver interventions to families, as described in Chapter 6. Web-based perinatal and postpartum depression interventions, for example, can be accessible in ways that make them well suited for the needs of expectant and new mothers. Although web-based programs and support sites are becoming available, there is very little evaluation of the effectiveness of these efforts. In one example, a pilot, randomized controlled trial is currently under way to evaluate a web-based version of the *Mamás y Bebés*/Mothers and Babies course, a cognitive-behavioral and psychoeducational intervention for prevention of postpartum depression (Muñoz et al., 2007; University of California, San Francisco, 2008).

The lack of high-quality research interventions in community settings is a major research gap. This gap could be addressed by more studies to examine the capacity for delivering interventions in these settings; to evaluate the implementation of existing evidence-based interventions not previously delivered in these settings; and to evaluate the effectiveness of programs already in place that have not been evaluated, taking into account that different measures are used to estimate depression in different community-based programs, which may lead to differences in the populations that are targeted and in outcomes.

RESEARCH GAPS

More research is needed on the prevention of adverse outcomes in families with depressed parents. Although there is preliminary support for interventions that prevent adverse effects for depressed parents and their children, most of these approaches need further evaluation, replication, and longitudinal studies before widespread implementation is warranted. Many of these studies target only a particular area (e.g., parenting or child development), and only a limited number of interventions have targeted both parents and their children. Additional research is needed to further support these existing preventive interventions for families with depressed parents. For the programs and practices that have already been found to be most promising in randomized trials, larger scale effectiveness studies and implementation and dissemination trials need to be pursued.

In addition, there is a need to develop new interventions targeted at the comprehensive needs of families with depression as well as adaptations or enrichments of more broad intervention approaches to enhance their effectiveness in these families. Because families with parental depression may present with depression as the primary problem or as part of a constellation of risk factors, more research is needed on identifying, engaging, and providing appropriate preventive interventions to such families not only in mental health services but in the variety of settings in which they may seek services. This is particularly relevant to low-income and ethnic-minority populations given that they are at increased risk for depression but are less likely to seek mental health services (Aguilar-Gaxiola et al., 2008).

Although these targeted approaches are likely to be most promising, more evidence is also needed to determine whether universal programs focused on wellness and mental health promotion can lead to reductions in depression in parents and the subsequent adverse effects in children.

The following types of programs need more research with attention to depression in parents:

- programs targeted at preventing depression in parents with children at all developmental stages;
- prevention programs targeted at improving parenting;
- prevention programs targeted at enhancing protective factors and reducing risk in children;
- multigenerational and multicomponent programs;
- prevention programs in settings in which families with depression and their children are readily accessed, such as schools and communities; and
- policy and social welfare interventions and other broad-based programs targeted at vulnerable families and children.

In all of these programmatic approaches, prevention research for families with parental depression needs to incorporate three major principles: (1) recognition and treatment of parental depression, (2) enhancement and support for parenting, and (3) a focus on the developmental outcomes of children.

A number of areas of focus are needed in these research efforts. First, programs designed to assist children when parents are depressed need to focus not only on symptoms and diagnoses in children but also on strength-based strategies that help them accomplish appropriate developmental tasks (staying in school, relationships, acquiring skills). In addition, intervention research is needed that can serve to identify the characteristics of parenting by depressed parents that is of sufficient quality (e.g., sufficient levels of warmth and structure) to reduce adverse outcomes in children.

For evidence-based preventive intervention strategies and prevention-focused service programs that are not specifically targeted to depressed families, future research needs to consider parental depression in intervention design, assess depression in families, and track outcomes in families with depression as a subgroup in their evaluations. Whenever possible, these interventions should examine effects on parental depression, on parenting, and on child outcomes. Additional research is also needed on the effectiveness of including specific intervention components to enrich the overall program for depressed parents. This research will elucidate how the effects of these interventions differ in families with depression and what adaptations or enhancements are needed to maximize the effectiveness of interventions for them.

Although attention to prevention is warranted for children of depressed parents at all developmental stages, because of the rapid course of brain development during the first 5 years of life, increased focus is needed on evaluations and implementation trials of interventions during this stage of development. This can include interventions in pregnancy and the postpartum period, parent-child interaction interventions in infancy and early childhood, home visitation, and early childhood education.

Finally, given the considerable evidence about the social determinants of health in general and its effects on parental depression in particular, it is important that intervention research to address depression in parents should assess relative effectiveness in low-income families, families in high-risk neighborhoods, families with unstable housing, and families from varied cultural and linguistic backgrounds as well as adaptations or enhancements to target these vulnerable populations. In addition, it is important to consider the effectiveness and possible adaptations or enhancements of interventions in families with co-occurring conditions, such as marital conflict, domestic violence, and exposure to trauma and coexisting mental and substance abuse disorders. Even when interventions are not designed to address these populations, population and socioeconomic demographics should be clearly reported so that studies can be placed in the proper context, the amount of risk properly assessed, and analyses of relative effectiveness in high-risk subpopulations conducted. Trials are also needed of specific ways to offer identification, outreach, engagement, and treatment and prevention services to vulnerable families who face multiple risks. This research will help elucidate the need to address these interrelated factors to successfully intervene to prevent and treat depression and improve parenting and child outcomes as well as the need to make other interventions for these vulnerable families more successful.

CONCLUSION

Given the high prevalence of depression in parents and the evidence for the effects of depression on parenting quality and on child outcomes, there is a pressing need to maximize the ability to improve outcomes for both depressed parents and their children. Approaches are needed that not only offer treatment of depression in the parent but also support parenting and healthy child development. The most effective prevention strategies are therefore likely to be those that incorporate multiple components and target both generations.

This conceptual basis has preliminary support from a small number of interventions that have targeted families with depressed parents and have demonstrated promise for improving outcomes for these families in at least one randomized trial (summarized in Table 7-1). They include interventions that prevent or improve depression in the parent, those that target the vulnerabilities of children of depressed parents, and those that improve parent-child relationships and parenting practices.

In some promising interventions, a two-generation approach is used to target both the parents and their children, and in some cases treatment of the parent has been combined with interventions targeted at parenting or child development. However, the data from most of these interventions designed for families with depression are limited, with mixed results for some intervention approaches, a limited number of trials, small sample sizes, a lack of outcome measures for both the parent and the child, and little longitudinal follow-up to demonstrate sustained effects.

There is, however, a broader and more robust evidence base for preventive interventions to support families and the healthy development of children, which has been reviewed in detail elsewhere (National Research Council and Institute of Medicine, 2009). Multiple safe and effective interventions are currently available that are targeted more generally at improving parent-child relations, teaching parenting skills, or supporting the healthy development of children. These interventions (or elements of these interventions) have the potential to be incorporated into multiple settings and to serve multiple populations across development, from pregnancy through childhood and adolescence.

Few of these broader prevention interventions specifically address families with depression. Nonetheless, these broadly robust prevention strategies hold promise for families with depression because, given the high prevalence of depression in parents, most prevention strategies that have been shown to be effective were evaluated in a population that probably included families with depression, even if there was no assessment of parents' mental health status.

Several approaches described in this chapter, both those targeted to families with parental depression and those more broadly targeted to prevention interventions, have already been demonstrated to be safe and effective. Therefore, they stand ready for evaluations to determine whether selected components of these interventions, in combination with approaches to identify and treat depression in parents, can be effective when delivered in a variety of real-world service settings as part of integrated, two-generation approaches to meet the needs of families with a depressed parent.

TABLE 7-1 Examples of Interventions Specifically Targeted to
Depression in Parents

Intervention	Description	Citation	Population and Demographics	Setting
Prevention of Parents' Depression				
ROSE Program (Reach Out, Stand Strong, Essentials for New Mothers)	Interpersonal psychotherapy-based group intervention	Zlotnick et al. (2001, 2006)	Nondepressed pregnant women with at least one risk factor for depression (assessed by risk survey)	Prenatal clinic
	Four weekly 60-minute group sessions delivered during pregnancy. Second trial included a 50-minute booster session after delivery		First trial n = 35 Age: 23.4 (mean) Race/ethnicity: 46% Caucasian 54% Non-Caucasian SES: Receiving public assistance Single-parent: 77% Exclusion/inclusion criteria not reported	
			Second trial n = 99 Age: 22.4 (mean) Race/ethnicity: 28% Caucasian 44% Hispanic 17% African American 2% Asian 8% Other SES: Receiving public assistance Single-parent: 67% Excluded: Substance abuse disorder; any current mental health treatment	

Parent Outcomes	Parenting Outcomes	Child Outcomes	Follow-up Time	Research Method
Fewer episodes of major depression at 3 months' postpartum (diagnosed by SCI-D)	Not assessed	Not assessed	3 months	Randomized trials

continued

TABLE 7-1 Continued

Intervention	Description	Citation	Population and Demographics	Setting
Peer support	Individualized telephone-based peer-support intervention Minimum of four peer-support phone sessions starting at 2 weeks' postpartum delivered by peer volunteers who had recovered from postpartum depression	Dennis et al. (2009)	Nondepressed women in the first 2 weeks' postpartum at high risk for depression (EPDS > 9) n = 701 Age: <20 – >35 (range) Race/ethnicity: 81% Canadian; 19% Other SES: Mixed Single-parent: 8% Excluded: Non-English speaking; currently taking antidepressant or antipsychotic medications	Telephone-based (Identified in standard postpartum care in seven health regions in Canada)
Infant Sleep	Behavior-modification program to improve infant sleep One-time consultation delivered by well-child nurses to mothers at infant ages 8 months to develop individualized sleep management plan with one follow-up visit after 2 weeks	Hiscock et al. (2007, 2008)	Mothers reporting a problem with their infants' sleep at 7 months n = 49 centers and 328 mother/infant pairs Age (mothers): 33 (mean) Age (children): 8 months Race/ethnicity: Not reported SES: Mixed low, middle, and high Single-parent: 3% Excluded: Non-English speaking	Maternal and Child Health centers in Australia

Parent Outcomes	Parenting Outcomes	Child Outcomes	Follow-up Time	Research Method
Fewer mothers with EPDS scores consistent with postpartum depression (EPDS > 12)	Not assessed	Not assessed	12 weeks	Randomized trial
Lower levels of depression symptoms (mean EPDS scores) at infant's age 10 months, 12 months, and 2 years Lower rates of EPDS scores consistent with postpartum depression (using EPDS > 9 and EPDS ≥ 13) at age 2 years	No differences in parenting practices	Reduced infant sleep problems at ages 10 months and 12 months; sleep problems resolved in both groups at age 2 years No differences in child mental health	2 months, 4 months, and 18 months	Randomized trial (randomized at center level)

continued

TABLE 7-1 Continued

Intervention	Description	Citation	Population and Demographics	Setting
Treatment of Parents' Depression				
STAR*D: Pharmacological treatment	Assessment of children of depressed mothers participating in a trial of pharmacological treatment for depression	Pilowsky et al. (2008) Weissman et al. (2006)	Depressed mothers participating in a treatment trial and their children n = 151 mother/child pairs entered in study n = 123 mother/child pairs completed child assessments during 1 year of follow-up Age (mothers): 37.7 (mean); 24–52 (range) Age (children): 11.7 years (mean); 6–17 years (range) Race/ethnicity: 37% African American 42% White 18% Hispanic 3% Other SES: Mixed but with a large proportion of low-income Single-parent: 56% Excluded: Adults with bipolar disorder, schizophrenia, or schizoaffective disorders; adults with any medical condition contraindicating one of the study medications	Primary care and psychiatric outpatient clinics

Parent Outcomes	Parenting Outcomes	Child Outcomes	Follow-up Time	Research Method
33% of mothers had remission of depression (HRSD ≤ 7) by 3 months and 57% by 1 year	Not assessed	32% of children had current DSM-IV diagnosis at baseline At 3 months: Larger decrease in children's diagnoses (K-SADS) and symptoms (CBCL) for mothers whose depression remitted; higher levels of maternal response to treatment (% change on HRSD compared to baseline) were associated with larger decrease in rates of children's diagnoses and symptoms At 1 year: Larger decrease in children's symptoms (K-SADS) for mothers whose depression remitted; during the year following initiation of maternal treatment, decreases in children's psychiatric symptoms (K-SADS) were associated with decreases in maternal depression severity (HRSD)	3 months' intervals up to 1 year	Ancillary study of a randomized trial

continued

TABLE 7-1 Continued

Intervention	Description	Citation	Population and Demographics	Setting
Treatment of dysthymia	Assessment of children of parents participating in a trial of pharmacotherapy, interpersonal psychotherapy, or a combination for treatment of dysthymia	Browne et al. (2002) Byrne et al. (2006)	Parents with dysthymia participating in a treatment trial and their children n = 353 children entered in study at baseline n = 145 parents and 260 children with assessments at 2-year follow-up Age (parents): 41.1 (mean) Age (children): 10.3 years (mean); 4–16 years (range) Race/ethnicity: Not reported SES: Mixed Single-parent: 22.1% Excluded: Acute suicide risk; bipolar disorder; schizophrenia or any psychotic disorder; clinically significant and unstable medical conditions	Suburban primary care group practice in Canada

Parent Outcomes	Parenting Outcomes	Child Outcomes	Follow-up Time	Research Method
66.9% of parents responded to treatment (≥ 40% reduction in baseline depressive symptoms on MADRS)	Not assessed	Improved emotional and behavioral symptoms (CBCL) in children whose parents responded to treatment	2 years	Ancillary study of a randomized trial

continued

TABLE 7-1 Continued

Intervention	Description	Citation	Population and Demographics	Setting
Psychological treatment of postpartum depression	Comparison of 3 psychological treatments (nondirective counseling, cognitive-behavioral therapy, psychodynamic therapy) or routine primary care Weekly therapy from 8 to 18 weeks' postpartum	Cooper et al. (2003) Murray et al. (2003)	Depressed postpartum women after their first pregnancy and their children n = 190 mother/child pairs <u>Age (mothers):</u> 27.7 (mean); 17–42 (range) <u>Race/ethnicity:</u> Not reported <u>SES:</u> Mixed; 21% high social disadvantage <u>Single-parent:</u> 12% <u>Excluded:</u> Premature delivery; congenital abnormality; English not first language	Home visits

Parent Outcomes	Parenting Outcomes	Child Outcomes	Follow-up Time	Research Method
Improved maternal mood with all three treatments at 4.5 months' postpartum (EPDS) Reduced rate of depression diagnosis (increased rate of remission) at 4.5 months with psycho-dynamic therapy (SCI-D); effects not maintained; no benefit of any treatment after 9 months' postpartum	Reduced maternal reports of early difficulties in relationships with infants with all three treatments at 4.5 months (maternal self-report scale) More sensitive early mother-infant relations with nondirective counseling in mothers with high social adversity at 4.5 months (global rating scale assessment of videotaped interactions) No persistent impact on parent-child relationship or behavioral management at 5 years	Better infant emotional and behavioral rating at 18 months with nondirective counseling (BSQ) No persistent impact on childhood attachment and cognitive outcomes at 5 years	4.5, 9, and 18 months and 5 years	Randomized trial

continued

TABLE 7-1 Continued

Intervention	Description	Citation	Population and Demographics	Setting
Psychological treatment of postpartum depression	Interpersonal psychotherapy Weekly 1-hour sessions for 12 weeks	Forman et al. (2007) O'Hara et al. (2000)	Depressed postpartum women and their children n = 120 Age (mothers): 29.6 (mean) Age (infants): 6 months Race/ethnicity: Predominantly White SES: Not reported Single-parent: 0% Excluded: Single parent; psychotic depression; history of bipolar disorder, schizophrenia, organic brain syndrome, mental retardation, or antisocial personality disorder; current diagnosis of alcohol or substance abuse, panic disorder, somatization disorder, 3 or more schizo-typal features, serious eating disorder, or obsessive-compulsive disorders	Clinic

Interventions for Children of Depressed Parents

Group CBT	Group cognitive-behavioral preventive intervention for youth at high risk of depression 15 1-hour group sessions delivered by master's-level therapist	Clarke et al. (2001)	Children of depressed parents (current episode or past 12 months) with subdiagnostic depressive symptoms (symptoms insufficient to meet DSM-III-R diagnostic criteria or CESD > 24) n = 94 Age (parent): 41.4 (mean) Age (children): 14.6 years (mean); 13–18 years (range) Race/ethnicity: not reported SES: Not reported Single-parent: 35% Excluded: Current and past psychiatric disorders were not excluded.	HMO clinic

Parent Outcomes	Parenting Outcomes	Child Outcomes	Follow-up Time	Research Method
Greater decrease in depressive symptoms (HRSD and BDI) Greater rate of remission (HRSD ≤ 6; BDI ≤ 9; no longer meeting DSM-IV criteria for major depressive disorder)	No impact on parent-child relationship Reduced parental stress, but treated depressed mothers still had higher levels of parental stress than nondepressed mothers (PSI)	No impact on child outcomes	12 weeks (all outcomes) and 18 months (parenting and child outcomes)	Randomized trial
Not assessed	Not assessed	Fewer symptoms of depression (CESD) Lower rate of major depression diagnoses at 12 months (K-SADS-E); this effect diminished by 24 months	2 years	Randomized trial

continued

TABLE 7-1 Continued

Intervention	Description	Citation	Population and Demographics	Setting
Interventions Targeted to Parent–Child Relationship or Parenting Skills				
Interaction Coaching for At-risk Parents (ICAP)	Coached behavioral intervention to promote maternal-infant responsiveness as an addition to home visiting services Three home visits took place between ages 4–18 weeks	Horowitz et al. (2001)	Mothers with depressive symptoms (EPDS ≥ 10) and their infants n = 117 Age (mothers): 31 (mean); 17–41 (range) Age (children): 4–8 weeks (range) Race/ethnicity: 68.9% European American or White 7.4% African American or Black 7.4% Latina or Hispanic 7.4% Mixed background 4% Other 3.3% Asian or Pacific Islander 1.6% Native American SES: Mixed Single-parent: Not reported Excluded: Not reported	Home visitation
Mother-baby interaction	Mother-baby intervention delivered by master's-level home visitors with training in prevention or health education Program components: modeling of parenting; cognitive restructuring; practical pedagogical support; and infant massage 8–10 home visits lasting 60–90 minutes on average	Van Doesum et al. (2008)	Depressed mothers receiving outpatient treatment and their infant children n = 71 Age (mothers): 30 years (mean) Age (children): 5.5 months (mean); 1–12 months (range) Race/ethnicity: 85% Dutch (Caucasian) 11% Other (Turkish, Moroccan, Surinamese, Portuguese, Australian) SES: Mixed Single-parent: 8% Excluded: Psychotic disorder; manic depression; substance dependence	Home visitation

Parent Outcomes	Parenting Outcomes	Child Outcomes	Follow-up Time	Research Method
No difference in level of depressive symptoms (decreased equally in intervention group and control group) (BDI-II)	Improved maternal-infant responsiveness (Dyadic Mutuality Code)	Not assessed	10 weeks	Randomized trial
No difference in level of depressive symptoms (decreased equally in intervention group and control group) (BDI)	Improved maternal-infant interaction, for four dimensions: maternal sensitivity, maternal structuring, child responsiveness, child involvement (EAS)	Improved attachment security (AQS) and socioemotional competence; no difference on externalizing, internalizing, or dysregulation measures (ITSEA)	6 months	Randomized trial

continued

TABLE 7-1 Continued

Intervention	Description	Citation	Population and Demographics	Setting
Mother's Assessment of the Behavior of her Infant (MABI)	Weekly assessments of infant's behavior by the mother for 1 month	Hart, Field, and Nearing (1998)	Depressed mothers (CESD ≥ 16) and their newborn infants n = 27 Age (mothers): 21.6 (mean); 15–30 (range) Age (children): Newborn Race/ethnicity: 68% Hispanic 30% African American 2% White SES: Low income Single-parent: Not reported Excluded: Not reported	Mothers trained in hospital maternity unit followed by use of assessment instrument at home
Parent-child focused comprehensive program	Multicomponent intervention delivered over 3 months Intervention included day care for the infants; social, educational, and vocational programs for the mothers; mood induction interventions for the mothers; infant massage therapy; and mother-infant interaction coaching	Field et al. (2000)	Adolescent mothers with depressive symptoms selected based on predictor variables and their infants; predictor variables: low interaction scores and elevated norepinephrine, serotonin, and cortisol at neonatal stage; increased right frontal EEG and low vagal tone at 3 months' postpartum n = 160 mother/infant pairs (96 selected for randomization) Age (mothers): 17.3 (mean) Age (children): 3 months Race/ethnicity: 60.9% African American 24.3% Hispanic 14.8% Non-Hispanic White SES: Low income Single-parent: Not reported Excluded: Not reported	Public vocational high school

Parent Outcomes	Parenting Outcomes	Child Outcomes	Follow-up Time	Research Method
No effect on maternal depression (CESD)	Not assessed	Improvements in social interaction and state organization (Neonatal Behavioural Assessment Scale)	1 month	Randomized trial
Reduced depressive symptoms at 6 and 12 months' postpartum (BDI)	Improved parent-child interactions (Interaction Rating Scale) at post-intervention.	Improved infant development at 6 and 12 months (Bayley Mental and Motor); improved responding and initiating at 12 months (Early Social Communication Scales)	6 months' (to 12 months' post-partum)	Randomized trial

continued

TABLE 7-1 Continued

Intervention	Description	Citation	Population and Demographics	Setting
Toddler-parent psychotherapy (TPP)	Joint therapy sessions for mothers and their toddlers to improve the mother-child interaction and maternal responsivity Average of 45 sessions delivered over an average of 58 weeks	Cicchetti, Toth, and Rogosch (2004) Toth et al. (2006)	Mothers with at least one major depressive episode since the birth of their toddler n = 130 Age (mothers): 31.68 (mean); 21–41 (range) Age (children): 20.34 months (mean) Race/ethnicity: 92.9% European American SES: Middle to high Single-parent: 12.1% Excluded: Bipolar disorder; low socioeconomic status	Research university

Interventions That Combine Components for Treating Parents, Improving Parenting, and/or Supporting Child Development

Intervention	Description	Citation	Population and Demographics	Setting
CBT family intervention	Cognitive therapy strategies to treat depression integrated with teaching of parenting skills compared with a behavioral family intervention for treatment of oppositional and disruptive behavior in children 12 weekly sessions delivered by trained therapists	Sanders and McFarland (2000)	Families with depressed mothers (DSM-IV diagnosis) and children with conduct disorder or oppositional-defiant disorder n = 47 Age (parents): 34.3 years (mean) Age (children): 4.39 years (mean); 3–9 years (range) Race/ethnicity: Not reported SES: Mixed Single-parent: 32% Excluded: Not reported	8 clinic sessions and 4 feedback sessions delivered in homes

Parent Outcomes	Parenting Outcomes	Child Outcomes	Follow-up Time	Research Method
No effect on mothers' depression	Not assessed	More secure attachment (strange situation)	To age 3 years	Randomized trial
At 6 months: better maintenance of reduced depressive symptoms (BDI); greater concurrent change in depressive symptoms (BDI) amd child disruptive behavior (PDR)	No difference between groups	At 6 months: greater concurrent change in child disruptive behavior (PDR) maternal depressive symptoms (BDI)	6 months	Randomized trial

continued

Intervention	Description	Citation	Population and Demographics	Setting
Family Talk Intervention	7-session (average) clinician-facilitated family intervention for parents and their children delivered by licensed social workers or clinical psychologists compared to 2-session lecture group discussion with parents	Beardslee et al. (1997, 2003, 2007)	Parents with a history of depression and their children Pilot families plus first trial families plus additional families combined for long-term follow-up: n = 105 families <u>Age (parents):</u> 43 (mean) <u>Age (children):</u> 12 years (mean); 8–15 years (range) <u>Race/ethnicity:</u> Predominantly White <u>SES:</u> Predominantly middle-class <u>Single-parent:</u> 19% <u>Excluded:</u> Parents acutely psychotic, acutely abusing substances, or in the midst of a divorce; or marital crisis. Children acutely depressed or with a history of depression; other psychiatric diagnoses not excluded	Most families recruited from HMO or referred from mental health providers
Family Talk Intervention	Adaptation of Family Talk Intervention for single, minority mothers	Podorefsky, McDonald-McDowdell, and Beardslee (2001)	Parents with a history of depression and their children n = 16 families <u>Age (parents):</u> Not reported <u>Age (children):</u> Not reported <u>Race/ethnicity:</u> 100% minority <u>SES:</u> Predominantly low-income <u>Single-parent:</u> 100% <u>Excluded:</u> Not reported	Most families recruited from health and community centers

Parent Outcomes	Parenting Outcomes	Child Outcomes	Follow-up Time	Research Method
Changes in parents' behaviors and attitudes toward their depression (interview ratings)	Increased family communication and parental attention to children's experience (interview ratings)	Increased understanding of parents' depression (interview ratings)	4.5 years	Randomized trials
Changes in parents' behaviors and report of global benefit of intervention (interview ratings)	Increased parental attention to children (interview ratings)		Post-intervention	Randomized trial

continued

Intervention	Description	Citation	Population and Demographics	Setting
Parenting and child coping skills	Cognitive-behavioral intervention; parenting skills training for parents and teaching children skills to cope with their parents' depression	Compas, Forehand, and Keller (presented at the Society for Research on Child Development in 2009)	Depressed parents (current or history of during the lifetime of their child) and their children n = 111 families (155 children) Age (parents): 42.8 (mean) Age (children): 11.4 years (mean); 9–15 years (range) Race/ethnicity: 79% European American 7.7% African American 3.2% Asian American 1.3% Hispanic 7.7% Mixed ethnicity SES: Mixed with high levels of low-income families Single-parent: 36% Excluded: Parent with history of bipolar I, schizophrenia, or schizoaffective disorder; children with history of autism spectrum disorders, mental retardation, bipolar I disorder or schizophrenia or who met criteria for conduct disorder or substance/alcohol abuse or dependence	Academic research setting

NOTES: The committee did not seek to systematically identify every study on existing interventions and program evaluations that target families with a depressed parent or that illustrate important conceptual principles for addressing these needs of these families; instead, whenever possible, the committee drew on existing meta-analyses and systematic reviews and whenever possible reviewed interventions that have been evaluated in at least one randomized trial. All outcomes reported in table are statistically significant.

AQS = Attachment Q Sort Version 3; BSQ = Behavioral Screening Questionnaire; BSID = Bailey Scale of Infant Development; BDI = Beck Depression Inventory; CBCL = Child Behavior Checklist; CBT = cognitive-behavioral therapy; CESD = Center for Epidemiologic Studies Depression Scale; DSM-IV = *Diagnostic and Statistical Manual of Mental Disorders*, fourth edition; EAS = Emotional Availability Scale, Infancy to Early Childhood Version; EEG = electroencephalogram; EPDS = Edinburgh Postnatal Depression Scale; HMO = health maintenance organization; HRSD = Hamilton Rating Scale for Depression; ITSEA = Infant Toddler Social and Emotional Assessment; KSADS = Kiddie-Schedule for Affective Disorders and Schizophrenia; KSADS-E = K-SADS, Epidemiological Version; MADRS = Montgomery Asberg Depression Rating Scale; PDR = Parent Daily Report; PSI = Parenting Stress Index; SCI-D = Structured Clinical Interview for DSM-IV; SES = socioeconomic status.

Parent Outcomes	Parenting Outcomes	Child Outcomes	Follow-up Time	Research Method
Reduced depressive symptoms at 2 months (BDI-II); not sustained at 6 or 12 months	Not assessed	At 12 months: improved children's self-reports of depressive symptoms and other internalizing and externalizing problems (CESD and Youth Self-Report); improved parents' reports of adolescents' externalizing symptoms (CBCL)	12 months	Randomized trial

REFERENCES

Administration for Children and Families. (2002). *Making a Difference in the Lives of Children and Families: The Impacts of Early Head Start Programs on Infants and Toddlers and Their Families.* Washington, DC: U.S. Department of Health and Human Services.

Agency for Healthcare Research and Quality. (2008). *Group Visits Focused on Prenatal Care and Parenting Improve Birth Outcomes and Provider Efficiency.* Available: http://www.innovations.ahrq.gov/content.aspx?id=1909 [accessed April 14, 2009].

Aguilar-Gaxiola, S., Elliott, K., Deeb-Sossa, N., King, R.T., Magaña, C.G., Miller, E., Sala, M., Sribney, W.M., and Breslau, J. (2008). *Engaging the Underserved: Personal Accounts of Communities on Mental Health Needs for Prevention and Early Intervention Strategies.* Sacramento: University of California, Davis Health System.

Altfeld, S. (2003). *The Chicago Doula Project Evaluation Final Report.* Chicago, IL: Ounce of Prevention Fund.

Barlow, J., Coren, E., and Stewart-Brown, S. (2008). Parenting-training programmes for improving maternal psychosocial health. *Cochrane Database of Systematic Reviews*, Art. No. CD002020.

Battle, C.L., and Zlotnick, C. (2005). Prevention of postpartum depression. *Psychiatric Annals, 35*, 590–598.

Baydar, N., Reid, M.J., and Webster-Stratton, C. (2003). The role of mental health factors and program engagement in the effectiveness of a preventive parenting program for Head Start mothers. *Child Development, 74*, 1433–1453.

Bayer, J.K., Hiscock, H., Hampton, A., and Wake, M. (2007). Sleep problems in young infants and maternal mental and physical health. *Journal of Paediatric and Child Health, 43*, 66–73.

Beardslee, W.R., and Podorefsky, D. (1988). Resilient adolescents whose parents have serious affective and other psychiatric disorders: Importance of self-understanding and relationships. *American Journal of Psychiatry, 145*, 63–69.

Beardslee, W.R., Gladstone, T.R., Wright, E.J., and Cooper, A.B. (2003). A family-based approach to the prevention of depressive symptoms in children at risk: Evidence of parental and child change. *Pediatrics, 112*, e119–e131.

Beardslee, W.R., Hosman, C., Solantaus, T., van Doesum, K., and Cowling, V. (in press). Children of mentally ill parents: An opportunity for effective prevention all too often neglected. In C. Hosman, E. Jane-Llopis, and S. Saxena (Eds.). *Prevention of Mental Disorders: Effective Interventions and Policy Options.* Oxford, England: Oxford University Press.

Beardslee, W.R., Salt, P., Versage, E.M., Gladstone, T.R., Wright, E.J., and Rothberg, P.C. (1997). Sustained change in parents receiving preventive interventions for families with depression. *American Journal of Psychiatry, 154*, 510–515.

Beardslee, W.R., Wright, E.J., Gladstone, T.R.G., and Forbes, P. (2007). Long-term effects from a randomized trial of two public health preventive interventions for parental depression. *Journal of Family Psychology, 21*, 703–713.

Beeber, L.S., Perreira, K.M., and Schwartz, T. (2008). Supporting the mental health of mothers raising children in poverty. *Annals of the New York Academy of Sciences, 1136*, 86–100.

Bodnar, L.M., and Wisner, K. (2005). Nutrition and depression: Implications for improving mental health among childbearing aged women. *Society of Biological Psychiatry, 58*, 679–685.

Browne, G., Steiner, M., Roberts, J., Gafni, A., Byrne, C., Dunn, E., Bell, B., Mills, M., Chalklin, L., Wallik, D., and Kraemer, J. (2002). Sertraline and/or interpersonal psychotherapy for patients with dysthymic disorder in primary care: 6-month comparison with longitudinal 2-year follow-up of effectiveness and costs. *Journal of Affective Disorders*, 68, 317–330.

Brugha, T.S., Wheatly, S., Taub, N.A., Culverwell, A., Freidman, T., Kirwan, P., Jones, D.R., and Shapiro, D.A. (2000). Pragmatic randomized trial of antenatal intervention to prevent postnatal depression by reducing psychosocial risk factors. *Psychological Medicine*, 30, 1273–1281.

Byrne, C., Bwone, G., Roberts, J., Mills, M., Bell, B., Gafni, A., Jamieson, E., and Webb, M. (2006). Changes in children's behavior and costs for service use associated with parents' response to treatment for dysthymia. *Journal of the American Academy of Child and Adolescent Psychiatry*, 45, 239–246.

Chazan-Cohen, R., Ayoub, C., Pan, B.A., Roggman, L., Raikes, H., McKelvey, L., Whiteside-Mansell, L., and Hart, A. (2007). It takes time: Impacts of Early Head Start that lead to reductions in maternal depression two years later. *Infant Mental Health Journal*, 28, 151–170.

Cicchetti, D., Rogosch, F.A., and Toth, S.L. (2000). The efficacy of toddler-parent psychotherapy for fostering cognitive development in offspring of depressed mothers. *Journal of Abnormal Child Psychology*, 28, 135–148.

Cicchetti, D., Toth, S.L., and Rogosch, F.A. (1999). The efficacy of toddler-parent psychotherapy to increase attachment security in off-spring of depressed mothers. *Attachment and Human Development*, 1, 34–66.

Cicchetti, D., Toth, S.L., and Rogosch, F.A. (2004). Toddler-parent psychotherapy for depressed mothers and their offspring: Implications for attachment theory. In L. Atkinson and S. Goldberg (Eds.), *Attachment Issues in Psychopathology and Intervention* (pp. 229–275). Philadelphia: Lawrence Erlbaum Associates.

Clapp, J.F. (2002). *Exercising Through Your Pregnancy*. Omaha, Nebraska: Addicus Books.

Clarke, G.N., Hawkins, W., Murphy, M., Sheeber, L.B., Lewinsohn, P.M., and Seeley, J.R. (1995). Targeted prevention of unipolar depressive disorder in an at-risk sample of high school adolescents: A randomized trial of a group cognitive intervention. *Journal of the American Academy of Child and Adolescent Psychiatry*, 34, 312–321.

Clarke, G.N., Hornbrook, M., Lynch, F., Polen, M., Gale, J., Beardslee, W., O'Connor, E., and Seeley, J. (2001). A randomized trial of a group cognitive intervention for preventing depression in adolescent offspring of depressed parents. *Archives of General Psychiatry*, 58, 1127–1134.

Compas, B.E., Forehand, R., and Keller, G. (2009). *Cognitive-Behavioral Prevention in Families of Depressed Parents: 12-Month Outcomes of a Randomized Trial*. Paper presented at the biannual meeting of the Society for Research on Child Development, Denver, CO.

Compas, B.E., Keller, G., and Forehand, R. (in press). Preventive intervention in families of depressed parents: A family cognitive-behavioral intervention. In T.J. Strauman, P.R. Costanzo, J. Garber, and L.Y. Abramson (Eds.), *Preventing Depression in Adolescent Girls: A Multidisciplinary Approach*. New York: Guilford Press.

Cooper, P.J., Murray, L., Wilson, A., and Romaniuk, H. (2003). Controlled trial of the short- and long-term effect of psychological treatment of post-partum depression. I. Impact on maternal mood. *British Journal of Psychiatry*, 182, 412–419.

Cuijpers, P., van Straten, A., Smit, F., Mihalopoulos, C., and Beekman, A. (2008). Preventing the onset of depressive disorders: A meta-analytic review of psychological interventions. *American Journal of Psychiatry*, 165, 1272–1280.

Cunningham, C.E., Bremner, R., and Boyle, M. (1995). Large group community-based parenting programs for families of preschoolers at risk for disruptive behaviour disorders: Utilization, cost-effectiveness, and outcome. *Journal of Child Psychology and Psychiatry and Allied Disciplines*, 36, 1141–1159.

D'Angelo, E.J., Llerena-Quinn, R., Shapiro, R., Colon, F., Rodriguez, P., Gallagher, K., and Beardslee, W.R. (2009). Adaptation of the preventive intervention program for depression for use with predominantly low-income Latino families. *Family Process, 48,* 260–291.

DeGarmo, D.S., Patterson, G.R., and Forgatch, M.S. (2004). How do outcomes in a specified parent training intervention maintain or wane over time? *Prevention Science, 5,* 73–89.

Dennis, C.-L. (2005). Psychosocial and psychological interventions for prevention of postnatal depression: Systematic review. *British Medical Journal, 331,* 15–22.

Dennis, C.-L., and Creedy, D. (2004). Psychosocial and psychological interventions for preventing postpartum depression. *Cochrane Database of Systematic Reviews,* Art. No. CD001134.

Dennis, C.-L., Hodnett, E., Kenton, L., Weston, J., Zupancic, J., Stewart, D.E., and Kiss, A. (2009). Effect of peer support on prevention of postnatal depression among high risk women: Multisite randomized controlled trial. *British Medical Journal, 338,* 280–284.

Emshoff, J.G., and Price, A.W. (1999). Prevention and intervention strategies with children of alcoholics. *Pediatrics, 103,* 1112–1121.

Epps, S.R., and Huston, A.C. (2007). Effects of a poverty intervention policy demonstration on parenting and child behavior: A test of the direction of effects. *Social Science Quarterly, 88,* 344–365.

Field, T., Grizzle, N., Scafidi, F., Abrams, S., Richardson, S., Kuhn, C., and Schanberg, S. (1996). Massage therapy for infants of depressed mothers. *Infant Behavior and Development, 19,* 107–112.

Field, T., Pickens, J., Prodromidis, M., Malphurs, J., Fox, N., Bendell, D., Yando, R., Schanberg, S., and Kuhn, C. (2000). Targeting adolescent mothers with depressive symptoms for early intervention. *Adolescence, 35,* 381–414.

Forman, D.R., O'Hara, M.W., Stuart, S., Gorman, L.L., Larsen, K.E., and Coy, K.C. (2007). Effective treatment for postpartum depression is not sufficient to improve the developing mother-child relationship. *Developmental Psychopathology, 19,* 585–602.

Garber, J., Clarke, G.N., Brent, D.A., Beardslee, W.R., Weersing, R., Gladstone, T.R.G., Debar, L., D'Angelo, E.J., and Hollon, S. (2007). *Preventing Depression in At-Risk Adolescents: Rationale, Design, and Preliminary Results.* Symposium 48, American Academy of Child and Adolescent Psychiatry, 54th Annual Meeting, Boston, MA.

Garber, J., Clarke, G.N., Weersing, V.R., Beardslee, W.R., Brent, D.A., Gladstone, T.R.G., DeBar, L.L., Lynch, F.L., D'Angelo, E., Hollon, S.D., Shamseddeen, W., and Iyengar, S. (2009). Prevention of depression in at-risk adolescents: A randomized controlled trial. *Journal of the American Medical Association, 301,* 2215–2224.

Gennetian, L.A., and Miller, C. (2002). Children and welfare reform: A view from an experimental welfare program in Minnesota. *Child Development, 73,* 601–620.

Greaves, D. (1997). The effect of rational-emotive parent education on the stress of mothers of children with Down Syndrome. *Journal of Rational-Emotive and Cognitive Therapy, 15,* 249–267.

Gross, D., Fogg, L., and Tucker, S. (1995). The efficacy of parent training for promoting positive parent-toddler relationships. *Research in Nursing and Health, 18,* 489–499.

Gunlicks, M.L., and Weissman, M.M. (2008). Change in child psychopathology with improvement in parental depression: A systematic review. *Journal of the American Academy of Child and Adolescent Psychiatry, 47,* 379–389.

Guyll, M., Spoth, R.L., Chao, W., Wickrama, K.A., and Russell, D. (2004). Family-focused preventive interventions: Evaluating parental risk moderation of substance use trajectories. *Journal of Family Psychology, 18,* 293–301.

Hagan, R., Evans, S.F., and Pope, S. (2004). Preventing postnatal depression in mothers of very preterm infants: A randomized controlled trial. *BJOG: An International Journal of Obstetrics and Gynaecology, 111,* 641–647.

Hart, S., Field, T., and Nearing, G. (1998). Depressed mothers' neonates improve following the MABI and a Brazelton demonstration. *Journal of Pediatric Psychology, 23*, 351–356.

Hiscock, H., Bayer, J., Gold, L., Hampton, A., Ukoumunne, O.C., and Wake, M. (2007). Improving infant sleep and maternal mental health: A cluster randomised trial. *Archives of Disease in Childhood, 92*, 952–958.

Hiscock, H., Bayer, J.K., Hampton, A., Ukoumunne, O.C., and Wake, M. (2008). Long-term mother and child mental health effects of a population-based infant sleep intervention: Cluster-randomized, controlled trial. *Pediatrics, 122*, e621–e627.

Honikman, J. (2002). *I'm Listening: A Guide to Supporting Postpartum Families*. Santa Barbara, CA: Studio E Books.

Horowitz, J.A., Bell, M., Trybulski, J., Munro, B.H., Moser, D., Hartz, S.A., McCordic, L., and Sokol, E.S. (2001). Promoting responsiveness between mothers with depressive symptoms and their infants. *Journal of Nursing Scholarship, 33*, 323–329.

Huston, A.C., McLoyd, V.C., Weisner, T.S., Duncan, G.J., Crosby, D.A., and Ripke, M.N. (2005). Impacts on children of a policy to promote employment and reduce poverty for low-income parents: New hope after 5 years. *Developmental Psychology, 41*, 902–918.

Ickovics, J.R., Kershaw, T.S., Wesdahl, C., Magriples, U., Massey, Z., Reynolds, H., and Rising, S.S. (2007). Group prenatal care and perinatal outcomes: A randomized controlled trial. *Obstetrics and Gynecology, 110*, 330–339.

Institute of Medicine. (1994). *Reducing Risks for Mental Disorders: Frontiers for Preventive Intervention Research*. P.J. Mrazek and R.J. Haggerty (Eds.). Washington, DC: National Academy Press.

Irvine, A.B., Biglan, A., Smolkowski, K., Metzler, C.W., and Ary, D.V. (1999). The effectiveness of parenting skills program for parents of middle school students in small communities. *Journal of Consulting and Clinical Psychology, 67*, 811–825.

Jacobs, F., Easterbrooks, M.A., Brady, A., and Mistry, J. (2005). *Healthy Families Massachusetts: Final Evaluation Report*. Medford, MA: Tufts University.

Jarrett, R., and Burton, L. (1999). Dynamic dimensions of family structure in low-income African American families: Emergent themes in qualitative research. *Journal of Comparative Family Studies, 30*, 177–187.

Jaser, S.S., Fear, J.M., Reeslund, K.L., Champion, J.E. Reising, M.M., and Compas, B.E. (in press). Maternal sadness and adolescents' responses to stress in offspring of mothers with and without a history of depression. *Journal of Clinical Child and Adolescent Psychology*.

Jaser, S.S., Langrock, A.M., Keller, G., Merchant, M.J., Benson, M.A., Reeslund, K.L., Champion, J.E., and Compas, B.E. (2005). Coping with the stress of parental depression II: Adolescent and parent reports of coping and adjustment. *Journal of Clinical Child and Adolescent Psychology, 34*, 193–205.

Kaminski, J.W., Valle, L.A., Filene, J.H., and Boyle, C.L. (2008). A meta-analytic review of components associated with parent training program effectiveness. *Journal of Abnormal Child Psychology, 36*, 567–589.

Kling, J.R., Liebman, J.B., and Katz, L.F. (2007). Experimental analysis of neighborhood effects. *Econometrica, 75*, 83–119.

Kling, J.R., Liebman, J.B., Katz, L.F., and Sanbonmatsu, L. (2004). *Moving to Opportunity and Tranquility: Neighborhood Effects on Adult Economic Self-Sufficiency and Health from a Randomized Housing Voucher Experiment*. (John F. Kennedy School of Government Working Paper No. RWPO4-035.) Cambridge, MA: Harvard University.

Langrock, A.M., Compas, B.E., Keller, G., Merchant, M.J., and Copeland, M.E. (2002). Coping with the stress of parental depression: Parents' reports of children's coping, emotional, and behavioral problems. *Journal of Clinical Child and Adolescent Psychology, 31*, 312–324.

Lieberman, A.F., Weston, D.R., and Pawl, J.H. (1991). Preventive intervention and outcome with anxiously attached dyads. *Child Development*, 62, 199–209.

Lumley, J., Watson, L., Small, R., Brown, S., Mitchell, C., and Gunn, J. (2006). PRISM (Program of Resources, Information and Support for Mothers): A community-randomized trial to reduce depression and improve women's physical health six months after birth. *BMC Public Health*, 6, 37.

Malphurs, J.E., Field, T.M., Larraine, C., Pickens, J., Pelaez-Nogueras, M., Yando, R., and Bendell, D. (1996). Altering withdrawn and intrusive interaction behaviors of depressed mothers. *Infant Mental Health Journal*, 17, 152–160.

Manson, S.M., and Brenneman, D.L. (1995). Chronic disease among older American Indians: Preventing depressive symptoms and related problems of coping. In D.K. Padgett (Ed.), *Handbook on Ethnicity, Aging, and Mental Health* (pp. 284–303). Westport, CT: Greenwood Press.

McGillicuddy, N.B., Rychtarik, R.G., Duquette, J.A., and Morsheimer, T. (2001). Development of a skill training program for parents of substance-abusing adolescents. *Journal of Substance Abuse Treatment*, 20, 59–68.

Miller, C., Huston, A.C., Duncan, G.J., McLoyd, V.C., and Weisner, T.S. (2008). *New Hope for the Working Poor: Effects After Eight Years for Families and Children*. New York: MDRC.

Morris, P., Duncan, G.J., and Clark-Kauffman, E. (2005). Child well-being in an era of welfare reform: The sensitivity of transitions in development to policy change. *Developmental Psychology*, 41, 919–932.

Muñoz, R.F., Le, H.N., Ghosh-Ippen, C., Diaz, M.A., Urizar, G., Soto, J., Mendelson, T., Delucchi, K., and Lieberman, A.F. (2007). Prevention of postpartum depression in low-income women: Development of the *Mamás y Bebés*/Mothers and Babies course. *Cognitive Behavioral Practice*, 14, 70–83.

Muñoz, R.F., Ying, Y.W., Bernal, G., Perez-Stable, E.J., Sorensen, J.L., Hargreaves, W.A., Miranda, J., and Miller, L.S. (1995). Prevention of depression with primary care patients: A randomized controlled trial. *American Journal of Community Psychology*, 23, 199–222.

Murray, L., Cooper, P.J., Wilson, A., and Romaniuk, H. (2003). Controlled trial of the short- and long-term effect of psychological treatment of post-partum depression: 2. Impact on the mother-child relationship and child outcome. *British Journal of Psychiatry*, 182, 420–427.

Napholz, L. (2005). An effectiveness trial to increase psychological well-being and reduce stress among African American blue-collar working women. In K.V. Oxington (Ed.), *Psychology of Stress* (pp. 17–34). Hauppauge, NY: Nova.

National Research Council and Institute of Medicine. (1999). *Revisiting Home Visiting: Summary of a Workshop*. N.G. Margie and D.A. Phillips (Eds.). Washington, DC: National Academy Press.

National Research Council and Institute of Medicine. (2009). *Preventing Mental, Emotional, and Behavioral Disorders Among Young People: Progress and Possibilities*. Committee on Prevention of Mental Disorders and Substance Abuse Among Children, Youth, and Young Adults: Research Advances and Promising Interventions. M.E. O'Connell, T. Boat, and K.E. Warner (Eds.). Board on Children, Youth, and Families, Division of Behavioral and Social Sciences and Education. Washington, DC: The National Academies Press.

Nelson, G., Westhues, A., and MacLeod, J. (2003). A meta-analysis of longitudinal research on preschool prevention programs for children. *Prevention and Treatment*, 6(3), Art. D31a.

Nixon, C.D., and Singer, G.H.S. (1993). Group cognitive-behavioral treatment for excessive parental self-blame and guilt. *American Journal on Mental Retardation*, 97, 665–672.

O'Hara, M.W., Stuart, S., Gorman, L., and Wenzel, A. (2000). Efficacy of interpersonal psychotherapy for postpartum depression. *Archives of General Psychiatry*, 57, 1039–1045.

Patterson, J., Barlow, J., Mockford, C., Klimes, I., Pyper, C., and Stewart-Brown, S. (2002). Improving mental health through parenting programmes: Block randomized controlled trial. *Archives of Disease in Childhood*, 87, 472–477.

Pelaez-Nogueras, M., Field, T.M., Hossain, Z., and Pickens, J. (1996). Depressed mothers' touching increases infants' positive affect and attention in still-face interactions. *Child Development*, 67, 1780–1792.

Phillips, R.S. (2000). Preventing depression: A program for African American elders with chronic pain. *Family and Community Health*, 22, 57–65.

Pilowsky, D.J., Wickramaratne, P.J., Talati, A., Tang, M., Hughes, C.W., and Garber J. (2008). Children of depressed mothers 1 year after the initiation of maternal treatment: Findings from the STAR*D-Child Study. *American Journal of Psychiatry*, 165, 1136–1147.

Pisterman, S., Firestone, P., McGrath, P., Goodman, J.T., Webster, I., Mallory, R., and Goffin, B. (1992). The effects of parent training on parenting stress and sense of competence. *Canadian Journal of Behavioural Science*, 24, 41–58.

Podorefsky, D.L., McDonald-Dowdell, M., and Beardslee, W.R. (2001). Adaptation of preventive interventions for a low-income, culturally diverse community. *Journal of the American Academy of Child and Adolescent Psychiatry*, 40, 879–886.

Priest, S., Henderson, J., Evans, S., and Hagan, R. (2003). Stress debriefing after childbirth: A randomized controlled trial. *Medical Journal of Australia*, 178, 542–545.

Quint, J.C., Bos, J.M., and Polit, D.F. (1997). *New Chance: Final Report on a Comprehensive Program for Young Mothers in Poverty and Their Children*. New York: MDRC.

Reid, M.J., Webster-Stratton, C., and Baydar, N. (2004). Halting the development of conduct problems in head start children: The effects of parent training. *Journal of Clinical Child and Adolescent Psychology*, 33, 279–291.

Reyno, S.M., and McGrath, P.G. (2006). Predictors of parent training efficacy for child externalizing behavior problems—A meta-analytic review. *Journal of Child Psychology and Psychiatry*, 47, 99–111.

Robert Wood Johnson Foundation. (2008). *Chicago Project Delivers Support to Young Mothers-to-Be*. Grant Results Report. Available: http://www.rwjf.org/pr/product.jsp?id=18096 [accessed April 16, 2009].

Sanders, M.F., and McFarland, M. (2000). Treatment of depressed mothers with disruptive children: A controlled evaluation of cognitive behavioural family intervention. *Behaviour Therapy*, 31, 89–112.

Sanders, M.R. (1999). Triple P-Positive Parenting Program: Towards an empirically validated multilevel parenting and family support strategy for the prevention of behavior and emotional programs in children. *Clinical Child and Family Psychology Review*, 2, 71–90.

Scott, M.J., and Stradling, S.G. (1987). Evaluation of a group programme for parents of problem children. *Behavioral Psychotherapy*, 15, 224–239.

Shaw, E., Levitt, C., Wong, S., and Kaczorowski, J. (2006). Systematic review of the literature on postpartum care: Effectiveness of postpartum support to improve maternal parenting, mental health, quality of life, and physical health. *Birth*, 33, 210–220.

Sheeber, L.B., and Johnson, J.H. (1994). Evaluation of a temperament-focused, parent-training program. *Journal of Clinical Child Psychology*, 23, 249–259.

Solantaus, T., and Toikka, S. (2006). The Effective Family Programme: Preventative services for the children of mentally ill parents in Finland. *International Journal of Mental Health Promotion*, 8, 37–43.

Spoth, R.L., Redmond, C., and Shin, C. (2001). Randomized trial of brief family interventions for general populations: Adolescent substance use outcomes 4 years following baseline. *Journal of Consulting and Clinical Psychology*, 69, 627–642.

Spoth, R.L., Redmond, C., Trudeau, L., and Shin, C. (2002). Longitudinal substance initiation outcomes for a universal preventive intervention combining family and school programs. *Psychology of Addictive Behaviors*, 16, 129–134.

Spoth, R., Shin, C., Guyll, M., Redmond, C., and Azevedo, K. (2006). Universality of effects: An examination of the comparability of long-term family intervention effects on substance use across risk-related subgroups. *Prevention Science, 7*, 209–224.

Sweet, M.A., and Appelbaum, M.I. (2004). Is home visiting an effective strategy? A meta-analytic review of home visiting programs for families with young children. *Child Development, 75*, 1435–1456.

Talati, A., Wickramaratne, P.J., Pilowsky, D.J., Alpert, J.E., Cerda, G., Garber, J., Hughes, C.W., King, C.A., Malloy, E., Sood, A.B., Verdeli, H., Trivedi, M.H., Rush A.J., and Weissman, M.M. (2007). Remission of maternal depression and child symptoms among single mothers. *Social Psychiatry and Psychiatric Epidemiology, 42*, 962–971.

Taylor, T.K., Schmidt, F., Pepler, D., and Hodgins, C.A. (1998). A comparison of eclectic treatment with Webster-Stratton's parents and children series in a children's mental health center: A randomized controlled trial. *Behavior Therapy, 29*, 221–240.

Tonge, B., Brereton, A., Kiomall, M., Mackinnon, A., King, N., and Rinehart, N. (2006). Effects on parental mental health of an education and skills training program for parents of young children with autism: A randomized controlled trial. *Journal of the American Academy of Child and Adolescent Psychiatry, 45*, 561–569.

Toth, S.L., Rogosch, F.A., Manly, J.T., and Cicchetti, D. (2006). The efficacy of toddler-parent psychotherapy to reorganize attachment in the young offspring of mothers with major depressive disorder: A randomized preventive trial. *Journal of Consulting and Clinical Psychology, 74*, 1006–1016.

University of California, San Francisco. (2008). *Mother and Babies Internet Project.* Available: http://HealthyPregnancy.ucsf.edu [accessed April 22, 2009].

van Doesum, K.T.M., Riksen-Walraven, J.M., Hosman, C.M.H., and Hoefnagels, C. (2008). A randomized controlled trial of a home-visiting intervention aimed at preventing relationship problems in depressed mothers and their infants. *Child Development, 79*, 547–561.

Van Voorhees, B.W., Walters, A.E., Prochaska, M., and Quinn, M.T. (2007). Reducing health disparities in depressive disorders outcomes between non-Hispanic whites and ethnic minorities: A call for pragmatic strategies over the life course. *Medical Care Research and Review, 64*.

Verduyn, C., Barrowclough, C., Roberts, J., Tarrier, T., and Harrington, R. (2003). Maternal depression and child behaviour problems. Randomised placebo-controlled trial of a cognitive-behavioural group intervention. *British Journal of Psychiatry, 183*, 342–348.

Webster-Stratton, C. (1998). Preventing conduct problems in Head Start children: Strengthening parenting competencies. *Journal of Consulting and Clinical Psychology, 66*, 715–730.

Webster-Stratton, C., Reid, M., and Hammond, M. (2001). Preventing conduct problems, promoting social competence: A parent and teacher partnership in Head Start. *Journal of Clinical Child Psychology, 30*, 283–302.

Weissman, M.M., Alpert, J.E., Fava, M., Trivedi, M.H., and Rush, A.J. (2006). Remission of maternal depression and children's psychopathology. *Journal of the American Medical Association, 296*, 1233–1234.

Zaslow, M.J., and Eldred, C.A. (1998). *Parenting Behavior in a Sample of Young Mothers in Poverty: Results of the New Chance Observational Study.* New York: MDRC.

Zlotnick, C., Johnson, S.L., Miller, I.W., Pearlstein, T., and Howard, M. (2001). Postpartum depression in women receiving public assistance: Pilot study of an interpersonal-therapy-oriented group intervention. *American Journal of Psychiatry, 158*, 638–640.

Zlotnick, C., Miller, I.W., Pearlstein, T., Howard, M., and Sweeney, P. (2006). A preventive intervention for pregnant women on public assistance at risk for postpartum depression. *American Journal of Psychiatry, 163*, 1443–1445.

8

Working from the Present to the Future: Lessons Learned from Current Practice

SUMMARY

- Clues emerging from the current research base point to an ideal evidence-based program for the identification, treatment, and prevention of depression among adults would integrate mental and physical health services. For those who are parents, it would strengthen and support parent-child relationships, offer developmentally appropriate treatment and prevention interventions for children, and provide comprehensive resources and referrals for other comorbidities associated with depression in multiple health care settings, including those that engage young children and families. Furthermore, this system of care would utilize more proactive approaches for prevention or early intervention of depression in parents in the context of a two-generation model and would be family-focused, culturally informed, and accessible to vulnerable populations.
- The existing health care and social services systems are far from implementing the ideal system of care for depressed adults and parents. Early efforts in the adoption, implementation, integration, and dissemination of various components of evidence-based depression care programs offer insight into the future development of key features of such an ideal system.

Quality Improvement Interventions

- Studies of interventions intended to improve the quality of the design and organization of primary care services for treating adults with depression have resulted in improved outcomes—including quality of care, individual clinical outcomes, cost-effectiveness, and employment status. The implementation of these interventions offers important lessons in designing new approaches for depressed parents.

Adding a Parent-Child Dimension

- Adding a parent-child dimension to adult depression care requires linkages of a range of services and systems integrated across a diverse range of settings.
- Existing exemplary strategies in individual service settings—primary care, home visitation, early childhood and parenting training programs, schools, the criminal justice system, and community-wide programs—offer important lessons regarding the challenges faced in implementing such strategies for depressed parents and their outcomes.

Federal-Level Initiatives

- Federal efforts in the identification, treatment, and prevention of depression among parents and its effects on children focus primarily on maternal depression that occurs during pregnancy or the postpartum period. Current efforts are scattered across several agencies in the U.S. Department of Health and Human Services and include data collection, health education, treatment, prevention, workforce development, and other research activities.

State-Level Initiatives

- A few state-level initiatives have developed and implemented strategies focused on the needs of depressed parents and their children—particularly targeted to women and other vulnerable populations. These initiatives have focused on the training of service providers, expanding access to screening and services, and promoting public awareness to help reduce the stigma associated with mental health disorders.

European Interventions

- Several system-wide, collaborative, and interdisciplinary approaches to preventive care in children of the mentally ill—using prevention professionals, master trainers, and family-oriented prevention interventions—and often specific to depression have been developed, implemented, and disseminated in a few European countries.

Supported by the research presented in the previous chapters, the long-term goal should be that evidence-based programs offer services for the identification, treatment, and prevention of depression among adults and would be available in multiple health care settings. These settings would integrate mental and physical health services, and for those who are parents, also strive to strengthen and support parent-child relationships during therapeutic treatment, offer developmentally appropriate treatment and preventive interventions for children and other family members, and provide comprehensive resources and referrals for other comorbidities that might be associated with the parent's depression (such as substance use, unemployment, unstable housing). Ideally, more proactive approaches to prevention and early intervention in depressed parents would also be available in multiple settings that engage young children and families, such as child care centers, home visitation programs, family support programs, and school-based programs. These treatment, prevention, and proactive approaches would be family-focused, culturally informed, and accessible to vulnerable populations, which often have difficulty in navigating transitions among health care, mental health, and community-based programs, and they would help overcome barriers to access to needed care. These interventions would emphasize the importance of treating depression in the context of a two-generation model, helping parents improve their parenting skills while coping with depression, and also offering enhanced supports for children who may be at risk of mental, emotional, and behavioral disorders because of a depressed parent.

Existing health care and social services systems are far from achieving this goal and realizing the vision of fully integrated two-generational programs. Yet initial efforts offer important clues in a variety of service settings regarding the nature, scope, quality, and costs of the development of key features of this ideal. These clues provide valuable guidance about the types of models that deserve further support and experimentation in building integrated, comprehensive, and two-generation service strategies to treat and prevent depression among parents and to mitigate its effects on their children.

This chapter begins with an overview of selected research studies associated with quality improvement efforts in the treatment of adult depression. Although few of these studies have focused on the parenting aspects of this disorder, they offer important insights into the types of enhancements that generate treatment effectiveness and improved outcomes for individual adult patients. Next, the chapter reviews major issues related to the adoption, implementation, integration, and dissemination of evidence-based depression care programs specifically for parents with depression and their children across a wide range of health care and other service settings. The chapter then reviews current federal initiatives intended to bolster the knowledge base to help develop programs and policies that enhance the response to depression among parents and early interventions for children. The final sections of this chapter examine different models of depression interventions for parents that have emerged in selected states as well as Europe. These models offer distinctive approaches to integrating health care and family-focused interventions with an explicit focus on identification, prevention, treatment, and expanded access for vulnerable populations. The chapter concludes with a set of recommendations that could advance the knowledge base associated with the design, experimentation, and implementation of different service models.

QUALITY IMPROVEMENT INTERVENTIONS AND THE TREATMENT OF ADULT DEPRESSION

A significant body of research has emerged demonstrating that despite the availability of evidence-based interventions and practice guidelines, the outcomes of adult patients with depression remain poor in primary care settings (Schoenbaum et al., 2001). These findings have prompted a search for improvements in the design and organization of primary care services, frequently evaluated through studies of quality improvement (QI), clinical effectiveness, and health care services research. Such studies have shown that certain quality improvement efforts—for example, the Partners in Care (PIC) model, which adds specialized training programs and resources in practice-based settings or the Improving Mood-Promoting Access to Collaborative Treatment (IMPACT), which includes a collaborative care model using a primary care physician, a care manager, a mental health specialist, consistent measurement, and stepped care treatment—have resulted in better outcomes as measured by improved quality of care, quality of life, clinical outcomes, and retention in employment over a 1-year follow-up (Schoenbaum et al., 2001; Unützer et al., 2002; Wells et al., 2000).

The QI interventions for the PIC model increased health care costs (compared with usual care). Such average increases were $419 for QI-meds and $485 for QI-therapy. However, the societal cost-effectiveness of such increases was comparable to other accepted medical interventions. The long-term cost-effectiveness of implementing the IMPACT model (for depression care later in life) lowered the mean total health care costs during 4 years compared with usual care (87 percent probability) (Unützer et al., 2008). The PIC and IMPACT evaluation studies have therefore demonstrated that QI efforts are feasible and cost-effective and can be implemented in "naturalistic" practice-based settings. Follow-up studies confirmed these findings for minorities and whites as well as for those with both depressive disorder and subthreshold depression.

The QI studies have reported cumulative prevention and treatment benefits beyond the short-term outcomes, especially for minorities. For example, comparison studies with usual care have demonstrated improvements in 5-year and 9-year outcomes after a 6-month intervention with the PIC model described above, including improved employment status (Wells et al., 2000); they also reduced stressful life events, equivalent to removing 6–12 deaths of a loved one over a 9-year interval (Sherbourne et al., 2008; Wells et al., 2005). Greater outcome improvements were reported for underserved minorities than whites (Miranda et al., 2003).

QI programs have also been successfully adapted to a variety of settings, populations, and those with co-occurring disorders. For example, the IMPACT model has been implemented in eight different health care systems (e.g., health maintenance organizations, fee for service, inner-city county hospitals, Veterans Administration clinics) and has been tested in African Americans, Latinos, and white patients. It has been tested as well in patients with and without comorbid medical illnesses (like diabetes and cancer) or anxiety disorders and in adults of all ages as well as adolescents (University of Washington, 2009). In all of these settings, populations, and conditions in which IMPACT has been adapted and implemented, it has been shown to be more effective in depression care than usual care (Ell et al., 2008; Grypma et al., 2006; Kinder et al., 2006; Richardson, McCauley, and Katon, 2009).

Although these QI programs focus on primary care settings, they should not be viewed as just health care interventions. Starting with patients who are receiving care in primary care settings, they then add a systems approach that often includes mental health specialists or outreach workers who can extend the program beyond primary care. The QI programs also adopt a user-friendly approach, supporting patient education and preferences in the choice of medications or therapeutic interventions, thus increasing the chances that patients will get the intervention they prefer (Dwight-Johnson et al., 2001).

It is important to note, however, that the existing QI studies do not differentiate outcomes based on the parental status of the individual adult patient. Nor do they address outcomes beyond those observed in the care setting or in assessing individual health and employment status. A significant opportunity exists, therefore, to identify and assess the impact of QI interventions (such as PIC and IMPACT) on adults who are parents of children of various ages. These assessments could examine outcomes associated with QI effects on parenting practices, parent-child relationships, and child outcomes. Such studies would need to disentangle multiple factors, however, such as the changes in parent-child relationships that might be attributable to improved health or improved employment, as well as the interactions among them.

ADDING A PARENT-CHILD DIMENSION TO DEPRESSION CARE INTERVENTIONS

The research on quality improvement suggests that multiple opportunities exist to incorporate evidence-based practices that enhance positive outcomes from the treatment of adult depression. Experience with the implementation of quality improvement interventions thus offers important lessons in designing new approaches that could focus on strengthening parent-child relationships as well as clinical effectiveness in treatment settings. But adding and implementing an explicit focus on parenting and parent-child relationships to different forms of screening, prevention, and treatment models for adults who struggle with depression (which we collectively term as "depression care") require resolution of multiple challenges. Such interventions need to be multidisciplinary, to be developmentally oriented (e.g., pregnant women, first-time parents, parents with multiple children or blended families), to include a two-generation approach that could include services for children of varying ages, to be culturally appropriate, to have multiple points of access, and to offer patient-centered choices among evidence-based components (such as medication or cognitive-behavioral therapy). Since parental depression frequently occurs in the context of a constellation of comorbid medical and mental health conditions, as well as social and economic risk factors and concurrent circumstances, adjunctive interventions may be required in addition to treatment of the depression and parenting interventions.

The committee recognizes that many of the challenges faced in adding and implementing a parent-child dimension to depression care are similar to the challenges faced with the identification, treatment, and prevention of other mental heath and substance use disorders and health care in general as described in the 2006 Institute of Medicine report, *Improving Quality of Health Care for Mental and Substance-Use Conditions*. However, it is unclear (as well as out of the scope of the committee's task) if specifically incorporating a two-generation, developmentally oriented model of care for other mental health and substance abuse disorders, other chronic health diseases, and health in general is appropriate and requires further exploration. Still, potential models of care for parents with depression may need to bridge a range of services and systems and integrate across a diverse range of settings.

SPECIAL ISSUES BY SERVICE SETTING

Individual service settings offer further insight and important lessons regarding the challenges that deserve systematic attention in implementing innovative strategies to strengthen, identify, treat, and prevent depression and improve parenting practices and parent-child relationships for depressed adults who are parents and their children. This section reviews the experience with exemplary strategies in such settings, including primary care, home visitation, early childhood and parent training programs, schools, the criminal justice system, and community-wide models.

Primary Care

Primary care practices figure prominently in efforts to improve depression care. Many of the more carefully crafted randomized controlled trials have focused on these practices as an important gateway to care (Dietrich et al., 2004; Katon et al., 2004; Wells et al., 2000). Although the evidence is fairly strong that integrated approaches through primary care can be effective in the management of depression (Gilbody et al., 2003, 2006; Minkovitz et al., 2007), there are many challenges in attempting to scale up these systems.

For physicians, time is a major constraint to adopting new roles and responsibilities. A number of studies have shown that practitioners may have difficulty making the time to effectively learn and reliably apply new practices (Horwitz et al., 2007; Olson et al., 2002; Østbye et al., 2005; Tai-Seale, McGuire, and Zhang, 2007). Although there is some contrary evidence (Cabana et al., 1999), the possibility of a ubiquitous time crunch is difficult to ignore, particularly as the body of applicable knowledge grows (Jones, 2009). When primary care physicians are asked, for example, to learn and apply new procedures for addressing depression among their patients, it may be hard for them to do so without considering the effect this will have on the overall learning they must do to stay up-to-date and preserve their self-image as a competent clinician as well as their ability to do their job.

In primary care settings, where most people encounter the health care system and are an important focus for screening and care for depressed parents, there are many competing demands (Stange et al., 1998). Depression inquiry, counseling, or treatment must compete with multiple clinician and patient priorities, such as treatment of acute illness, provision of preventive services, and response to patient requests (Klinkman, 1997). These competing demands make individual and organizational learning, as well as incorporation of evidence-based care, more difficult. For example, visits to family physicians typically involve more than three health care problems or conditions, and such visits may involve nearly five for people with chronic diseases (Beasley et al., 2004). Nearly one in five visits also includes concerns or care related to someone other than the primary patient (Flocke, Goodwin, and Stange, 1998). Although family medicine's capacity for caring for multiple family members is a benefit in dealing with depressed parents and their children, depression care innovations that do not explicitly take comorbidity and family members into account may be less easily integrated into practice.

Financial considerations are also likely to be an inhibitory factor in the assimilation and use of depression care models by primary care physicians, since most of these models appear to add to the gross costs of practice (e.g., for an integrated care manager) (Gilbody, Bower, and Whitty, 2006; Gilbody et al., 2003; Mattke, Seid, and Ma, 2007; Simon et al., 2001). Mental health care has been financially carved out of primary care by many payers over the past 20 years and remains so for many Medicaid programs (Horvitz-Lennon, Kilbourne, and Pincus, 2006). Where they still persist, mental health carve-outs remain a financial barrier to better depression screening and care in primary care by keeping the mental health sector and the general health sector systematically fragmented.

The frequent separation of care for adult parents (generally mothers) and their children in primary care settings may make implementation of new policies or tools related to parental depression effects for children more difficult. Some pediatricians do screen mothers for depression, especially in the first few months after delivering a baby. But others may feel that parents are not their patients, or they choose not to screen because they don't know how or have few options for referring parents for treatment. Pediatricians also lack tools for screening children for the effects of depression in parents since no validated tools currently exist. The American Academy of Pediatrics and the American College of Obstetrics and Gynecology encourage obstetricians/gynecologists to screen for maternal depression, particularly in the weeks after delivery (American Academy of Pediatrics and American College of Obstetrics and Gynecology, 2007). However, these providers may not consider infants and children as their patients, or like other primary care providers, may not know that children may need to be evaluated for effects of parental depression. Efforts to implement and disseminate new policies and tools to improve identification and treatment of children affected by parental depression will need to engage clinicians who care for both children and parents and help them understand the role they can play.

Although it has not been carefully examined yet as a solution to the problem of getting effective depression care to the people who need it, the conversion of family physician practices into "medical homes" for patients is an idea in good currency that might provide a way to reach a large proportion of the population who could benefit from such care (Freudenheim, *New York Times*, July 21, 2008; Sia et al., 2004; Starfield and Shi, 2004). Through this arrangement, a doctor assumes full responsibility for a patient's medical care, either providing it directly or coordinating access to it. The closer relationship that develops between doctor and patient as a result may increase the likelihood of depression being discussed or symptoms being disclosed (Starfield and Shi, 2004). When physicians receive additional compensation for functioning as a "medical home," they may also be able to hire more staff to help manage patient care. Physicians who serve as medical homes may thus develop greater interest and capacity to assimilate and use new developments in depression care.

Home Visitation

Home visitation programs for young families represent another possible avenue for the identification, treatment, and prevention of depression in parents. A number of home visitation models that serve high-risk populations have been widely implemented. These programs largely serve low-income, young mothers with few resources or social supports, a demographic group that tends not to use center-based services for themselves or their families. These families also experience high levels of associated risk factors, including histories of child maltreatment, domestic violence, and substance abuse.

Most home visitation programs include standardized assessments conducted by the home visitor for the purposes of determining eligibility for and level of services. Depression screens have been incorporated into routine assessments by several state-based home visiting programs (e.g., Ohio, Connecticut). Most home visitation program models perform some case management functions and rely on referrals to community services to provide specialized forms of care as necessary. Home visitation programs are therefore potentially able to screen and refer associated comorbidities, such as substance abuse, for appropriate services.

Home visitation programs are well positioned to address one of the missing elements in services for depressed and at-risk parents: child development and parenting training. Preliminary studies indicate that successful treatment of maternal depression is not sufficient to improve parenting and child outcomes in depressed mother-child dyads (Forman et al., 2007).

However, a small, randomized trial of a home visiting–based parenting intervention for depressed mothers demonstrated significant improvements in attachment security (as measured by the Attachment Q-Set), maternal sensitivity, and child socioemotional competence (van Doesum et al., 2008).

The Nurse-Family Partnership (NFP) has drawn a significant amount of attention and support owing to the high quality and persuasiveness of the evidence for its effectiveness on the basis of three, well-designed, randomized controlled trials and long-term findings (Isaacs, 2007; Karoly, Kilburn, and Cannon, 2005; Partnership for America's Economic Success, 2008). In this program, nurse home visitors are trained to screen first-time mothers for depression and to make appropriate referrals for treatment. Louisiana was one of the early adopters of the NFP model and has tested a supplemented version that couples nurse visitor teams with an infant mental health specialist, usually a social worker, to help identify and treat parental, mostly maternal, mental health issues (Boris et al., 2006). A consortium of local agencies in the Cincinnati area called Every Child Succeeds, which operates both the Nurse-Family Partnership and another home visiting program, Healthy Families America, have tested, with some success, the use of cognitive behavioral therapy with participating mothers diagnosed with depression (Ammerman et al., 2005).

Early Childhood and Parent Training Programs

A system with enormous potential for reaching parents with or at risk of depression is the array of programs and services that have taken shape to support the early development of children and parenting. By far the largest and most prominent of these programs is Head Start. Like many early childhood interventions, Head Start is designed to address the needs of children and, to some extent, their parents. In recent years, federal performance standards for Head Start have heavily emphasized the program's responsibility for readying children for school, with relatively less weight given to the program's role in helping and engaging parents.

This has been counterbalanced to some extent by the emergence of Early Head Start, a program for children from birth to age 3 years and their families. Early Head Start is actually a set of program options from which local Head Start agencies may choose: center-based care for children, home visiting for children and their families, or a combination of the two. Although initial findings from the 17-site randomized trial of Early Head Start did not show any impact on parental depression, more recent evidence suggests that the program may have had a delayed inoculatory effect (Chazan-Cohen et al., 2007). The downstream incidence of depression (i.e., delaying the impact on maternal depression) among parents in the treatment group has been significantly lower than those in the control condition.

Head Start, because of its size and sustained support and dissemination, would appear to be an attractive vehicle for reaching a large number of disadvantaged parents, but there are questions about the capability of local Head Start agencies to take on more responsibility. Even though Head Start is striving to improve the quality of local agency staff, the overall level of education and experience remains relatively low and turnover can be a problem (consistent with the general experience in early childhood education) (Barnett, 2002; Bryant et al., 1994; Currie and Neidell, 2007; Early et al., 2007; Gallagher and Clifford, 2000; Pai-Samant et al., 2005). Nor are the effects of staff quality on outcomes entirely clear (Currie and Niedell, 2007). Nonetheless, Head Start's 40 years of durability—a remarkable feat among nonentitlement social programs—makes it a credible target of opportunity for extending the reach of effective depression care.

Beardslee and colleagues (in press-a) have developed an adaptation of programs generally used in Head Start centers called Family Connections. Given that the rate of depression in parents of children attending these centers is high and in one Early Head Start study was 48 percent, Beardlee's approach is to provide education about depression and work closely in a staff development approach to increase teachers' competence in dealing with depression and related mental health difficulties in parents and children (Knitzer, Theberge, and Johnson, 2008). This approach was chosen because of the very high rates of depression noted in studies of parents in Head Start and Early Head Start. Given the high prevalence, Head Start and Early Head Start teachers encounter depression daily in the parents of children they deal with and undoubtedly also see the effects of depression in the children (Beardslee et al., in press-a). The core approach was to combine trainings in which all of the staff participated around key issues in mental health, such as how to engage difficult parents, how to build resilience in youngsters, and how to understand depression with onsite consultation over a 3-year period. The central goal of the program was to increase teachers' self-reflection and shared reflection and their understandings of how to take care of themselves. It also aimed to promote self-reflection and self care in parents. This approach was developed in partnership with Head Start providers in the Boston area, particularly Action for Boston Community Development. Working in a single site over 3 years, the investigators showed that the trainings were well received, as was the consultation model, and that in qualitative interviews with teachers and staff and assessor observation, substantial teacher growth occurred. Through this work, they have advanced the thesis that it is necessary to consider depression's impact at four levels: the individual level, the family level, the caregiving system level, and the community level. Correspondingly, it is necessary to identify resilience and strength and ways to cope with depression at each of these four levels.

Family Connections provides a consultant who works with teachers, children, and parents, with a primary focus on teachers' concerns to address depression and related adversities. This consultation is paired with staff group trainings about key issues in mental health: how to build resilience in the face of depression, what is depression, how to engage difficult parents, how to build resilience in parents and children in the face of depression, and the importance of self-reflection both for parents and teachers. The trainings are conducted by the consultant, who works in the center and is therefore able to address any concerns that a parent, teacher, or child may have and to apply the content of the trainings to everyday challenges. A set of materials for parents, teachers, and workshop leaders has been developed and includes brief documents for parents and teachers about the key issues as well as a workshop leader's guide to how to conduct trainings and lessons learned. These materials are available on the Head Start website to all Head Start centers (Avery et al., 2008). Initial evaluation of the approach shows that teachers value the training and consultation and report that it influences their practice; parents also report positive responses (Beardslee et al., in press-a).

In addition to Head Start, a variety of other evidence-based, family-focused programs have slowly been gaining wider application and are able to connect directly with vulnerable parents. Investigations show that well-designed parent training programs can reduce parental depression while also improving parenting skills (DeGarmo, Patterson, and Forgatch, 2004; Kaminski et al., 2008), at least for a period of time (Barlow, Coren, and Stewart-Brown, 2003). Even when such programs do not directly affect depression, they may still enable gains in parenting knowledge and ability (Baydar, Reid, and Webster-Stratton, 2003; Olds et al., 2003). Parent training is also part of the responsibility of the public child welfare system at the state and local levels. However, the quality of the training programs used by child welfare agencies varies widely, and there is little evidence on how effective even the higher quality programs are in practice (Barth et al., 2005).

School-Based Services

Schools offer the potential to provide integrated parent-child depression services, especially for teenage parents. Many schools have school nurses or nurse aids who could be trained to screen for depression (Centers for Disease Control and Prevention, 2006), but these and other school employees (i.e., school counselors) have a range of other duties. However, only a minority of schools have a school-based health clinic where additional capacity might be situated to deal with a range of identified mental health needs. Less than a fifth of these clinics report offering mental health services (Brener et al., 2007). By and large, schools do not actively engage in detecting, attempting to treat, or making efforts to prevent depression (Foster et al., 2005). Their approaches tend to be passive and reactive, and, to the extent that they respond to mental health situations, an orientation to short-term, crisis intervention appears to predominate (Foster et al., 2005).

Schools are a challenging environment for depression care for at least three reasons. First, schools are semi-closed systems, meaning that they are to a degree designed to be impervious to external influence (Ringeisen, Henderson, and Hoagwood, 2003). And they are not organized to address two-generation depression issues. Second, the work cultures of schools and mental health providers differ; the words and concepts they use and the outcomes on which they focus, while sharing some points of intersection, differ enough to make communication and collaboration difficult (Hoagwood and Johnson, 2003; Kutash, Duchnowski, and Lynn, 2006).

Third, even when cultural differences can be reconciled, trying to add work or change practices inside schools has been shown to require time-consuming and careful planning and extensive and often expensive support, to integrate new activities with the old (Gottfredson and Gottfredson, 2002). Programs and practices to improve mental health that cannot be readily integrated into the curriculum and what goes on in classrooms—that is, cannot be amalgamated with the core technology of schools—may stand little chance of broad and effective use (Hawkins et al., 1999; Hoagwood et al., 2007). Even when integration is possible, limited headway may be made without strong and consistent support from the school principal (Kam, Greenberg, and Walls, 2003; Ringwalt et al., 2003).

Criminal Justice System

Another possibility to consider involves organizations in the criminal justice system, given the disproportionate representation of persons with mental illness in county and state jails and prisons and the especially high rates of depression among incarcerated women (Kane-Mallik and Visher, 2008). The opportunity to infuse improvements in depression care into this system would seem beneficial for a couple of reasons. One is the slow but growing use of programs to divert low-risk and youthful offenders, including those with mental health problems, from incarceration into treatment programs (Steadman and Naples, 2005). Mental health courts have emerged in some jurisdictions to facilitate and support diversion (Boothroyd et al., 2005; Grudzinskas et al., 2005). In some cases, both mental health and regular courts have diverted youth into evidence-based treatments, such as multisystem therapy, functional family therapy, and treatment foster care (Cuellar, McReynolds, and Wasserman, 2006).

Another reason is the recently elevated policy interest in community reentry of offenders who have completed their sentences (e.g., P.L. 110-199, the Second Chance Act of 2007) (Conway and Hutson, 2007; Re-entry Policy Council, 2005). No actual system exists yet for this purpose. However, through mostly federal and philanthropic support, several reentry programs have been or are being tested. One notable, recently completed demonstration involved the use of small and medium-sized urban churches in partnership with local juvenile justice authorities and social service agencies (Bauldry, 2006; Bauldry and Hartmann, 2004; Branch, 2002). Although the churches were highly committed, they lacked the formal structures, staffing capabilities, and discipline needed to be effective without substantial and sustained amounts of training and technical assistance from outside experts. Interestingly enough, this research found that mentoring seemed to prevent depression among participating youth, although there were doubts that it would be as effective with already depressed youth (Bauldry, 2006).

It may be worth noting that the criminal justice system has been one of the more active arenas for the implementation of evidence-based practices and programs (Aos, Miller, and Drake, 2006; National Research Council, 2007). Research indicates that prisons may be more likely than jails and probation and parole offices to use evidence-based practices (Henderson, Taxman, and Young, 2008). And community-based organizations may be more likely than either prisons or jails to implement programs and practices of known effectiveness (Friedmann, Taxman, and Henderson, 2007).

In all cases, the experiences and beliefs of administrators have emerged as an important moderating factor (Friedmann, Taxman, and Henderson, 2007; Henderson, Taxman, and Young, 2008). There is also evidence that criminal justice organizations tend to implement clusters of complementary practices rather than one practice at a time (Henderson, Taxman, and Young, 2008). However, among evidence-based practices, developmentally appropriate and research-supported forms of treatment appear to be the least likely for criminal justice entities to use (Henderson, Taxman, and Young, 2008), perhaps because these do not fit neatly into their core social technology, namely, incarceration (Thompson, 1967). Evidently, most jails provide some form of mental health screening and are equipped to administer psychotropic medications (Soloman et al., 2008). Slightly under half offer mental health counseling, but only about a fourth help offenders find mental health services after they have been released (Soloman et al., 2008).

Community-Level Models

Although not specific to depression care, the Communities That Care model of local collaboration may turn out to be an effective means of mobilizing and sustaining support for evidence-based interventions. In this risk and protective factors approach, stakeholders come together to review data about youth problems in the community and then to select available evidence-based programs to address the problems they determine to be most salient (Hawkins, Catalano, and Associates, 1992). Early results from an ongoing randomized clinical trial show that communities using the model are experiencing greater reductions in youth problem behavior (Hawkins et al., 2008). Evaluation of implementation suggests some of the reasons why participating communities may be doing better than nonparticipating ones, but the methods used have not been robust or precise enough to link implementation activities causally to outcomes (Brown et al., 2007; Fagan et al., 2008). Nor has the cost-effectiveness of the Communities That Care approach been determined.

Surveys of community primary care and mental health providers have found that concurrent treatment of depressed patients is common in the community, but these treatments are less interactive and collaborative than the treatment models proven effective in randomized controlled trials. Researchers think that colocation of these providers would improve the collaboration and effectiveness (Valenstein et al., 1999). There are good real-world models of colocation and collaboration that work well (Druss et al., 2001); however, disseminating such models more broadly would require organizational and financial integration, as well as removal of policy barriers (Horvitz-Lennon, Kilbourne, and Pincus, 2006).

Collaboration seems applicable to the variety of integrated depression care models that have been evaluated. The evidence, though favorable, may be less persuasive because it is derived from clinical trial experience rather than real-world performance. Effect sizes demonstrate that collaborative care is significantly better than usual practice, but effects may be too narrowly targeted or may not rise to the level needed to compel adoption, other than among a minority of practitioners or organizations (Mattke, Seid, and Ma, 2007; Pfeffer and Sutton, 2006). Often with multisite trials, evidence is aggregated across sites, raising questions about whether some sites did notably better than others and thus leading to the possibility that unidentified factors may lie behind good performance (Rosenheck, 2001). Data on costs may be missing or incomplete or based on studies using samples that are not large enough to ensure validity (Briggs and Gray, 1998; Gardiner, Sirbu, and Rahbar, 2004; Sturm, Unützer, and Katon, 1999).

FEDERAL-LEVEL INITIATIVES

Federal efforts in the United States to treat and prevent depression among parents and to mitigate the effects of a parent's depression on children currently include data collection; health education; treatment, prevention, and workforce development; and research activities. These activities, currently scattered across several agencies in the U.S. Department of Health and Human Services, provide a basis for the development of more intensive and collaborative programs and policies to enhance state-based and professional responses to depression in parents and early interventions for children whose parents may be affected by this disorder. At present, federal efforts focus primarily on maternal depression that occurs during pregnancy or the postpartum period. Although one of the strategic goals of the U.S. Department of Health and Human Services is to "promote and encourage preventative health care, including mental health, lifelong healthy behaviors, and recovery" (U.S. Department of Health and Human Services, n.d.), efforts to coordinate programmatic, policy, and research efforts targeted to depression in parents have not emerged as a national priority.

Agency for Healthcare Research and Quality

A 2005 report for the Agency for Healthcare Research and Quality (AHRQ), *Perinatal Depression: Prevalence, Screening, Accuracy, and Screening Outcomes* (Gaynes et al., 2005), observed that depression is as common in women during pregnancy as it is after they give birth. The report defined perinatal depression as a condition that encompasses major and minor depressive episodes that occur either during pregnancy or within the first 12 months after delivery, noting that this disorder may affect as many as 5 to 25 percent of new mothers. The AHRQ report indicates that these repercussions are of significant public health concern and concludes that perinatal depression is the leading cause of disease-related disability among women, resulting in depressive episodes and negatively affecting their children and families.

To assist health care providers and community planners, AHRQ has also developed a guide to adopting innovations that provides generic advice on the issues and steps that potential adopters should consider and whether or not a given innovation will address their needs and is feasible (Brach et al., 2008). Further details of this report are provided in Chapter 10.

Centers for Disease Control and Prevention

The Centers for Disease Control and Prevention (CDC) initiated the Pregnancy Risk Assessment Monitoring System (PRAMS) in 1987. The program "identifies and monitors selected maternal experiences and behaviors before, during, and after pregnancy." This effort surveys indicators associated with the incidence of infant mortality and low birth weight, and includes self-reports (by mothers) regarding postpartum depression. CDC does not specifically collect data regarding the incidence or severity of depression during other stages of parenting, the identification of paternal depression, or the impact of parental depression on children; however one of the leading health indicators—mental health—identified in Healthy People 2010 led to a number of objectives including "increase the proportion of adults with recognized depression who receive treatment" and "increase the proportion of persons with co-occurring substance abuse and mental disorders who receive treatment for both disorders." It also contains objectives intended to increase access to quality health services, with topics including insurance, preventive and behavioral services, and competencies as well as racial and ethnic disparities for health providers (U.S. Department of Health and Human Services, 2000).

Health Resources and Services Administration

The Health Resources and Service Administration (HRSA) has created a public education website that provides comprehensive information related to maternal and peripartum depression. The Maternal and Child Health Bureau (MCHB) in HRSA has produced a free booklet that describes common concerns of peripartum women and offers guidance (including recommendations and information about other relevant organizations) about how best to deal with the symptoms of depression that may occur during pregnancy. A related website includes the same content with accompanying hyperlinks. Publications include *Depression During and After Pregnancy: A Resource for Women, Their Families, and Friends* (Health Resources and Services Administration, 2006). HRSA officials have sought to incorporate findings from the 2005 AHRQ report noted above into state-based planning and professional development efforts, through such activities as the DataSpeak web conference series organized by the Maternal and Child Health Information Resource Center (see, for example, http://mchb.hrsa. gov/mchirc/dataspeak/events/june_05/index.htm).

Healthy Start is another HRSA-funded program that draws on evidence-based interventions in community-based contexts, striving to reduce the infant mortality rate—especially among women who are statistically more likely to have infants die prematurely. Women enrolled in Healthy Start are linked to a medical home from the moment of conception until 2 years postpartum. Health providers routinely screen for signs of perinatal depression and other mental and physical challenges that prenatal women may face.

HRSA and MCHB also support research to explore health service system factors that may contribute to perinatal depression. One such study explores how the health-seeking and resilient behaviors of recent immigrants coping with maternal depression compare with the experiences of the majority population (Huang, 2007). This study will also use national survey data to explore the role of selected social influences as moderators or mediators of maternal depression.

MCHB is addressing the need to increase the number of individuals trained to provide mental health services for people with depression, and in particular peripartum depression, by means of investigators and programs that purport to achieve that goal. For example, a grant was awarded to a program administered by the School of Public Health at the University of California, Berkeley that aimed to increase the capacity to screen, assess, and treat mental health disorders in peripartum women. The program organized convening activities of relevant leaders and stakeholders to develop and evaluate a continuing educational curriculum to be offered to relevant health professionals (Guendelman, 2008). MCHB has also awarded grants to institutions that increase the competence of physicians to render depression-related services to all adults, regardless of gender (Bureau of Health Professions, n.d.).

National Institutes of Health

Several institutes of the National Institutes of Health (NIH), most notably the National Institute of Mental Health, sponsor research studies investigating biological and environmental factors associated with maternal, postpartum, and generalized forms of adult depression. A noteworthy example, as described in Chapter 7, includes an analysis of the STAR*D findings, which reported in 2006 that when women treated for depression become symptom-free, their children are less likely to be diagnosed with depression (Weissman et al., 2006). The study alerts health professionals and patients to the need for vigorous identification and treatment of depressed mothers as well as the evaluation of their children for symptoms.

At present, no systematic effort is available to coordinate the findings from NIH studies about parental depression or to integrate these research findings into programmatic and state-based programs in HRSA, AHRQ, CDC, or the Substance Abuse and Mental Health Services Administration (SAMHSA).

Substance Abuse and Mental Health Services Administration

SAMHSA is tasked with setting national mental health policy, conducting translational research, and delivering mental health services. Its National Mental Health Information Center provides access to multiple public and private resources focused on maternal depression as well as highlighting the impact of parental depression on children (Substance Abuse and Mental Health Services Administration, 2000). These publications and online resources offer links to governmental centers and nongovernmental organizations that offer assistance to women dealing with mental illness.

SAMHSA also coordinates and provides a National Registry of Evidence-based Programs and Practices. This self-nominating, peer-reviewed, and rated registry is a searchable database of interventions for the prevention and treatment of mental and substances use disorders. It aims to improve access to information on tested programs and practices that can be readily disseminated by individuals, agencies, and organizations in their communities (Substance Abuse and Mental Health Services Administration, 2009).

In addition, the SAMHSA Center for Mental Health Services (CMHS) has for 35 years provided financial support for people who are ethnic minorities to pursue mental health professions–related careers (Substance Abuse and Mental Health Services Administration, 2008). This mission helps to address the need to increase the number of individuals trained to provide mental health services to people with depression.

The CMHS center in SAMHSA also includes the Child, Adolescent, and Family Branch (CAFB).[1] This branch promotes and ensures that the mental health needs of children and their families are addressed by a "community-based system of care." The systems of care framework highlights the importance of meeting the mental health needs of children, adolescents, and their families in their home, school, and community environments. The framework also rests on the principles of being child-centered, family-driven, strength-based, and culturally competent and involving interagency collaboration.

CAFB has launched several major initiatives that provide a basis for extending its work with a more explicit focus on parental depression. These include

- Caring for Every Child's Mental Health Campaign
- Child and Adolescent Mental Health and Substance Abuse State Infrastructure Grants
- Circles of Care
- Comprehensive Community Mental Health Services Program for Children and Their Families
- Council on Coordination and Collaboration
- Partnerships for Youth Transition
- Statewide Family Network Grant Program

---

[1]See http://mentalhealth.samhsa.gov/publications/allpubs/KEN95-0016/default.asp.

Office of the Surgeon General

The Office of the Surgeon General (OSG) identifies priority areas of focus in addressing public health concerns. Currently, these include disease prevention, eliminating health disparities, public health preparedness, and improving health literacy. Those specifically related to improving the quality of care for depressed parents and their children include eliminating health disparities and public health preparedness. To help eliminate health disparities the OSG is expanding programs like Community Health Centers and the State Children's Health Insurance Program, helping to increase public awareness and outreach, as well as conducting additional research to help inform policy and activities to increase the access to health information, health insurance, and health services. To improve the public health preparedness of the nation, one of the OSG's priorities is mental health and resilience. Specifically, it has been targeting parents, teachers, and emergency relief workers to provide guidance on coping with fear and anxiety as a result of trauma and disaster. Past efforts of the OSG included the publications that asserted that mental health is a public health problem and that striking disparities in access, quality, and availability of mental health services exist for racial and ethnic minorities in the United States (U.S. Surgeon General, 1999, 2001).

Office of Women's Health

The Office of Women's Health (OWH) has a Women's Mental Health Initiative, which strives to provide an understanding of mental health in physical health care, promoting awareness of mental health, and advising health providers and consumers. This office has convened stakeholders (including decision makers, advocates, and consumers) following a 2005 workshop on women's mental health organized by the Office of the U.S. Surgeon General. OWH has published several reports to enhance public education and consumer-directed initiatives, but such publications do not address parenting roles, nor do they examine the impact of depression among women on their children.

STATE-LEVEL INITIATIVES

A few states have made significant attempts to develop system-wide strategies that are focused on the needs of depressed parents and their children. Current state policy strategies are relatively limited and have not been systematically evaluated. However, they provide insight into the opportunities and barriers that emerge in developing more integrated, comprehensive, community-based, and multigenerational approaches in meeting the needs of vulnerable populations.

Two strategies have emerged that deserve attention. First, several states have developed comprehensive initiatives that typically combine professional training of service providers (i.e., to educate them about prevalence, causes, and consequences) with access to expanded screening and services in nontraditional settings. These multipronged efforts are state-initiated and rely primarily on state funds. Some states have successfully expanded their use of Medicaid funds, particularly to pay for maternal screening and other preventive services. Second, several states have adopted state legislation (and funding) to reduce the stigma of mental health disorders and to promote public awareness, particularly focused on perinatal depression. These state policy reforms are especially important in reducing barriers to seeking care and providing services among vulnerable populations that may be unable to afford private services or are reluctant to engage with community programs.

State-Led Comprehensive Initiatives

Illinois

Illinois has several initiatives that are primarily directed at improving outcomes for pregnant women and young children. These include

- The Perinatal Mental Health Consultation Service, operated by the University of Illinois at Chicago and the state,[2] in partnership with the Illinois Chapter of the Academy of Pediatrics and the Academy of Family Physicians, offers provider consultative services and education and training to clinicians across disciplines to develop competencies in assessment and treatment of maternal depression. The education and quality improvement initiatives also include a pilot to develop a stepped care model; it includes self-care kits to be disseminated statewide that provide information on when and where to access resources. The state is also piloting a tool to assess risk at the preconception and interconception stages. The initiative also includes support for postpartum depression crisis intervention through hotlines.
- Through a contract with its managed care organizations and its primary care case management network, Illinois requires prenatal and postpartum depression screening using an approved, validated,

---

[2] The state agencies involved are the Department of Human Services, the Department of Healthcare and Family Services, the Department of Public Health, the Department of Financial and Professional Regulation, and the Medical Licensing Board.

standardized tool,[3] referral, and treatment, as well as ongoing monitoring and tracking for enrollees. A complementary state law requires that women and their families be educated about perinatal mental health disorders in prenatal and labor and delivery settings, and that women be invited to take an assessment questionnaire in prenatal, postnatal, and pediatric care settings.

- Screening for perinatal depression using an approved instrument is reimbursable for women enrolled in health care and family services, from pregnancy through 1 year after delivery. If women are screened by a provider during their infant's well-child and episodic visits, the screening can be reimbursed through the infant's coverage. Infants and toddlers of mothers with mental health diagnoses (including depression) are automatically eligible for the early intervention program.

Iowa

In Iowa, the Department of Public Health is working to improve provider knowledge and capacity as well as consumer knowledge and ease of access.

- In collaboration with three other state departments, a statewide advocacy organization and the University of Iowa sponsor a statewide train-the-trainer program that to date has trained an estimated 100 trainers. The program trains program staff in early childhood, maternal health, case management, and mental health programs, as well as Special Supplemental Nutrition Program for Women, Infants, and Children (WIC), nursing, and home visiting staff. It includes a mentorship component, requires agency-level commitment to screening, and reimburses agencies for staff time.
- In collaboration with the University of Iowa, the state has developed a web-based training for physicians known as STEP, Support and Train to Enhance Primary Care. It contains a consultation component and is designed to enhance the state's capacity in primary care to appropriately identify and treat perinatal depression.
- The state also produced a pocket guide for health care professionals, that is, a reference book that includes information on treatment, coding, and billing. It is anticipated that this will be widely distributed through the major health care provider associations.
- Iowa also established a provider and consumer website providing

---

[3]Depression Screening Tools: Use in Perinatal Populations, see http://www.psych.uic.edu/research/perinatalmentalhealth/pdf/screening_assessment.pdf.

referral information that identifies mental health providers in all 99 counties, including details of their payment requirements and their specific training in perinatal depression. Primary care providers who access this service can also get free consultation with a University of Iowa–based mental health clinician.

To improve screening, the state added two depression screening questions (from the Patient Health Questionnaire, a standardized assessment) to the Department of Human Services–approved Prenatal Risk Assessment tool required for all providers. The state funds a toll-free telephone resource and referral information line.

New Jersey

The New Jersey initiative focuses on a legislatively mandated perinatal care network and the use of state dollars to pay for treatment for those who would otherwise not have access (Cooper, 2008). The development of the perinatal care network has also facilitated improved data collection and accountability. Through the state's e-birth certificate program, mandated screenings for maternal depression can be tracked (between 80–85 percent of the screenings are now in the database). The other components include

- Six grants to private, nonprofit, maternal and child health consortia whose geographic reach extends across the state. Each regional consortium customizes its approach to providing family support activities.
- State subsidy for treatment of postpartum depression through community behavioral health services, providing a crucial access point irrespective of insurance status.

New Jersey also recently awarded a grant to a pediatric entity to work with pediatricians to improve screening and referral capacity, and the state supports a crisis hotline for providers.

North Carolina

In North Carolina the state effort has focused on creating a supportive Medicaid fiscal framework to support expanded screening and treatment of depression for both children and women.

- State Medicaid policy requires that pediatric practices use a formal, standardized developmental screening tool during well-child visits and that parents be screened for depression by the child's primary care provider.

- The state has expanded Medicaid coverage to reimburse for up to 26 mental health visits for children, 6 of which can be used by the parents to see primary care providers, social workers, and psychologists.

Ohio

The Ohio Departments of Health and Mental Health have launched a statewide, county-based home visitation program. This program, titled Help-Me-Grow, includes an emphasis on screening and referrals for parental depression among the participating mothers in collaboration with local mental health agencies.

- Help-Me-Grow home visitors administer the Edinburgh Postnatal Depression Scale (EPDS) to new mothers with infants ages 4 to 20 weeks. EPDS scores and demographic data are entered into a web-based data system that prompts the home visitor to make a referral for mothers who score above selected cut-off points. The client's score and pertinent referral information are made available to the local mental health agency, and the program database automatically prompts a monitor to review client interactions with the mental health agency to see if appointments were made and kept. Currently operating in 17 Ohio counties, the program is scheduled to increase to 40 counties in 2010. Unpublished results indicate that 20 percent of screened mothers met the EPDS clinical threshold, 68 percent of positive screens accepted mental health referral offers, and 37 percent of referred mothers kept their mental health appointments at 30 days after referral. No data are collected on treatment outcomes.

Rhode Island

In Rhode Island, a specific initiative targets a subpopulation, those receiving public assistance.

- The Work Towards Wellness Program, a telephone care management strategy to address depression, has demonstrated early signs of success among individuals with depression in the Temporary Assistance for Needy Families Program. Nearly 98 percent of the largely female participants with depression have children, and one-third of the children are under age 5. The telephone care management strategy is modeled after a quality initiative for depression in primary care. To date, more than 75 percent of the participants enrolled in the treatment component of the study experienced a reduction in symptoms, and, among two-fifths of these individuals with depression, symptoms were reduced by more than 50 percent (Bloom et al., 2007).

This effort, however, is linked with and builds on other work that Rhode Island has carried out through the Department of Public Health to reduce the impact of high-risk parental conditions on young children.

State-Led Specific Public Awareness Activities

In addition to the more comprehensive initiatives highlighted above, several states also have made efforts to promote public awareness and to reduce the stigma attached to parental depression.

In both Washington and New Jersey, Speak Up When You Are Down is a multilingual public education campaign to increase awareness of postpartum depression funded through a legislative appropriation. In Iowa, an extensive public information and antistigma campaign was launched by the state that included fact sheets on maternal depression and infant mental health for legislators, a display board and booth at the state fair, and articles in the local media. In Minnesota, state legislation passed in 2005 requires that all hospitals and health care providers provide parents and families of newborns with information about postpartum depression. Providers are also required to make available information about postpartum depression to pregnant women and their families. The state developed multilingual fact sheets and brochures on postpartum depression and information on best practices for care management. There is, however, no research on the effectiveness of these campaigns, particularly when they are not linked to further supports for providers or improved access to treatment.

It should also be noted that, through a variety of special, often foundation-funded initiatives, such as the Assuring Better Child Health and Development (ABCD) project supported by the Commonwealth Fund (Pelletier and Abrams, 2003), states are engaging in strategic analysis and fiscal planning to improve their use of Medicaid and other federal dollars to improve developmentally appropriate health care and better support for positive social and emotional outcomes in young children. This major effort, through several different cohorts, now involves close to half of the states.

Finally, as an indication of the sustainability of program implementation, Project THRIVE at the National Center for Children in Poverty has documented the progress of states implementing the Early Childhood

Comprehensive Systems—a program targeting early intervention for young children at risk of developmental delays and serious emotional disturbances and their families—to develop policy commitments and relationships between the state agencies and the local service delivery systems (Johnson and Theberge, 2007a, 2007b; Johnson et al., 2008). These demonstration grants, supported by federal agencies, have also found that states vary in their ability to make commitments and sustain them over time.

EUROPEAN PREVENTIVE INTERVENTIONS WITH PARENTS AND CHILDREN

Several European countries have developed useful and novel approaches to preventive work with children of the mentally ill, often with a specific focus on depression (Beardslee et al., in press-b). The work in these European countries goes far beyond the state-level initiatives described above by focusing on experimentation with system-wide approaches as well as collaborative interdisciplinary efforts. None of these multisectoral strategies has been rigorously evaluated; however, they demonstrate strong interest among care providers in collaborating with new service models that focus on the complex dimensions and family relationships that are an integral part of responding to the needs of children and parents who are coping with depression in their household. These examples further demonstrate how a national health policy that explicitly focuses on prevention as well as treatment can stimulate and enhance the formation of provider training programs, multiple partnerships, and innovative efforts in local communities.

The Netherlands

In the 1970s the Netherlands began to develop a network of prevention and health promotion teams that were located in multiple service sectors (public health services, mental health services, addiction clinics, and several others) supported by prevention-oriented national institutes and research centers. Preventionists have a specific role and title, and many have been educated in Dutch academic and training programs that feature a particular focus on prevention, health education, and health promotion. The work is part of a national health policy, and about 5–10 percent of the budgets of community mental health centers are spent on prevention of mental disorders, much of it to support the work of prevention experts, although it also supports the part-time involvement of mental health professionals.

Five main priorities of prevention have been identified: (1) depression, (2) stress in the workplace, (3) child abuse, (4) children of mentally ill parents, and (5) chronically mentally ill patients and their networks. The approach is to make the care of children of mentally ill parents a regular part of the systems of care, not an isolated activity. If someone comes in for care for an adult mental illness, they are routinely asked if they have children. If children are present, the family automatically qualifies for services. Informal home visits and an array of prevention services from which parents and children can choose are offered.

Over the past 15 years, a comprehensive array of services for children of mentally ill parents have been developed, including play and talk groups, information support groups, online work websites, brochures, videos, school-based education, and a buddy system for children and for parents, home-based mother-baby interventions, parent training, and others. This is accompanied by extensive postgraduate training. Using the existing network of preventionists in community health centers, over 80 preventionists have been trained in the use of the Family Talk Intervention devised by Beardslee and colleagues and has used it in their regular practice.

In the Netherlands, a group of professionals also has been certified to do preventive care. It allows for the adoption and dissemination of related evidence-based programs when they become available. The preventionists are subject to continuous improvement and modification. They have a network in which they collaborate with research institutes, and the structure of support is thought to be essential to making preventive intervention a regular part of care. They have emphasized that it is important to consider preventive care for children of the mentally ill as an integral part of the mental health and primary health care system. They have also emphasized that adequate support for time and the development of services is required as new services become available, with a need for a constant interplay between research and practice (Beardslee et al., in press-a).

Finland

In Finland, starting in 2001 under the leadership of Tytti Solantaus, a nationwide program has been developed effectively in a stepwise fashion. The Finnish Child Welfare Act states that, if a parent is identified as receiving treatment, the needs of children should be addressed. The aim of the Efficient Family Program is to build care of patients' children into routine practice, with every parent receiving support. This was deliberately conceived as a change from an individual and treatment-centered program to a family and prevention-centered one. Mass media campaigns, national and local conferences, and seminars were offered, and the clinics' leadership and the clinicians were eager to learn. Training began with extensive training of master trainers, who then trained many others. Initially, over a 2-year period, over 40 master trainers were trained. Two master trainers from each site were trained with a commitment from the clinic leadership that they would return to their original sites and be able to use the preventive services and train others in their clinics (Beardslee et al., in press-b; Solantaus and Toikka, 2006; Toikka and Solantaus, 2006).

The program involves a family of interventions, including the Family Talk Intervention, a 1- to 2-session intervention using a book for parents, the Let's Talk About Children discussion, peer groups, and a group intervention. Thus, in thinking of large-scale public health interventions, having multiple vehicles to deliver the same content is important. In addition, a network meeting was introduced in which either clinicians or parents involved with either the care of children or in their own care could call for a meeting of all professionals involved in the care of a child and devise a coordinated plan. This network meeting was also an attempt to address the long-standing lack of integration between services for children and services for adults. The groups served by the intervention have been expanded to include families with serious medical illness, families facing substance abuse problems, and families with court-related matters.

The program is now being used in all of the health districts in Finland. Over 80 master trainers and over 700 clinicians have been trained. A randomized trial comparing the Family Talk Intervention with the Let's Talk About Children discussion is under way. Initial findings from parents are that both interventions are safe and feasible in the Finnish setting, with a greater effect for the more intensive Family Talk Intervention.

From a public health point of view, the idea that every professional working with mentally ill parents is responsible for initiating child preventive services is an important contribution. The program has shown that nurses, doctors, psychologists, social workers, and therapists can master the Let's Talk About Children discussion and that a countrywide strategy can be successful. There are many advantages to proceeding first by training those who can train others and then in a stepwise fashion over a number of years, ensure the dissemination of a program. The program has demonstrated that flexibility in the delivery of these strategies and their application to the kinds of conditions beyond depression with which parents wrestle are valuable. It is also important to note that, in contrast to the Dutch system, the program does not use special preventionists, but rather all clinicians have responsibility for preventive services.

Investigators in Finland, Iceland, Norway, Sweden, and Denmark have formed a coalition named the Nordic Forum. A 3-day meeting is held annually in which those countries developing programs for children of the mentally ill meet together in mutual support. Iceland, Norway, and Sweden have chosen to include the Family Talk Intervention as part of their regular array of services, and both Norway and Sweden are in the process of developing national programs.

RESEARCH GAPS

While evidence is emerging about ways to improve and strengthen the quality of treatment programs for depressed adults, little is known about the extent to which these quality improvement efforts apply to the particular needs of adults who are parents or to their children. Furthermore, research presented in the preceding chapters suggests that children are directly affected by a parent's depression. Their needs are not addressed in a care system that focuses solely on improving treatment effectiveness without regard for the vulnerable persons (especially very young children) whose care and relationships may be disrupted by the disorder.

Research is therefore needed to examine how quality improvement efforts contribute to enhancing the relationships and outcomes of parents and their children when compared with the general population of nonparenting adults who participate in treatment programs, and it should incorporate three major principles—recognition and treatment of parental depression, enhancement and support for parenting, and a focus on the developmental outcomes of children. Research resources should be dedicated to understanding common as well as unique problems in designing treatment services for parents with children at different stages of development, including infants, toddlers, school-age children, and adolescents. Once optimal strategies are identified, research is needed for the dissemination of these programs into the care settings that match these developmental stages.

Further, many individuals who screen positive for depression decline mental health services. For widespread implementation of programs that are shown to be effective for families with depression, there is a need for more work on issues of engagement and barriers to access to services as most families with depressed parents do not receive adequate intervention. Research on depression care models should therefore identify characteristics of individuals who accept services and individuals who decline them to determine how well a given model fits with the cultural and socioeconomic characteristics of the relevant community. Research opportunities may exist to engage individuals in treatment that is directly relevant to distinct stages of parenting, such as those noted above: preconception, prenatal, postpartum, and later stages, as well as comparing the outcomes of first-time parents with those who are raising older children or children in blended families The comparative effectiveness of treatment strategies that are targeted on these developmental stages deserves to be tested in designing future quality improvement research studies. Interventions centered on parenting are particularly compelling because engagement is a crucial step to effectively intervening in families with depression. Programs that address parenting needs offer great promise as a highly effective way to engage parents and, when needed, trigger services that can address their depression, parenting, and prevention of adverse outcomes in children. Trials are also needed of specific ways to offer additional identification, outreach, engagement, and treatment and prevention services to those vulnerable families who face multiple risks.

Finally, families with depressed parents are most likely to be recognized in a variety of settings. As described in Chapter 7, targeted intervention approaches are likely to be most promising. Therefore, in addition to interventions for parents who present with depression for mental health services, research is needed on how best to identify parental depression and provide services within a range of settings in which families at high risk for depression seek services (such as Head Start, WIC, preschool). Thus, resources need to be available in these settings to identify parental depression and to assist families in getting treatment and prevention services. This is most relevant to low-income and ethnic-minority populations given that they are at increased risk for depression but are less likely to seek mental health services.

CONCLUSION

The size of the problem and the enormous number of families at risk of the effects of parental depression ideally call for experimentation with interventions that can be implemented at multiple sites in existing systems and deployed with planned variations on regional levels and for culturally diverse populations. A wide range of settings are now available for identifying, treating, and preventing depression in parents and its consequences for children. Existing strategies and evidence suggest opportunities in primary care, home visitation programs, early childhood care and education programs, schools, the criminal justice system, and community-based programs. Primary care, home visitation, and early childhood settings, in particular, offer valuable opportunities for identification of depression in parents and its outcomes, the encouragement of sustained relationships and high levels of trust, and reduction of barriers for low-income populations at higher risk of parental depression. Each setting, however, requires different implementation approaches that frequently involve innovative service strategies to address complex interactions between depression, parenting practices, and parent and child engagement with services. It is important to note as well that each setting frequently has difficulty in establishing strong linkages with mental health services.

Some of the most successful depression care programs have been implemented in quality improvement efforts in primary care settings. However, physicians in particular face competing demands for their time and attention, as the average office visit requires them to address multiple health care problems and complaints. Mental health carve-outs as well as the potential increase in gross costs present financial barriers to adoption for many primary care practices. Medical homes, however, offer an attractive environment with potential remuneration and improved physician-patient rapport, which should facilitate screening and interventions for parental depression.

Home visitation programs provide a service setting in which high-risk parents and families can be readily screened for depression in the comfort of their own homes. In addition to screening and mental health referrals, home visitors can provide parenting interventions to depressed parents and screen for developmental delays and emotional problems in their children. Early childhood and parent training programs also offer ready access to high-risk families and the opportunity to provide services to both parents and children.

Schools provide another venue in which to engage both parents and children, although their semiclosed nature and absence of a mental health orientation present significant challenges. Criminal justice systems, while often overlooked, may provide important opportunities to reach individuals with high rates of depression and mental illness. The criminal justice system as a whole has been in the forefront of adopting evidence-based practices. However, a variety of institutional and legal constraints limit the ability to research the success of these efforts.

Communities interested in developing comprehensive integrated depression care screening, prevention, or treatment components in one or more the settings will need to wrestle with the complexity inherent to coordination and communication among multidisciplinary, multisystem components. Getting started in one or two settings, such as a primary care clinic or a Head Start program, may offer more opportunity and be easier to initiate than launching a comprehensive community effort. But an innovative parental depression program will have to compete with other routine demands in selected service settings. It will require a passionate leader and team members who can organize group commitment and find resources for treatment or treatment referral options for identified parents and children. It will also require new forms of data collection to monitor client characteristics, services, and outcomes. The experience with single-setting programs can reveal the scope of the problem and offer treatment success stories that could lead to more comprehensive community efforts for treating parental depression with a two-generation lens in settings particular to diverse and vulnerable populations.

Multiple agencies scattered across the U.S. Department of Health and Human Services are working to provide a basis for the development of programs and policies to enhance responses to depression among parents through data collection, health education, workforce development, and other research activities. Most of these efforts focus on maternal depression during pregnancy and the postpartum period and have not been coordinated across the agencies.

Finally, selected states form the vanguard for demonstration efforts by revising programs and policies to introduce more comprehensive and family-focused interventions for parents with depression. These efforts seek to raise the professional training of care providers as well as educate the public about the causes and consequences of depression, striving to reduce stigma associated with this disorder and to improve child outcomes. Such efforts are especially laudable in calling attention to the multidimensional nature of depression and highlighting approaches that require innovative strategies and collaborative efforts. In addition, a number of European countries have developed extensive national programs and mental health prevention teams. Children of mentally ill parents often routinely qualify for services. Prevention professionals, the use of master trainers, and family-oriented prevention interventions are important components in these system-wide, collaborative, interdisciplinary programs.

RECOMMENDATIONS

This chapter describes the components of an ideal evidence-based program for the care of depressed adults who are parents. Although the current system of care is far from being ready to implement this ideal, a variety of initiatives for improving the quality of services for depressed parents and their children have emerged at the community, state, and federal level, as well as internationally in a variety of service settings. Based on the opportunities (and challenges) that have emerged in implementing these initiatives, the committee makes three recommendations intended to build on them and to improve the outreach and delivery of services in different settings for diverse populations of children and families.

Improve Awareness and Understanding

Recommendation 1: The Office of the U.S. Surgeon General should identify depression in parents and its effects on the healthy development of children as part of its public health priorities focused on mental health and eliminating health disparities.

To implement this recommendation, the U.S. Surgeon General should encourage individual agencies, particularly the National Institutes of Health, HRSA, CDC, and SAMHSA, to support the Healthy People 2020 overarching goal of achieving health equity and eliminating health disparities by including the importance of identification, treatment, and prevention of depression and its potential impact on the healthy development of children of depressed parents. These agencies should pay particular attention to groups and populations that have historically and currently experience barriers in receiving quality health care, including for behavioral health. Efforts should be made to ensure that effective strategies are employed to increase the participation and engagement of these vulnerable populations in critical research studies and clinical trials. New research methods and innovative models that partner with vulnerable communities should be supported. Particular focus should be directed at prevention and early intervention efforts that are community based and culturally appropriate so that the high burden of disability currently associated with depression in populations experiencing health disparities can be reduced.

> **Recommendation 2: The Secretary of the U.S. Department of Health and Human Services, in coordination with state governors, should launch a national effort to further document the magnitude of the problem of depression in adults who are parents, prevent adverse effects on children, and develop activities and materials to foster public education and awareness.**

To implement this recommendation, first, the Secretary of the U.S. Department of Health and Human Services should encourage individual agencies, particularly the National Institute of Mental Health, HRSA, CDC, and AHRQ, to identify the parental status of adults and add reliable and valid measures of depression to ongoing longitudinal and cross-sectional studies of parents and children and national health surveys, in ways that will support analyses of prevalence, incidence, disparities, causes, and consequences. Second, CDC should develop guidelines to assist the states in their efforts to collect data on the incidence and prevalence of the number of depressed adults who are parents and the number of children at risk to adverse health and psychological outcomes. Finally, using this information, the U.S. Department of Health and Human Services should encourage agencies, most notably HRSA, to develop a series of public education activities and materials highlighting what is known about the impact of depression in parents. These activities and materials should specifically target the public and individuals who make decisions about care for a diverse population of depressed parents and their children in a variety of settings (e.g., state and county leadership, state health directors, state mental health agencies, and state maternal and child health services).

Support Innovative Strategies

> **Recommendation 3: Congress should authorize the creation of a new national demonstration program in the U.S. Department of Health and**

Human Services that supports innovative efforts to design and evaluate strategies in a wide range of settings and populations to identify, treat, and prevent depression in parents and its adverse outcomes in their children. Such efforts should use a combination of components—including screening and treating the adult, identifying that the adult is a parent, enhancing parenting practices, and preventing adverse outcomes in the children. The results of the new demonstration program should be evaluated and, if warranted, Congress should subsequently fund a coordinated initiative to introduce these strategies in a variety of settings.

To implement this recommendation, agencies in the U.S. Department of Health and Human Services should prepare a request for proposals for community-level demonstration projects. Such demonstration projects

- should test ways to reduce barriers to care by using one or more empirically based strategies to identify, treat, and prevent depression in parents in heterogeneous populations (i.e., race/ethnicity, income level), those in whom depression is typically underidentified, and those with risk factors and co-occurring conditions (e.g., trauma, anxiety disorders, substance use disorders);
- should call attention to effective interventions in which screening and assessment are linked to needed care of parents with depression, that support training in positive parenting, and that encourage strategies to prevent adverse outcomes in their children;
- could identify multiple opportunities to engage parents who are depressed as well as to identify children (at all ages) who are at risk because their parents are depressed;
- could include the Healthy Start Program, the Head Start Program, the Nurse-Family Partnership, home visiting, schools, primary care, mental health and substance abuse treatment settings, and other programs that offer early childhood interventions;
- would ideally use more than one strategy and could use funds to test state-based efforts that experiment with different service strategies and service settings and to strengthen the relationship between mental health services and parental support programs;
- could test ways to reduce the stigma and biases frequently associated with depression, address cultural and racial barriers and disparities in the mental health services system, and explore opportunities to strengthen formal and informal supports for families that are consistent with cultural traditions and resources; and
- should include state mental health agencies and local government (e.g., counties), at least in an advisory capacity.

Finally SAMSHA should promote interagency collaboration with other U.S. Department of Health and Human Services agencies—CDC, HRSA, the National Institute on Drug Abuse, the National Institute on Alcohol Abuse and Alcoholism, the National Institute of Mental Health, the National Institute on Nursing Research, and the National Institute of Child Health and Human Development—to develop coordinated strategies that support the design and evaluation of these demonstration projects. SAMHSA could identify an interagency committee to pool information about programs that are affected by parents with depression, programs that offer opportunities to engage parents and children in the treatment and prevention of this disorder, and research and evaluation studies that offer insight into effective interventions. SAMHSA could develop opportunities to introduce effective interventions in both community-based systems of care frameworks and in integrated behavioral and mental health services in a variety of settings, including primary care and substance abuse treatment settings.

REFERENCES

American Academy of Pediatrics and American College of Obstetrics and Gynecology. (2007). *Guidelines for Perinatal Care* (6th ed.). Elk Grove Village, IL: American Academy of Pediatrics.

Ammerman, R.T., Putnam, F.W., Stevens, J., Holleb, L.J., Novak, A.L., and Van Ginkel, J.B. (2005). In-home cognitive behavior therapy for depression: An adapted treatment for first-time mothers in home visitation. *Best Practices in Mental Health*, *1*, 1–14.

Aos, S., Miller, M., and Drake, E. (2006). *Evidence-Based Public Policy Options to Reduce Future Prison Construction, Criminal Justice Costs, and Crime Rates*. Olympia: Washington State Institute for Public Policy.

Avery, M.R., Beardslee, W.R., Ayoub, C.C., and Watts, C.L. (2008). *Family Connections Materials: A Comprehensive Approach in Dealing with Parental Depression and Related Adversities*. Available: http://eclkc.ohs.acf.hhs.gov/hslc/ecdh/Mental%20Health/Resources%20and%20Support%20for%20Families/Parent%20Support%20and%20Resources/FamilyConnection.htm#TrainingModules [accessed April 24, 2009].

Barlow, J., Coren, E., and Stewart-Brown, S.S.B. (2003). Parent-training programmes for improving maternal psychosocial health. *Cochrane Database of Systematic Reviews*, (4) Art. no. CD002020.

Barnett, W.S. (2002). Early childhood education. In A. Molnar (Ed.), *School Reform Proposals: The Research Evidence* (pp. 1–26). Greenwich, CT: Information Age.

Barth, R.P., Landsverk, J. Chamberlain, P., Reid, J.B., Rolls, J.A., Hurlburt, M.S., Farmer, E.M.Z., James, S., McCabe, K.M., and Kohl, P.L. (2005). Parent-training programs in child welfare services: Planning for a more evidence-based approach to serving biological parents. *Research on Social Work Practice*, *15*, 353–371.

Bauldry, S. (2006). *Positive Support: Mentoring and Depression among High-Risk Youth*. Philadelphia: Public/Private Ventures.

Bauldry, S.G., and Hartmann, T.A. (2004). *The Promise and Challenge of Mentoring High-Risk Youth: Findings from the National Faith-Based Initiative*. Philadelphia: Public/Private Ventures.

Baydar, N., Reid, M.J., and Webster-Stratton, C. (2003). The role of mental health factors and program engagement in the effectiveness of a preventive parenting program for Head Start mothers. *Child Development, 74,* 1433–1453.

Beardslee, W.R., Avery, M.W., Ayoub, C., and Watts, C.L. (in press-a). Family Connections: Helping Early Head Start/Head Start staff and parents make sense of mental health challenges. *Journal Zero to Three.*

Beardslee, W.R., Hosman, C., Solantaus, T., van Doesum, K., and Cowling, V. (in press-b). Children of mentally ill parents: An opportunity for effective prevention all too often neglected. In C. Hosman, E. Jane-Llopis, and S. Saxena (Eds.), *Prevention of Mental Disorders: Effective Interventions and Policy Options.* Oxford, England: Oxford University Press.

Beasley, J.W., Hankey, T.H., Erickson, R., Stange, K.C., Mundt, M., Elliott, M., Wiesen, P., and Bobula, J. (2004). How many problems do family physicians manage at each encounter? A WReN study. *Annals of Family Medicine, 2,* 405–410.

Bloom, D., Redcross, C., Hsueh, J., Rich, S., and Martin, V. (2007). *Four Strategies to Overcome Barriers to Employment: An Introduction to the Enhanced Services for the Hard-to-Employ Demonstration and Evaluation Project.* New York: MDRC.

Boothroyd, R.A., Mercado, C.C., Poythress, N.G., Christy, A., and Petrila, J. (2005). Clinical outcomes of defendants in mental health court. *Psychiatric Services, 56,* 829–834.

Boris, N.W., Larrieu, J.A., Zeanah, P.D., Nagle, G.A., Steier, A., and McNeill, P. (2006). The process and promise of mental health augmentation of nursing home-visiting programs: Data from the Louisiana Nurse-Family Partnership. *Infant Mental Health Journal, 27,* 26–40.

Brach, C., Lensfestey, N., Rouseel, A., Amoozegar, J., Sorenson, A. (2008). *Will It Work Here?: A Decisionmaker's Guide to Adopting Innovations.* (AHRQ Pub. No. 08-0051.) Rockville, MD: Agency for Healthcare Research and Quality.

Branch, A.Y. (2002). *Faith and Action: Implementation of the National Faith-Based Initiative for High-Risk Youth.* Philadelphia: Public/Private Ventures.

Brener, N.D., Weist, M., Adelman, H., Taylor, L., and Vernon-Smiley, M. (2007). Mental health and social services: Results from the school health policies and programs study 2006. *Journal of School Health, 77,* 486–499.

Briggs, A.H., and Gray, A.M. (1998). Power and sample size calculations for stochastic cost-effectiveness analysis. *Medical Decision Making, 18,* S81–S92.

Brown, E.C., Hawkins, J.D., Arthur, M.W., Briney, J.S., and Abbott, R.D. (2007). Effects of Communities That Care on prevention services systems: Findings from the Community Youth Development Study at 1.5 years. *Prevention Science, 8,* 180–191.

Bryant, D.M., Burchinal, M., Lau, L.B., and Sparling, J.J. (1994). Family and classroom correlates of Head Start children's developmental outcomes. *Early Childhood Research Quarterly, 9,* 289–309.

Bureau of Health Professions. (n.d.). *Residency Training in Primary Care: FY 2005 Grant Summaries.* Available: http://bhpr.hrsa.gov/medicine-dentistry/05summaries/residency.htm [accessed March 27, 2009].

Cabana, M.D., Rand, C.S., Powe, N.R., Wu, A.W., Wilson, M.H., Abboud, P.C., and Rubin, H.R. (1999). Why don't physicians follow clinical practice guidelines: A framework for improvement. *Journal of the American Medical Association, 282,* 1458–1465.

Centers for Disease Control and Prevention. (2006). *School Health Policies and Programs Study: Changes Between 2000 and 2006.* Atlanta: Author.

Chazan-Cohen, R., Ayoub, C., Pan, B.A., Roggman, L., Raikes, H., McKelvey, L., Whiteside-Mansell, L., and Hart, A. (2007). It takes time: Impacts of Early Head Start that lead to reductions in maternal depression two years later. *Infant Mental Health Journal, 28,* 151–170.

Conway, T., and Hutson, R.Q. (2007). Parental incarceration: How to avoid a "death sentence" for families. *Clearinghouse Review Journal of Poverty Law and Policy, 41,* 212–221.

Cooper, J.L. (2008). *Towards Better Behavioral Health for Children, Youth and Their Families: Financing That Supports Knowledge.* New York: National Center for Children in Poverty, Columbia University Mailman School of Public Health.

Cuellar, A.E., McReynolds, L.S., and Wasserman, G.A. (2006). A cure for crime: Can mental health treatment diversion reduce crime among youth? *Journal of Policy Analysis and Management, 25,* 197–214.

Currie, J., and Neidell, M. (2007). Getting inside the "black box" of Head Start quality: What matters and what doesn't. *Economics of Education Review, 26,* 83–99.

DeGarmo, D.S., Patterson, G.R., and Forgatch, M.S. (2004). How do outcomes in a specified parent training intervention maintain or wane over time? *Prevention Science, 5,* 73–89.

Dietrich, A.J., Oxman, T.E., Williams, J.W., Schulberg, H.C., Bruce, M.L., Lee, P.W., Barry, S., Raue, P.J., Lefever, J.J., Heo, M., Rost, K., Kroenke, K., Gerrity, M., and Nutting, P.A. (2004). Re-engineering systems for the treatment of depression in primary care: Cluster randomised controlled trial. *British Medical Journal, 329,* 602–605.

Druss, B.G., Rohrbaugh, R.M., Levinson, C.M., and Rosenheck, R.A. (2001), Integrated medical care for patients with serious psychiatric illness: A randomized trial. *Archives of General Psychiatry, 58,* 861–868.

Dwight-Johnson, M., Unutzer, J., Sherbourne, C., Tang, L.Q., and Wells, K.B. (2001). Can quality improvement programs for depression in primary care address patient preferences for treatment? *Medical Care, 39,* 934–944.

Early, D.M., Maxwell, K.L., Burchinal, M., Bender, R.H., Ebanks, C., Henry, G.T., Iriondo-Perez, J., Mashburn, A.J., Pianta, R.C., Alva, S., Bryant, D., Cai, K., Clifford, R.M., Griffin, J.A., Howes, C., Jeon, H.-J., Peisner-Feinberg, E., Vandergrift, N., and Zill, N. (2007). Teachers' education, classroom quality, and young children's academic skills: Results from seven studies of preschool programs. *Child Development, 78,* 558–580.

Ell, K., Xie, B., Quon, B., Quinn, D.I., Dwight-Johnson, M., and Lee, P.J. (2008). Randomized controlled trial of collaborative care management of depression among low-income patients with cancer. *Journal of Clinical Oncology, 26,* 4488–4496.

Fagan, A.A., Hanson, K., Hawkins, J.D., and Arthur, M.W. (2008). Bridging science to practice: Achieving prevention program implementation fidelity in the community youth development study. *American Journal of Community Psychology, 41,* 235–249.

Flocke, S.A., Goodwin, M.A., and Stange, K.C. (1998). The effect of a secondary patient on the family practice visit. *Journal of Family Practice, 46,* 429–434.

Forman, D.R., O'Hara, M.W., Stuart, S., Gorman, L.L., Larsen, K.E., and Coy, K.C. (2007). Effective treatment for postpartum depression is not sufficient to improve the developing mother-child relationship. *Development and Psychopathology, 19,* 585–602.

Foster, S., Rollefson, M., Doksum, T., Noonan, D., Robinson, G., and Teich, J. (2005). *School Mental Health Services in the United States, 2002–2003.* Rockville, MD: U.S. Department of Health and Human Services, Substance Abuse and Mental Health Services Administration, Center for Mental Health Services.

Freudenheim, M. (2008, July 21). Trying to save by increasing doctors' fees. *New York Times,* P1.

Friedmann, P.D., Taxman, F.S., and Henderson, C.E. (2007). Evidence-based treatment practices for drug-involved adults in the criminal justice system. *Journal of Substance Abuse Treatment, 32,* 267–277.

Gallagher, J., and Clifford, R. (2000). The missing support infrastructure in early childhood. *Early Childhood Research and Practice, 2.*

Gardiner, J.C., Sirbu, C.M., and Rahbar, M.H. (2004). Update on statistical power and sample size assessments for cost-effectiveness studies. *Expert Review of Pharmacoeconomics and Outcomes Research*, 4, 89–98.

Gaynes, B.N., Gavin, N., Meltzer-Brody, S., Lohr, K.N., Swinson, T., Gartlehner, G., Brody, S., and Miller, W.C. (2005). Perinatal depression: Prevalence, screening and accuracy, and screening outcomes. In *Evidence Report/Technology Assessment No. 119*. (AHRQ Pub. No. 05-E006-2.) Rockville, MD: Agency for Healthcare Research and Quality.

Gilbody, S., Bower, P., and Whitty, P. (2006). Costs and consequences of enhanced primary care for depression: Systematic review of randomized economic evaluations. *British Journal of Psychiatry*, 189, 297–308.

Gilbody, S., Bower, P., Fletcher, J., Richard, D., and Sutton, A. (2006). Collaborative care for depression: A cumulative meta-analysis and review of long-term outcomes. *Archives of Internal Medicine*, 166, 2314–2321.

Gilbody, S., Whitty, P., Grimshaw, J., and Thomas, R. (2003). Educational and organizational interventions to improve the management of depression in primary care: A systematic review. *Journal of the American Medical Association*, 289, 3145–3151.

Gottfredson, D.C., and Gottfredson, G.D. (2002). Quality of school-based prevention programs: Results from a national survey. *Journal of Research in Crime and Delinquency*, 39, 3–35.

Grudzinskas, A.J., Jr., Clayfield, J.C., Roy-Buynowski, K., Fisher, W.H., and Richardson, M.H. (2005). Integrating the criminal justice system into mental health service delivery: The Worcester diversion experience. *Behavioral Sciences and the Law*, 23, 277–293.

Grypma, L., Little, S., Haverkamp, R., and Unützer, J. (2006). Taking an evidence-based model of depression care from research to practice: Making lemonade out of depression. *General Hospital Psychiatry*, 28, 101–107.

Guendelman, S. (2008). *The Regents of the University of California*. Available: http://mchb. hrsa.gov/training/project_info.asp?id=307 [accessed March 30, 2009].

Hawkins, J.D., Brown, E.C., Oesterle, S., Arthur, M.W., Abbott, R.D., and Catalano, R.F. (2008). Early effects of Communities That Care on targeted risks and initiation of delinquent behavior and substance use. *Journal of Adolescent Health*, 43, 15–22.

Hawkins, J.D., Catalano, R.F., Jr., and Associates. (1992). *Communities That Care: Action for Drug Abuse Prevention*. San Francisco: Jossey-Bass.

Hawkins, J.D., Catalano, R.F., Kosterman, R., Abbott, R., and Hill, K.G. (1999). Preventing adolescent health-risk behaviors by strengthening protection during childhood. *Archives of Pediatric and Adolescent Medicine*, 153, 226–234.

Health Resources and Services Administration. (2006). *Depression During and After Pregnancy: A Resource for Women, Their Families, and Friends*. Washington, DC: U.S. Department of Health and Human Services.

Henderson, C.E., Taxman, F.S., and Young, D.W. (2008). A Rasch model analysis of evidence-based treatment practices used in the criminal justice system. *Drug and Alcohol Dependence*, 93, 163–175.

Hoagwood, K., and Johnson, J. (2003). School psychology: A public health framework. I. From evidence-based practices to evidence-based politics. *Journal of School Psychology*, 41, 3–21.

Hoagwood, K.W., Olin, S.S., Kerker, B.D., Kratochwill, T.R., Crowe, M., and Saka, N. (2007). Empirically based school interventions targeted at academic and mental health functioning. *Journal of Emotional and Behavioral Disorders*, 15, 66–92.

Horvitz-Lennon, M., Kilbourne, A.M., and Pincus, H.A. (2006). From silos to bridges: Meeting the general health care needs of adults with severe mental illnesses. *Health Affairs*, 25, 659–669.

Horwitz, S.M., Kelleher, K.J., Stein, R.E.K., Storfer-Isser, A., Youngstrom, E.A., Park, E.R., Heneghan, A.M., Jensen, P.S., O'Connor, K.G., and Hoagwood, K.E. (2007). Barriers to the identification and management of psychosocial issues in children and maternal depression. *Pediatrics, 119*, e208–e218.

Huang, Z.J. (2007). *Maternal Depression, Mental Health Seeking Pattern, and Child Development in U.S. Immigrant Families.* Available: http://mchb.hrsa.gov/research/project_info. asp?ID=71 [accessed March 30, 2009].

Institute of Medicine. (2006). *Improving the Quality of Health Care for Mental and Substance-Use Conditions: Quality Chasm Series.* Committee on Crossing the Quality Chasm: Adaptation to Mental Health and Addictive Disorders. Board on Health Care Services. Washington, DC: The National Academies Press.

Isaacs, J.B. (2007). *Cost-Effective Investments in Children.* Washington, DC: Brookings Institution.

Johnson, K., and Theberge, S. (2007a). *Local Systems Development: Short Take No. 6.* New York: National Center for Children in Poverty, Columbia University Mailman School of Public Health.

Johnson, K., and Theberge, S. (2007b). *State of the States' ECCS Initiatives: Short Take No. 5.* New York: National Center for Children in Poverty, Columbia University Mailman School of Public Health.

Johnson, K., Davidson, L., Theberge, S., and Knitzer, J. (2008). *State Indicators for Early Childhood: Short Take No. 7.* New York: National Center for Children in Poverty, Columbia University Mailman School of Public Health.

Jones, B.F. (2009). The burden of knowledge and the "Death of the Renaissance Man": Is innovation getting harder? *Review of Economic Studies, 76*, 283–317.

Kam, C.-M., Greenberg, M.T., and Walls, C.T. (2003). Examining the role of implementation quality in school-based prevention using the PATHS curriculum. *Prevention Science, 4*, 55–63.

Kaminski, J.W., Valle, L.A., Filene, J.H., and Boyle, C.L. (2008). A meta-analytic review of components associated with parent training program effectiveness. *Journal of Abnormal Child Psychology, 36*, 567–589.

Kane-Mallik, K., and Visher, C.A. (2008). *Health and Prisoner Reentry: How Physical, Mental, and Substance Abuse Conditions Shape the Process of Reintegration.* Washington, DC: Urban Institute.

Karoly, L.A., Kilburn, M.R., and Cannon, J.S. (2005). *Early Childhood Interventions: Proven Results, Future Promise.* Santa Monica, CA: RAND.

Katon, W.J., Von Korff, M., Lin, E.H.B., Simon, G., Ludman, E., Russo, J., Ciechanowski, P., Walker, E., and Bush, T. (2004). The Pathways Study: A randomized trial of collaborative care in patients with diabetes and depression. *Archives of General Psychiatry, 61*, 1042–1049.

Kinder, L., Katon, W., Russo, J., Simon, G., Lin, E.H., Ciechanowski, P., Von Korff, M., and Young, B. (2006). Improving depression care in patients with diabetes and multiple complications. *Journal of General Internal Medicine, 21*, 1036–1041.

Klinkman, M.S. (1997). Competing demands in psychosocial care: A model for the identification and treatment of depressive disorders in primary care. *General Hospital Psychiatry, 19*, 98–111.

Knitzer, J., Theberge, S., and Johnson, K. (2008). *Reduce Maternal Depression and Its Impact on Young Children: Toward a Responsive Early Childhood Policy Framework.* New York: National Center for Children in Poverty, Columbia University Mailman School of Public Health.

Kutash, K., Duchnowski, A.J., and Lynn, N. (2006). *School-Based Mental Health: An Empirical Guide for Decision Makers.* Tampa: University of South Florida, Louis de la Parte Florida Mental Health Institute, Department of Child and Family Studies, Research and Training Center for Children's Mental Health.

Mattke, S., Seid, M., and Ma, S. (2007). Evidence for the effect of disease management: Is $1 billion a year a good investment? *American Journal of Managed Care, 13,* 670–676.

Minkovitz, C.S., Strobino, D., Mistry, K.B., Scharfstein, D.O., Grason, H., Hou, W., Ialongo, N., and Guyer, B. (2007). Healthy steps for young children: Sustained results at 5.5 years. *Pediatrics, 120,* e658–e668.

Miranda, J., Duan, N., Sherbourne, C., Schoenbaum., M., Lagomasino, I., Jackson-Triche, M., and Wells, K.B. (2003). Improving care for minorities: Can quality improvement interventions improve care and outcomes for depressed minorities? Results of a randomized, controlled trial. *Health Services Research, 38,* 613–630.

National Research Council. (2007). *Parole, Desistance from Crime, and Community Integration.* Committee on Community Supervision and Desistance from Crime. Committee on Law and Justice, Division of Behavioral and Social Sciences and Education. Washington, DC: The National Academies Press.

Olds, D.L., Hill, P.L., O'Brien, R., Racine, D., and Moritz, P. (2003). Taking preventive intervention to scale: The Nurse-Family Partnership. *Cognitive and Behavioral Practice, 10,* 278–290.

Olson, A.R., Kemper, K.J., Kelleher, K.J., Hammond, C.S., Zuckerman, B.S., and Dietrich, A.J. (2002). Primary care pediatricians' roles and perceived responsibilities in the identification and management of maternal depression. *Pediatrics, 110,* 1169–1175.

Østbye, T., Yarnall, K.S.H., Krause, K.M., Pollack, K.I., Gradison, M., and Michener, J.L. (2005). Is there time for management of patients with chronic diseases in primary care? *Annals of Family Medicine, 3,* 209–214.

Pai-Samant, S., DeWolfe, J., Caverly, S., Boller, K., McGroder, S., Zettler, J., Mills, J., Ross, C., Clark, C., Quinones, M., and Gulin, J. (2005). *Measurement Options for the Assessment of Head Start Quality Enhancements: Final Report Volume II.* Princeton, NJ: Mathematica Policy Research.

Partnership for America's Economic Success. (2008). *Long-Term Economic Benefits of Investing in Early Childhood Programs: Proven Programs Boost Economic Development and Benefit the Nation's Fiscal Health.* Washington, DC: Author.

Pelletier, H., and Abrams, M. (2003). *ABCD: Lessons from a Four-State Consortium.* New York: The Commonwealth Fund.

Pfeffer, J., and Sutton, R.I. (2006). Evidence-based management. *Harvard Business Review, 84,* 62–74.

Re-entry Policy Council. (2005). *Charting the Safe and Successful Return of Prisoners to the Community.* New York: Council of State Governments.

Richardson, L., McCauley, E., and Katon, W.J. (2009). Collaborative care for adolescent depression: A pilot study. *General Hospital Psychiatry, 3,* 36–45.

Ringeisen, H., Henderson, K., and Hoagwood, K. (2003). Context matters: Schools and the "research to practice gap" in children's mental health. *School Psychology Review, 32,* 153–168.

Ringwalt, C.L., Ennett, S., Johnson, R., Rohrbarch, L.A., Simons-Rudolph, A., Vincus, A., and Thorne, J. (2003). Factors associated with fidelity to substance use prevention curriculum guides in the nation's middle schools. *Health Education and Behavior, 30,* 375–391.

Rosenheck, R. (2001). Stages in the implementation of innovative clinical programs in complex organizations. *Journal of Nervous and Mental Disease, 189,* 812–821.

Schoenbaum, M., Unützer, J., Sherbourne, C., Duan, N., Rubenstein, L.V., Miranda, J., Meredith, L.S., Carney, M.F., and Wells, K. (2001). Cost-effectiveness of practice-initiated quality improvement for depression: Results of a randomized controlled trial. *Journal of the American Medical Association, 286*, 1325–1330.

Sherbourne, C.D., Edelen, M.O., Zhou, A., Bird, C., Duan, N., and Wells, K.B. (2008). How a therapy-based quality improvement intervention for depression affected life events and psychological well-being over time: A 9-year longitudinal analysis. *Medical Care, 46*, 78–84.

Sia, C., Tonniges, T.F., Osterhus, E., and Taba, S. (2004). History of the medical home concept. *Pediatrics, 113*, 1473–1478.

Simon, G.E., Manning, W.G., Katzelnick, D.J., Pearson, S.D., Henk, H.J., and Helstadd, C.P. (2001). Cost-effectiveness of systematic depression treatment for high utilizers of general medical care. *Archives of General Psychiatry, 58*, 181–187.

Solantaus, T., and Toikka, S. (2006). The Effective Family Programme: Preventative services for the children of mentally ill parents in Finland. *International Journal of Mental Health Promotion, 8*, 37–44.

Solomon, A.L., Osborne, J.W.L., LoBuglio, S.F., Mellow, J., and Mukamal, D.A. (2008). *Life After Lockup: Improving Re-Entry from Jail to the Community*. Washington, DC: Urban Institute.

Stange, K.C., Zyzanski, S.J., Jaén, C.R., Callahan, E.J., Kelly, R.B., Gillanders, W.R., Shank, J.C., Chao, J., Medalie, J.H., Miller, W.L., Crabtree, B.F., Flocke, S.A., Gilchrist, V.J., Langa, D.M., and Goodwin, M.A. (1998). Illuminating the "black box": A description of 4,454 patient visits to 138 family physicians. *Journal of Family Practice, 46*, 377–389.

Starfield, B., and Shi, L. (2004). The medical home, access to care, and insurance: A review of evidence. *Pediatrics, 113*, 1493–1498.

Steadman, H.J., and Naples, M. (2005). Assessing the effectiveness of jail diversion programs for persons with serious mental illness and co-occurring substance use disorders. *Behavioral Sciences and the Law, 23*, 163–170.

Sturm, R., Unützer, J., and Katon W. (1999). Effectiveness research and implications for study design: Sample size and statistical power. *General Hospital Psychiatry, 21*, 274–283.

Substance Abuse and Mental Health Services Administration. (2000). *Women and Depression Fast Facts*. Available: http://mentalhealth.samhsa.gov/publications/allpubs/fastfact6/default.asp [accessed March 27, 2009].

Substance Abuse and Mental Health Services Administration. (2008). *Request for Applications (RFA): Minority Fellowship Program*. Available: http://www.samhsa.gov/Grants/2008/sm_08_006.aspx [accessed March 27, 2009].

Substance Abuse and Mental Health Services Administration. (2009). *National Registry of Evidence-Based Programs and Practices*. Available: http://nrepp.samhsa.gov/index.asp [accessed March 30, 2009].

Tai-Seale, M., McGuire, T.G., and Zhang, W. (2007). Time allocation in primary care office visits. *Health Services Research, 42*, 1871–1894.

Thompson, J.D. (1967). *Organizations in Action*. New York: McGraw-Hill.

Toikka, S., and Solantaus, T. (2006). The Effective Family Programme II: Clinicians' experiences of training in promotive and preventative child mental health methods. *International Journal of Mental Health Promotion, 8*, 4–10.

University of Washington. (2009). *Evidence for IMPACT*. Available: http://impact-uw.org/about/research.html [accessed March 26, 2009].

Unützer, J., Katon, W.J., Callahan, C.M., Williams, J.W., Hunkeler, E., Harpole, L., Hoffing, M., Della Penna, R.D., Hitchcock-Noël, P., Lin, E.H.B., Areán, P.A., Hegel, M., Tang, L., Belin, T., Oishi, S., and Langston, C. (2002). Collaborative care management of late-life depression in the primary care setting: A randomized controlled trial. *Journal of the American Medical Association, 288,* 2836–2845.

Unützer, J., Katon, W.J., Fan, M.Y., Schoenbaum, M.C., Lin, E.H.B., Della Penna, R.D., and Powers, D. (2008). Long-term cost effects of collaborative care for late-life depression. *American Journal of Managed Care, 14,* 95–100.

U.S. Department of Health and Human Services. (n.d.). *H.H.S. Strategic Plan Goals and Objectives: FY 2007–2012.* Available: http://www.hhs.gov/strategic_plan/ [accessed March 27, 2009].

U.S. Department of Health and Human Services. (2000). *Healthy People 2010, Volume I* (2nd ed). Washington, DC: U.S. Government Printing Office.

U.S. Surgeon General. (1999). *Mental Health: A Report of the Surgeon General.* Washington, DC: U.S. Department of Health and Human Services.

U.S. Surgeon General. (2001). *Mental Health: Culture, Race, Ethnicity-Supplement.* Washington, DC: U.S. Department of Health and Human Services.

Valenstein, M., Klinkman, M., Becker, S., Blow, F.C., Barry, K.L., Sattar, A., and Hill, E. (1999). Concurrent treatment of patients with depression in the community: Provider practices, attitudes, and barriers to collaboration. *Journal of Family Practice, 48,* 180–187.

van Doesum, K.T.M., Riksen-Walraven, J.M., Hosman, C.M.H., and Hoefnagel, C. (2008). A randomized controlled trial of a home-visiting intervention aimed at preventing relationship problems in depressed mothers and their infants. *Child Development, 79,* 547–561.

Weissman, M.M., Alpert, J.E., Fava, M., Trivedi, M.H., and Rush, A.J. (2006). Remission of maternal depression and children's psychopathology. *Journal of the American Medical Association, 296,* 1233–1234.

Wells, K.B., Sherbourne, C., Duan, N., Unützer, J., Miranda, S., Schoenbaum, M., Ettner, S.L., Meredith, L.S., and Rubenstein, L. (2005). Quality improvements for depression in primary care: Do patients with subthreshold depression benefit in the long run? *American Journal of Psychiatry, 162,* 1149–1157.

Wells, K.B., Sherbourne, C., Schoenbaum, M., Duan, N., Meredith, L., Unützer, J., Miranda, J., Carney, M.F., and Rubenstein, L.V. (2000). Impact of disseminating quality improvement programs for depression in managed primary care: A randomized controlled trial. *Journal of the American Medical Association, 283,* 212–220.

9

Strengthening Systemic, Workforce, and Fiscal Policies to Promote Research-Informed Practices

SUMMARY

Systemic Challenges

- A variety of systemic policies act as a barrier to implement research-informed practices to improve the quality care needed for depressed parents and their children. These challenges include, creating a two-generation response, meeting the need of vulnerable populations as well as those who experience depression with other comorbidities and family adversities, and developing complex interventions that can be adopted in a variety of settings.

Workforce Capacity and Competency

- Evidence shows that a variety of workforce issues remain as a barrier to implement research-informed practices to care for depressed parents and their children. These issues include mental health and primary care provider shortages; a lack of comfort with clinical skills, capacity, and awareness for dealing with depression and its co-occurring conditions in families; and a lack of effective training models to help providers learn and take on multiple roles.

Fiscal Policies

- A variety of financial challenges exist in implementing research-informed practices to improve the quality of care for depressed parents and their children. These challenges include a lack of or inadequate insurance coverage, reimbursement practices and policies that are inconsistent with the research base, and a lack of funding streams to pay for two-generation, research-informed prevention and parenting interventions as well as early interventions for children.

This chapter provides an overview of the policy environments that can resolve systemic, workforce, and fiscal policy challenges associated with implementing innovative and research-informed practices to improve outcomes for depressed parents and their children. It concludes by highlighting policy recommendations that support bolder federal and state responses to the problem of parental depression.

Three broad issues must be addressed to create a more responsive policy framework to increase access to research-based prevention, screening, and treatment through a family-focused lens for those coping with parental depression: (1) systemic barriers, (2) workforce capacity and competence, and (3) fiscal barriers.

SYSTEMIC OPPORTUNITIES

Building a comprehensive policy and service response to parental depression that includes attention to impacts on adults, on children (especially young children), and on parent-child relationships, as described in Chapter 8, requires refocusing program strategies through a family lens. Right now, few, if any, policy models exist for delivering family-focused mental health services. Systemic barriers across health, mental health, and other systems will have to be overcome to provide the range and intensity of research-informed prevention, treatment, and parenting support services discussed in this report.

Below we highlight four of the most important systemic policy and services frameworks challenges to overcome to implement these strategies:

1. creating a two-generation response to parental depression;
2. responding to the needs of vulnerable populations, particularly low-income and culturally and ethnically diverse families;
3. responding to families experiencing depression along with other comorbidities and family adversities; and
4. developing complex interventions that build on collaborative, integrated, and comprehensive service models.

Family-Focused Two-Generation Issues

A central gap across the relevant systems is the difficulty of implementing screening and services responsive not just to adults or to children, but to both, taking into account the family context. Barriers to a responsive family-focused perspective from the adult mental health system, for example, include the failure to require in protocols or administrative regulations that adults in treatment for any mental health issues are asked whether they are parents and what the impact of the illness is on the children. A recent study found that only 12 states report that they systematically inquire as to whether adults with any mental illness under their care are parents and provide some parenting services (Biebel et al., 2006). Similarly, the child mental health system lacks the capacity to provide either treatment or parenting interventions to parents with depression.

Furthermore, despite evidence about the importance of addressing the risks that parental depression poses to children, particularly young children, most children's mental health agencies lack the resources (or the legal mandate) to serve children at risk of developing mental health problems and instead focus all resources on those with diagnosed problems (Cooper et al., 2008). Financing for services and supports for children without a diagnosis remains limited. Nor are we aware of states that explicitly set forth referral priorities for children. This is further compounded for the youngest children because only a handful of states permit an early childhood diagnostic classification system, known as DC-03, as a basis for reimbursement for Medicaid (Stebbins and Knitzer, 2007), although it is widely recognized that there is a lack of fit with the *Diagnostic and Statistical Manual of Mental Disorders*, 4th edition (DSM-IV) for this age group. Similarly, there are still some states that do not permit family therapy for children under age 3 years, although according to a Kaiser Permanente study, 1 in 10 children from birth to age 3 has a parent with diagnosed depression or depressive symptoms (Dietz et al., 2007).

Taking the family context into account requires policy and administrative remedies to resolve several challenges. Introducing a responsive family-focused perspective from the adult mental health system, for example, will require changes in protocols or administrative regulations so that adults in treatment for any mental health issues are asked about their parental status and are invited to describe the impact of their illness on their children.

Responding to the Needs of Low-Income and Minority Families

A responsive policy framework for parental depression has to be flexible enough to support different approaches focused on different populations. For example, given that depression disproportionately impacts low-income populations, a supportive parental depression policy agenda must be able to provide incentives to implement effective outreach and engagement strategies known to enhance treatment, as well as efforts to adapt research-informed practices to diverse families. It is also important in crafting a policy framework responsive to low-income parents, particularly single parents, to take into account their need for other supportive benefits to reduce the stresses and hardship related to poverty that can in fact trigger or exacerbate depression.

One study shows that depressed mothers on welfare were more likely to report food insecurity, to have food stamps sanctioned or reduced, or to lose their welfare benefit than mothers who were not depressed (Casey et al., 2004), compounding the hardship to their families. Particularly for low-income and culturally diverse populations, interventions are often best delivered in nonclinical, community-based settings that children, youth, and families frequent and trust. Prevention, screening, treatment, and parenting support services therefore need to be available in a range of community-based settings that include not only obstetrics-gynecology, pediatric offices, and community health care settings, but also early childhood programs such as Head Start and Early Head Start and public assistance programs (e.g., Temporary Assistance to Needy Families, the Special Supplemental Nutrition Program for Women, Infants, and Children, or WIC). This means that clinicians must acquire experience in delivering services in these settings, as well as in homes, particularly for infants and toddlers, where the family and service providers can be linked to home visiting programs. State policies that prohibit services in nonclinical settings represent an important area for change to support these new collaborative approaches.

Co-Occurring Conditions

Depression rarely occurs in isolation. Chapter 3 on etiology of depression, for example, notes that adult depression typically occurs in a context of chronic and acute stress and includes multiple co-occurring hardships, such as social disadvantage, exposure to violence, low social support, and comorbid psychiatric, substance, and medical problems.

This constellation of risk factors may be essential to understanding the problems in children of depressed parents. The associated features also may be essential in identifying approaches to treating parents' depression and also improving the quality of parenting and children's outcomes. Such recognition might involve, at a minimum, assessing the constellation of risk factors and also evaluating the relative contribution of the multiple disorders to the problems with parenting and with child functioning. These risk factors may also affect how and where services can best be provided.

Multiple initiatives to promote integrated care approaches have emerged in diverse settings (as discussed in Chapter 8) but they are often stymied by policy, institutional, and practice barriers (Dausey et al., 2007). Rather than providing incentives for treatment strategies that recognize comorbidities, the policy environment often sets up barriers. Thus, for the most part, even the limited empirical knowledge about how best to treat adults with comorbid conditions remains largely unexploited (Drake et al., 1998).

One striking example involves the absence of strategies that can respond effectively to depressed parents who are also substance abusers. While it is known that 24 percent of adults with depression have a co-occurring substance use disorder (Kessler et al., 2003), less than 19 percent of individuals with co-occurring depression and substance use disorders receive treatment (Mark, 2003). This is fewer than the 30 percent of individuals with either disorder alone. For those individuals with co-occurring disorders (depression and alcohol addiction) that are treated, treatment is more costly, 68–80 percent higher than treatment for either disorder alone (Mark, 2003). Many parents, particularly low-income parents, experience not just depression, but depression and trauma, substance abuse, domestic violence, and other conditions that impair effective parenting (Cooper et al., 2007; Flynn and Chermack, 2008). Furthermore, evidence suggests that when parents experience multiple risk factors, this is reflected in negative cognitive and behavioral outcomes for children, particularly very young children (Whitaker, Orzol, and Kahn, 2006).

Complexity of Interventions

Many model programs tested in controlled trials and found to be effective for parental depression prevention and care involve complex strategies such as integrated services, coordinated programs, and comprehensive care, and strive to align the complexity of an intervention or organization with the complexity of the environment in which it functions (Dietrich et al., 2004; Katon et al., 2004; Wells et al., 2000). This approach, an example of the concept of requisite variety in systems theory, involves more of the variables that can affect a problem, but at the cost of increased difficulties in replicating complex solutions in new settings (Ashby, 1958; Bodenheimer, Wagner, and Grumbach, 2002; Pfeffer and Sutton, 2006). The limited evidence available on the implementation of depression care interventions, either after clinical trials or in nontrial settings, has shown increased variation in performance (Fisher, Goodman, and Chandra, 2008; Pearson et al., 2005; Pincus et al., 2005), which could be owing to many factors. But certainly the multiple working parts of these interventions—that is, their complexity—may be among the relevant influences.

The limited available evidence casts collaboration in depression care in a promising light (Bluthenthal et al., 2006; Wells et al., 2006). But the evidence is not yet sufficient to support confident interpretation that success can be attributed to generalizable factors rather than idiosyncrasies (e.g., a particular leader or a particular agency). In studies of the chronic care model, community collaboration has been found to be the least successful of the model's components, suggesting the inherent challenges of forging reliable and effective operational linkages across organizational boundaries and multiple providers (Pearson et al., 2005). For the most part, people and organizations will not adopt a practice or program if they cannot see it as an appropriate response to problems they care about. The intervention needs to have enough resonance with their existing beliefs and values to seem at least a little bit familiar (Hargadon and Douglas, 2001). Prevention models may fail to spread because they differ markedly from the usual practices carried out in communities (Gottfredson and Gottfredson, 2002).

In most diffusion research, the complexity of an intervention has been found to be a deterrent to adoption (Damanpour and Schneider, 2006; Rogers, 1995; Rye and Kimberly, 2007). However, the likelihood of implementing a complex intervention may be enhanced if the intervention is clearly perceived by its audience as a better solution than its rivals to a salient problem, if the audience has relatively high levels of absorptive capacity, or if an intervention is supported by an ample funding source (Knudsen and Roman, 2004).

The health care and human services literature often refers to making the business case for innovations (Green et al., 2006; Unützer et al., 2006). In an environment in which insurers and policy makers wish to control costs, the uptake of improvements in depression care may depend on whether such improvements can be shown over time to save more than they cost, will be cost-neutral, or will achieve major gains in quality and health outcomes for patients for a modest net increase in costs. At this point, cost-benefit and cost-effectiveness studies on some parental depression interventions show mixed results (Gilbody, Bower, and Whitty, 2006; Neumeyer-Gromen et al., 2004; Ofman et al., 2004). Moreover, costs are frequently more certain than the expected effects or benefits, especially when the latter are based on the carefully controlled and somewhat unreal conditions of clinical trial investigations. Many of the benefits to the children of depressed parents are only realized far into the future and may be difficult to account for in the usual cost-benefit analysis.

In addition to these aggregate cost issues, the question of incentives that would facilitate the adoption of evidence-based depression care procedures by clinicians deserves attention. Here, again, the evidence is mixed (Armour et al., 2001; Chaix-Couturier et al., 2000). By and large, bonus payments to induce behavior change have not been successful among physicians, perhaps because the bonuses are not large enough to be meaningful (Armour et al., 2001; Epstein, Lee, and Hamel, 2004; Town et al., 2005). Other, nonpecuniary inducements, such as public recognition and more attractive health care quality contracts with health plans, have seemed to have better success, although, in at least one study, less so for depression than other chronic diseases (Casalino et al., 2003).

WORKFORCE CAPACITY AND COMPETENCY

Workforce challenges—both provider shortages to meet the demand of those who need treatment and a poor fit between provider capacity and the skills that are needed to deliver effective, research-informed services, including those related to parental depression—are at the root of many mental health policy challenges (Annapolis Coalition, 2007; Institute of Medicine, 2006). Although this report does not focus on these workforce issues, they are a part of the context for the committee's depression-specific recommendations. One study reported that more than half of all counties in the United States lack a practicing mental health clinician (Pion et al., 1997). In primary care settings, pediatricians and other practitioners have indicated that the lack of community-based mental health capacity severely undermines their ability and confidence to appropriately identify and refer for mental health treatment, including family depression (Leaf et al., 2004; Nicholson et al., 2004). In addition, a lack of training in cultural competence is frequently cited. Among mental health professionals, providers from underrepresented minority communities are less than 25 percent of psychiatrists, 20 percent of social workers and psychiatric nurses, and 10 percent of psychologists (Duffy et al., 2004). Furthermore, among providers from the majority community, many lack the cultural and linguistic competence to adequately serve diverse communities (New Freedom Commission on Mental Health, 2003). As the U.S. population becomes more diverse—1 in 3 Americans are now from one of the four major racial/ethnic minority groups (U.S. Census Bureau, 2008)—the implications of these disparities widen.

Specific to maternal depression, a recent survey by the state of Iowa found that, among nursing programs in the state, on average, fewer than 3 hours of curriculum-based instruction were devoted to perinatal depression and to infant mental health (Montgomery and Trusty, n.d.). Research also shows that many practitioners and clinicians lack the skills to screen or treat parental depression, resulting in inappropriate responses (Horowitz et al., 2007; Leaf et al., 2004). These include not knowing how to respond to fears on the part of mothers that they may lose custody of their children as well as an inability or unwillingness to discuss depression with their patients (Busch and Redlich, 2007; Nicholson et al., 2004; Park, Solomon, and Mandell, 2006). Thus, the lack of clinician skills or understanding can contribute to stigma and discourage parents with depression from seeking care. Among clinicians and staff that attend to individuals with co-occurring disorders, there is a similar disconnect between the body of knowledge about effective practices and their implementation in everyday settings (Flynn and Brown, 2008). Cross-system training is limited or inadequate and undermines efforts to improve the quality of integrated care. One study of mental health professionals revealed that less than 40 percent had any formal training in substance use disorders or addiction services (Harwood, Kowalski, and Ameen, 2004). Only half had any exposure to substance abuse issues during their training, and only 7 percent were dually certified in substance abuse and mental health (Harwood, Kowalski, and Ameen, 2004). The problem of lack of training is exacerbated by uneven preparation and entry standards (Gallon, Gabriel, and Knudsen, 2003). The research does not even address the clinicians' lack of knowledge of the impact of parental comorbidities on children.

Onsite training requirements are dictated by multiple factors, including training resources, availability of staff time, model complexity, levels of differentiation of provider roles, data collection, and model fidelity requirements. Models of moderate to greater complexity cannot be effectively learned through on-the-job experience alone (Feltovich, Prietula, and Ericsson, 2006; Taatgen, Huss, and Anderson, 2006; Velmahos et al., 2004) or by reading manuals or information received through the mail (Ellis et al., 2005). Indeed, even the simplest models (e.g., brief depression screens) may be difficult to execute properly just by reading up on them. Their implementers are likely to need to be trained to minimize the probability of biased interpretations (Chi and Ohlsson, 2005).

Although formal training or education appears to be fairly common in research-informed practices and programs, including some of the more mature and sophisticated depression care models (e.g., Cole et al., 2000; Kilbourne et al., 2004; Wells et al., 2000), the adequacy of these training systems remains largely unknown. Specific descriptions of training are rare in the literature. In the field of training research, advances have been made in identifying factors that may contribute to training effectiveness (e.g., Burke and Hutchins, 2007; Clark and Elen, 2006; Merrill, 2002; Paas et al., 2005; Van Merrienboer and Kirschner, 2007). However, there is little indication that this knowledge has been or is being applied to the training associated with research-informed interventions (but see Cole et al., 2000).

While training may be necessary in learning how to operate a new practice or program, it is often not sufficient, given the context-dependence of learning (Anderson, Reder, and Simon, 1996; Ellis et al., 2005; Fixsen et al., 2005; Joyce and Showers, 2002). When clinicians learn in a formal training program, they are learning in that context, which will differ to a greater or lesser degree from the work context in which they will need to apply what they have learned. Evidence suggests that the knowledge acquired through training decays fairly rapidly unless it is used (Salas and Cannon-Bowers, 2001; Tunney, 2003; Wexley and Latham, 2002), and use depends on a context that will encourage and support it socially (Burke and Hutchins, 2007) as well as financially (Bachman et al., 2006).

People in supervisory roles and external sources of technical aid or coaching may need to be readily available to provide guidance and to help troubleshoot problems (Burke and Hutchins, 2007; Fixsen et al., 2005; Smith-Jentsch, Salas, and Brannick, 2001). Systems may need to be in place that provide regular, objective feedback on performance (Dunning, 2005; Ericsson, Krampe, and Tesch-Romer, 1993; Kluger and DeNisi, 1998; Webb and Sheeran, 2006). For especially complex interventions, developing proficiency may take a considerable period of time (Ericsson, 2003; Norman, 2005), during which the supportiveness of the context may be as important as individual ability in determining success.

Early training to prepare new entrants into the health care workforce is an important way to integrate parental depression care competencies, but it is even more important for general learning and collaboration skills. Doctors, nurses, pharmacists, and other health professionals are not being adequately prepared to provide the *highest* quality and *safest* medical care possible, and there is insufficient assessment of their ongoing proficiency (Institute of Medicine, 2003). In 2003, the Institute of Medicine made 10 recommendations designed to move training toward five interdisciplinary core competencies that support the goals of enhancing the quality and safety of care. Most of these recommendations have never been enacted, and training has not moved toward this aspiration.

Promising parental depression program models often involve multiple tasks, such as screening, referral, counseling or treatment, and ancillary social services. These different roles must either be performed by program staff with the appropriate skills or provided through referrals to a network of specialists and services partnering with the parental depression program. The necessity of covering multiple roles, either in the parental depression program or through collaboration with other providers, poses significant training, communication, funding, and sustainability challenges for parental depression programs.

For parental depression models in which all services are provided by staff that are primarily charged with delivering another service (e.g., home visitation, pediatric well-child visits, child care, etc.), training represents an additional burden of time and effort in addition to the paperwork and supervision required by the model. Staff tasked with multiple roles often face conflicting priorities in terms of which services take precedent over other roles. In such cases, good supervision informed by clear priorities is essential.

For parental depression models involving coordination among multiple providers (e.g., a risk screening program with facilitated referrals for mental health, a prevention program that addresses associated comorbidities), it may be necessary to cotrain all parties in the overall model and process to reduce misunderstandings about roles and responsibilities, identify program interfaces and potential problems, and to develop working relationships. It can be difficult to schedule staff from multiple systems for common training unless times have been preestablished.

Significant workforce challenges—including provider shortages, lack of skills and competencies, and lack of comprehensive training programs—remain a barrier to and offer opportunities for implementing research-informed strategies and improving the quality of care for parents who are depressed as well as support services for their children. In addition, opportunities for improving the quality of care exist in the fiscal policy environment.

FISCAL CHALLENGES

The foundation of a strong policy framework to address parental depression is largely based on who does and does not have insurance and what can and cannot be funded through the insurance. The problems fall into three large categories: (1) lack of insurance, (2) reimbursement practices and policies that are inconsistent with the evidence base of how best to respond to parental depression, and (3) funding gaps. For lower income families, under the current system, this is largely (although not exclusively) shaped at the federal level, particularly through Medicaid and the State Children's Health Insurance Program (CHIP), although states also have often unrecognized degrees of freedom (Rosenthal and Kaye, 2005; Stebbins and Knitzer, 2007). Furthermore, the majority of the payments made for mental health care are made by public sources (Institute of Medicine, 2006). However, it is also important to note the role that private-sector payers and purchasers play on the purchasing of services that are covered, including carve-out arrangements, that can be deleterious to insurance coverage for and the quality of mental health services. In general, there is a lack of publically accessible information on any specific barriers in implementing a family-focused, research-informed model of depression, but when such information is available we highlighted it in this section. The fiscal challenges identified below compound and exacerbate the workforce challenges just discussed.

Lack of or Adequate Insurance

Having health insurance is associated with better health outcomes for adults. Further population groups that most often lack stable health insurance coverage, including racial and ethnic minorities and lower income adults, would be likely to benefit most from increased health insurance coverage, and such coverage would probably reduce some of the disparities in health among these groups (Institute of Medicine, 2002). For both children and adults, the lack of insurance, including underinsurance (in which benefit packages lack comprehensive mental health coverage), is a major problem that limits access to treatment and supportive strategies related to parental depression. Overall, it is estimated that 11.1 million parents and 9 million children are uninsured (Henry J. Kaiser Family Foundation, 2009; Holahan, Cook, and Dubay, 2007). Most of those who are insured are covered through private insurance. For example, 18 percent of women in the general population are uninsured (16.7 million), another 10 percent are covered by Medicaid, and 64 percent are covered through their (or their spouse's) job (Henry J. Kaiser Family Foundation, 2008). A total of 29 million children are enrolled in Medicaid and 7 million in CHIP (Henry J. Kaiser Family Foundation, 2009).

One major concern is the parents whose income is too high for Medicaid but who lack private insurance, particularly parents with incomes between 100 and 300 percent of the official poverty level: for example, 11 states permit eligibility at or above 200 percent of the federal poverty level for working families, and 20 states permit eligibility at or above this level for pregnant women. But half of the states have an income eligibility requirement that is at or below the official poverty level (Stebbins and Knitzer, 2007). It is estimated that 6.2 million parents have incomes that fall below 300 percent of the official poverty level (Holahan, Cook, and Dubay, 2007).

Recent parity legislation was adopted after completion of the committee's deliberations, and therefore this report includes no analysis of its potential impact on access to appropriate services for parental depression. Although the new parity law could potentially improve treatment for adults and children with mental health and substance abuse problems, it does not tackle the fundamental problem that the committee is addressing—that children of parents with depression as well as parenting supports are not addressed by the payment system.

Funding Restrictions Inconsistent with Research-Informed Practice

Below we cite examples of how funding restrictions work to create barriers to implementing family-focused, research-informed prevention and treatment strategies related to parental depression.

One major problem is that, when clinicians are trained and want to implement research-informed practices, in most states the appropriate reimbursement mechanisms do not exist. Current billing mechanisms that facilitate payment for services in most states do not fit many research-informed practices. The billing procedures are designed for single provider types and service units constructed based on time increments, thus presenting a mismatch with research-informed practices. In particular, the crucial work done by case managers and other qualified providers to support treatment often is not reimbursed. Making adjustments to accommodate research-informed practices is administratively cumbersome (Cooper, 2008). Furthermore, billing procedures for Medicaid in some states prohibit same-day billing for multiple services or providers, even when those providers and the services rendered are delivering services under the same provider organization (Kautz, Mauch, and Smith, 2008)

Another example is the difficulty of paying for two-generation screening and interventions through Medicaid, which is very complex. Even when both parents and children have access to Medicaid or CHIP, there are limited policy mechanisms to pay for screening and follow-up. Low reimbursement rates, lack of benefit coverage to assess for maternal depression, prohibitions against pediatricians to assess parents, and a restricted range of eligible providers that are reimbursed in some states stymie the ability to use the Medicaid program as a vehicle of addressing maternal depression in a comprehensive manner. Fewer than 15 percent of state Medicaid programs report that they reimburse for maternal depression screening delivered in pediatric settings (Rosenthal and Kaye, 2005; Weissman et al., 2006). Medicaid-related limitations to facilitating two-generation strategies to address depression for the Medicaid-enrolled child include failure to reimburse for children at risk for social emotional delay (i.e., form close relationships, develop capacity to experience and regulate emotions) and failure to pay for all of the elements of research-informed, intergenerational interventions (Rosenthal and Kaye, 2005). Furthermore, although states can also pay for screening through early and periodic screening, diagnosis, and treatment programs, many do not (Cooper, 2008; Rosenthal and Kaye, 2005). Nor do federal Medicaid guidelines require the use of validated tools for the assessment of children.

There are also problems with eligibility cutoffs for women that limit access to services for postpartum depression. Even if mothers have access to Medicaid, for new mothers, eligibility is extended for only 2 months after the baby's birth in most states. The reauthorization of CHIP in 2009 established new options for states to cover pregnant women (instead of the unborn child); however, it limits current coverage of adults: Some states that currently receive waivers to cover parents instead will be establishing a set-aside separate from CHIP to cover parents (Henry J. Kaiser Family Foundation, 2009). Given that research shows that the average duration of a depressive episode is 6 months, if a mother is diagnosed as having postpartum depression, this is not enough time to provide treatment (Hasin et al., 2005). The failure to extend Medicaid coverage for up to a year for both parents and children in some states is not only undermining the treatment received, but it is also inefficient. Research shows that individuals with depression who lose Medicaid coverage are more costly to treat and have been linked to more intensive care, including emergency department care, and greater number of inpatient days (Harman, Hall, and Zhang, 2007).

It is very difficult in some states to pay for screening and services delivered in nonmental health settings. This has a particularly chilling effort on taking to scale interventions that target low-income families or are culturally and linguistically relevant. Research shows that a variety of interventions can be delivered in settings that families, particularly low-income families, trust, thus potentially reducing stigma, improving access, and reducing attrition (Ammerman et al., 2007; also see Chapter 7). These settings potentially include home visiting, prekindergarten, Head Start and Early Head Start programs, and community centers. To date, efforts have been funded only through research and demonstration projects, and there are still mental health agencies (for both children and adults) that do not pay for treatment in nonmental health settings on a routine basis.

In recent years, federal Medicaid policy has discouraged reimbursement for interventions in nonclinical settings. There is also a more recent effort to restrict payment for what is seen as nonmedical treatment or treatment that may impact domains other than mental health. In other words, Medicaid will not pay if the service system would need to provide that service anyway. This particularly threatens case management and support services, such as transportation. The proposed regulations, which are slated to go into effect, will also restrict Medicaid reimbursement for mental health services delivered in child welfare, child care, and educational settings (Cooper, 2008).

It is also difficult to pay for enriched or enhanced therapies, such as phone outreach, child care, and transportation, which research suggests are necessary to engage low-income adults, reduce attrition, and achieve positive outcomes with research-informed strategies. Evidence shows that for more traditional, clinic-based treatment to be effective with low-income families, it is necessary to invest in engagement and outreach strategies, but typically it is difficult to fund these activities (Miranda et al., 2004). Indeed, a number of demonstration projects highlight the importance of these enhanced approaches to traditional treatment, although there is limited capacity to take them to scale (Cardemil et al., 2005). This is so even though recent studies of culturally adapted treatments for different ethnic groups demonstrated improved outcomes and cost-effectiveness when measured against traditional treatment as usual (Cabassa and Hansen, 2007).

Although parental depression is often comorbid with other conditions that together pose risks to children, paying for integrated services is very challenging. Paying for treatment in a manner that recognizes the complexity of treating co-occurring disorders requires flexibility to incorporate different approaches that address both conditions either sequentially or simultaneously and with different levels of intensity. Current fiscal policy is generally unresponsive to this type of integrated treatment model. For example, programs with dual diagnosis capacity, or enhanced dual diagnosis services, cost more than programs that provide addiction or mental health services only. Yet neither Medicaid nor private insurance (which has even more limited benefits for substance use disorders) provides fiscal incentives to increase the capacity to address dual diagnosis. Indeed, there are fiscal policies that undermine an integrated approach to addressing co-occurring disorders. Even in Medicaid, mental health and addiction services are not covered evenly. For example, while all Medicaid programs cover assessment and treatment for mental health, many will not do so if they are done by primary care providers, and a handful of states do not cover substance abuse–related assessment and treatment (Robinson et al., 2003). Only half of states cover extensive outpatient services, and only a quarter of states cover case management for individuals with substance use conditions, both vital components of the service array of an integrated treatment approach (Robinson et al., 2003). Reimbursement rates for mental health services are generally higher than addiction services and credentialing and certification requirements also differ (O'Brien and Wilford, 2003). Finally, the chronic nature of depression and substance use disorders necessitates financing that is responsive to monitoring and support to prevent or manage relapse (Flynn and Brown, 2008). Again, across the board, both Medicaid and private insurance remain restricted.

Funding Gaps

There are three related and major funding gaps in supporting research-informed practices for depressed parents and their children. One is the absence of an ongoing federal funding stream to pay for two-generation, research-informed prevention and parental support activities to improve outcomes for children and their parents who are at risk of depression and its consequences. Addressing parental depression often requires parent-focused or parent and child–focused strategies. Some of these are directly linked to treatment, but others are linked to a range of other parenting supports, including prevention efforts to reduce risk factors (e.g., isolation, high stress levels linked to poverty); parent support groups; and even parent training interventions that take into account parental depression. And yet there is no dedicated federal funding stream that allows mental health providers to meet the needs of parents whose children are at high risk of developing problems related to parental depression. Specifically, neither Medicaid nor the only targeted funds for children's mental health, through the Mental Health Services for Children and Families Community Program, allow for family-focused prevention or early intervention services.

The second funding gap results from the fact that it is very difficult to pay for early intervention services for children, particularly young children, who show signs of problematic behavior that falls below the clinical threshold of diagnosable disorders. In some states, Medicaid does pay for children at risk of problems, but there is no accurate count of how many. More typically, even for infants and toddlers, children whose developmental and social and emotional behavior is problematic, cannot, in most states, access services. The federal Part C Early Intervention program of the Individuals with Disabilities Education Act, which provides services to infants and toddlers with identified developmental delays and, in theory, allows states to cover babies and toddlers at risk of such delays, does not work as it should, largely because it is inadequately funded. Today, only six states currently allow for the youngest children who are at risk to be served.

The third major funding gap is the lack of training resources available at all levels of the system. As described earlier, workforce capacity and competence are major barriers to implementing research-informed practices to care for depressed parents and their children. As described in Chapter 8, there are a limited number of funding sources available through federal initiatives—namely the Maternal and Child Health Bureau and the Center for Mental Health Services—that target training and workforce development for those who provide mental health services.

CONCLUSION

Adoption of the core recommendations of this report will involve significant changes in the current policy framework to develop systemic strategies as well as the workforce and fiscal resources necessary to implement research-informed prevention, screening, treatment, and parent support services for parents experiencing or at risk of experiencing depression and their children.

RECOMMENDATIONS

This chapter examines the systemic, workforce, and fiscal challenges associated with implementing innovative and research-informed practices to improve outcomes for parents who are depressed and their children. The committee recognizes that some of these challenges are problems faced by the general health care system; however, the care of depressed parents has a number of distinctive characteristics, including identifying, treating, and preventing the effects on parenting practices and their children's health and development, providing resources and referrals for comorbidities associated with depression, and supporting parent-child relationships. None of the recommendations below will fully address the systemic, workforce, and fiscal-related policy challenges in the health care system, and each involves a unique set of costs, benefits, and practical considerations. The committee nonetheless makes three recommendations intended to support bolder federal, state, and private-sector responses to improve the outreach and delivery of services in different settings for diverse populations of families with a depressed parent. They are meant to complement current local, state, and federal efforts to improve education, awareness, and development of innovative strategies.

Develop and Implement Systemic, Workforce, and Fiscal Policies

Recommendation 4: State governors, in collaboration with the U.S. Department of Health and Human Services, should support an inter-agency task force within each state focused on depression in parents. The task force should develop local and regional strategies to support collaboration and capacity building to prepare for the implementation of evidence-based practices, new service strategies, and promising programs for the identification, treatment, and prevention of depression in parents and its effects in children.

The wide variation in state resources and structures for providing mental health services and family support resources suggests that broad experimentation with different service strategies may be necessary to implement two-generation interventions for the treatment and prevention of depression in parents, to support parenting practices, and to prevent physical, behavioral, and mental health and problems in youth. First, state governors should designate a joint task force of state and local agencies to coordinate local efforts (e.g., counties) and to build linkages and the infrastructure that can support a strategic planning process; refine service models and delivery systems through collaboration among diverse agencies; prepare to incorporate an array of programs for different sites, settings, and target populations; prepare model plans that include multiple entry points in a variety of service sectors; and prepare for a stepwise rollout with ongoing or interim evaluation.

Second, the state strategies should include policy protocols and fiscal strategies that offer incentives across multiple systems (including health and education) to expand the state's capacity to respond to parental depression through a family-focused lens. These protocols and strategies could be supported by the efforts funded and coordinated by the U.S. Department of Health and Human Services (HHS) through its agencies that include the Substance Abuse and Mental Health Services Administration and the Health Resources and Services Administration. Third, the state strategies should offer flexible responses that can be adapted to the needs of urban and rural communities. Finally, states should be required to provide a biannual report to a designated office in HHS that describes their strategic plans as well as the challenges and barriers that affect their capacity to address depression in a family context for children of all ages. These reports should be shared to encourage states to learn from each other's initiatives.

> **Recommendation 5: The Substance Abuse and Mental Health Services Administration and the Health Resources and Services Administration, in collaboration with relevant professional organizations and accrediting bodies, should develop a national collaborative training program for primary, mental health care, and substance abuse treatment providers to improve their capacity and competence to identify, treat, and prevent depression in parents and mitigate its effects on children of all ages.**

For this recommendation to be realized, the national collaborative training program should strengthen a workforce that is informed about and prepared to address parenting issues associated with depression and the effects of adult disorder on children in a diverse society. This program should explore opportunities to enhance attention to interactions between depression and parenting in ongoing mental health and primary care training and continuing education programs, such as activities funded by Title VII and Title VIII of section 747 of the Public Health Service Act. Training efforts should include an emphasis on developmental issues, exploring the impact of depression and the combination of depression and its commonly co-occurring disorders (e.g., anxiety disorders, parental substance use disorders) on children of different ages, from pregnancy through adolescent development. Options for such training programs could include cross-disciplinary training with an emphasis on parental depression, parenting, and developmentally based, family-focused concerns that arise in the treatment of depression. Such training programs should call attention to identifying children at risk to adverse health and psychological outcomes. Training programs should also include efforts to build a more diverse and culturally competent workforce.

> **Recommendation 6: Public and private payers—such as the Centers for Medicare and Medicaid Services, managed care plans, health maintenance organizations, health insurers, and employers—should improve current service coverage and reimbursement strategies to support the**

implementation of research-informed practices, structures, and settings that improve the quality of care for parents who are depressed and their children.

Public and private payers should consider the following options for implementing this recommendation:

- The Centers for Medicare and Medicaid Services (CMS) could extend services and coverage of mothers to 24 months postpartum, which includes a critical period of early child development when interaction with parental care is especially important. Long-term coverage for parents would be optimal. CMS could remove restrictions on Medicaid's rehabilitation option and other payment options (including targeted case management and home visitation programs) that could reimburse services and supports in nonclinical settings and enhance access to quality care; allow same-day visit reimbursement for mental health and primary care services; reimburse primary care providers for mental health services; and remove prohibitions on serving children without medical diagnoses, thereby covering health promotion services for children at risk before diagnosis.
- States could work with CMS to implement financing mechanisms to support access to treatment and supportive services for depressed parents, through clarifying existing coverage, billing codes, or encouraging the use of research-informed practices. This would complement local and regional strategies developed by the states. Similarly, private health plans and self-insured employers could cover parental depression screening and treatment and support the implementation of effective models.

REFERENCES

Ammerman, R.T., Bodley, A.L., Putnam, F.W., Lopez, W.L., Holleb, L.J., Stevens, J., and Van Ginkel, J.B. (2007). In-home cognitive behavior therapy for a depressed mother in a home visitation program. *Clinical Case Studies, 6*, 161–180.

Anderson, J.R., Reder, L.M., and Simon, H.A. (1996). Situated learning and education. *Educational Researcher, 25*, 5–11.

Annapolis Coalition. (2007). *An Action Plan for Behavioral Health Workforce Development: A Framework for Discussion.* (SAMHSA/DHHS Pub. No. 280-02-0302.) Rockville, MD: Substance Abuse and Mental Health Services Administration, Department of Health and Human Services.

Armour, B.S., Pitts, M.M., MacLean, R., Cangialose, C., Kishel, M., Imai, H., and Etchason, J. (2001). The effective of explicit financial incentives on physician behavior. *Archives of Internal Medicine, 161*, 1261–1266.

Ashby, W.R. (1958). Requisite variety and its implications for the control of complex systems. *Cybernetica, 1*, 83–99.

Bachman, J., Pincus, H.A., Houtsinger, J.K., and Unützer, J. (2006). Funding mechanisms for depression care management: Opportunities and challenges. *General Hospital Psychiatry, 28*, 278–288.

Biebel, K., Nicholson, J., Geller, J., and Fisher, W. (2006). A national survey of state mental health authority programs and policies for clients who are parents: A decade later. *Psychiatric Quarterly, 77*, 119–128.

Bluthenthal, R., Jones, L., Fackler-Lowrie, N., Ellison, M., Booker, T., Jones, F., McDaniel, S., Moini, M., Williams, K.R., Klap, R., Koegel, P., and Wells, K.B. (2006). Witness for wellness: Preliminary findings from a community-academic participatory research mental health initiative. *Ethnicity and Diseases, 16*, 18–34.

Bodenheimer, T., Wagner, E.H., and Grumbach, K. (2002). Improving primary care for patients with chronic illness. *Journal of the American Medical Association, 288*, 1775–1779.

Burke, L.A., and Hutchins, H.M. (2007). Training transfer: An integrative literature review. *Human Resource Development Review, 6*, 263–296.

Busch, A., and Redlich, A.D. (2007). Patients' perception of possible child custody or visitation loss for nonadherance to psychiatric treatment. *Psychiatric Services, 58*, 999–1002.

Cabassa, L.J., and Hansen, M.C. (2007). A systematic review of depression treatment in primary care for Latino adults. *Research on Social Work Practice, 17*, 494–503.

Cardemil, E.V., Kim, S., Pinedo, T., and Miller, I.W. (2005). Developing a culturally appropriate depression prevention program: The Family Coping Skills Program. *Cultural Diversity and Ethnic Minority Psychology, 11*, 99–112.

Casalino, L., Gillies, R.R., Shortell, S.M., Schmittdiel, J.A., Bodenheimer, T., Robinson, J.C., Rundall, T., Oswald, N., Schauffler, H., and Wang, M.C. (2003). External incentives, information technology, and organized processes to improve health care quality for patients with chronic diseases. *Journal of the American Medical Association, 289*, 434–441.

Casey, P., Goolsby, S., Berkowitz, C., Frank, D., Cook, J., Cutts, D., Black, M.M., Zaldivar, N., Levenson, S., Heeren, T., Meyers, A., and the Children's Sentinel Nutritional Assessment Program Study Group. (2004). Maternal depression, changing public assistance, food security, and child health status. *Pediatrics, 113*, 298–304.

Chaix-Couturier, C., Durand-Zaleski, I., Jolly, D., and Durieux, P. (2000). Effects of financial incentives on medical practice: Results from a systematic review of the literature and methodological issues. *International Journal for Quality in Health Care, 12*, 133–142.

Chi, M.T.H., and Ohlsson, S. (2005). Complex declarative learning. In K.J. Holyoak and R.G. Morrison (Eds.), *Cambridge Handbook of Thinking and Reasoning*. New York: Cambridge University Press.

Clark, R.E., and Elen, J. (2006). When less is more: Research and theory insights about instruction for complex learning. In R.E. Clark, and J. Elen (Eds.), *Handling Complexity in Learning Environments: Research and Theory* (pp. 289–295). London: Elsevier.

Cole, S., Raju, M., Barrett, J., Gerrity, M., and Dietrich, A. (2000). The MacArthur Foundation Depression Education Program for Primary Care Physicians: Background, participant's workbook, and facilitator's guide. *General Hospital Psychiatry, 22*, 299–358.

Cooper, J.L. (2008). *Towards Better Behavioral Health for Children, Youth and Their Families: Financing That Supports Knowledge*. New York: National Center for Children in Poverty, Columbia University Mailman School of Public Health.

Cooper, J.L., Aratani, Y., Knitzer, J., Douglas-Hall, A., Masi, R., Banghart, P., and Dababnah, S. (2008). *Unclaimed Children Revisited: The Status of Children's Mental Health Policy in the United States*. New York: National Center for Children in Poverty, Columbia University Mailman School of Public Health.

Cooper, J.L., Masi, R., Dababnah, S., Aratani, Y., and Knitzer, J. (2007). *Strengthening Policies to Support Children, Youth, and Families Who Experience Trauma*. New York: National Center for Children in Poverty, Columbia University Mailman School of Public Health.

Damanpour, F., and Schneider, M. (2006). Phases of the adoption of innovation in organizations: Effects of environment, organization, and top managers. *British Journal of Management, 17*, 215–236.

Dausey, D.J., Pincus, H.A., Herrell, J.M., and Rickards, L. (2007). States' early experience in improving systems-level care for persons with co-occurring disorders. *Psychiatric Services, 58*, 903–905.

Dietrich, A.J., Oxman, T.E., Williams, J.W., Jr., Schulberg, H.C., Bruce, M.L., Lee, P.W., Barry, S., Raue, P.J., Lefever, J.J., Heo, M., Rost, K., Kroenke, K., Gerrity, M., and Nutting, P.A. (2004). Re-engineering systems for the treatment of depression in primary care: Cluster randomised controlled trial. *British Medical Journal, 329*, 602.

Dietz, P.M., Williams, S.B., Callaghan, W.M., Bachman, D.J., Whitlock, E.P., and Hornbrook, M.C. (2007). Clinically identified maternal depression before, during, and after pregnancy. *American Journal of Psychiatry, 164*, 1515–1520.

Drake, R.E., Mercer-McFadden, C., Mueser, K.T., McHugo, G.J., and Bond, G.R. (1998). Review of integrated mental health and substance abuse treatment for patients with dual disorders. *Schizophrenia Bulletin, 24*, 589–608.

Duffy, F.F., West, J.C., Wilk, J., Narrow, W.E., Hales, D., Thompson, J., Reiger, D.A., Kohout, J., Pion, G.M., Wicherski, M., Bateman, N., Whitaker, T., Merwin, E.I., Lyon, D., Fox, J.C., Delaney, K.R., Hanrahan, N., Stockton, R., Kaladow, J., Clawson, T.W., Smith, S.C., Ambrose, J.P., Blankertz, L., Thomas, A., Sullivan, L.D., Dwyer, K.P., Fleisher, M.S., Goldsmith, H.F., Henderson, M.J., Atay, J.E., and Manderscheid, R.W. (2004). Mental health practitioners and trainees. In R.W. Manderscheid and M.J. Henderson (Eds.), *Mental Health, United States, 2002* (pp. 327–368). Rockville, MD: Substance Abuse and Mental Health Services Administration, U.S. Department of Health and Human Services.

Dunning, D. (2005). *Self-Insight: Roadblocks and Detours on the Path to Knowing Thyself*. New York: Psychology Press.

Ellis, P., Ciliska, D., Sussman, J., Robinson, P., Armour, T., Brouwers, M., O'Brien, M.A., and Raina, P. (2005). A systematic review of studies evaluating diffusion and dissemination of selected cancer control interventions. *Health Psychology, 24*, 488–500.

Epstein, A.M., Lee, T.H., and Hamel, M.B. (2004). Paying physicians for high-quality care. *New England Journal of Medicine, 350*, 406–410.

Ericsson, K.A. (2003). Deliberate practice and the acquisition and maintenance of expert performance in medicine and related domains. *Academic Medicine, 79*, S70–S81.

Ericsson, K.A., Krampe, R.T., and Tesch-Romer, C. (1993). The role of deliberate practice in the acquisition of expert performance. *Psychology Review, 100*, 363–406.

Feltovich, P.J., Prietula, M.J., and Ericsson, K.A. (2006). Studies of expertise from psychological perspectives. In K.A. Ericsson, N. Charness, P.J. Feltovich, and R.R. Hoffman (Eds.), *Cambridge Handbook of Expertise and Expert Performance*. New York: Cambridge University Press.

Fisher, E.S., Goodman, D.C., and Chandra, A. (2008). *Disparities in Health and Health Care Among Medicare Beneficiaries: A Brief Report of the Dartmouth Atlas Project*. Princeton, NJ: Robert Wood Johnson Foundation.

Fixsen, D.L., Naoom, S.F., Blasé, K.A., Friedman, R.M., and Wallace, F. (2005). *Implementation Research: A Synthesis of the Literature*. Tampa: University of South Florida.

Flynn, H.A., and Chermack, S.T. (2008). Prenatal alcohol use: The role of lifetime problems with alcohol, drugs, depression, and violence. *Journal of Studies on Alcohol and Drugs, 69*, 500–509.

Flynn, P.M., and Brown, B.S. (2008). Co-occurring disorders in substance abuse treatment: Issues and prospects. *Journal of Substance Abuse Treatment, 34*, 36–47.

Gallon, S.L., Gabriel, R.M., and Knudsen, J.R.W. (2003). The toughest job you'll ever love: A Pacific Northwest treatment workforce survey. *Journal of Substance Abuse Treatment, 24*, 183–196.

Gilbody, S., Bower, P., and Whitty, P. (2006). Costs and consequences of enhanced primary care for depression: Systematic review of randomized economic evaluations. *British Journal of Psychiatry, 189*, 297–308.

Gottfredson, D.C., and Gottfredson, G.D. (2002). Quality of school-based prevention programs: Results from a national survey. *Journal of Research in Crime and Delinquency, 39*, 3–35.

Green, L.W., Orleans, T., Ottoson, J.M., Cameron, R., Pierce, J.P., and Bettinghaus, E.P. (2006). Inferring strategies for disseminating physical activity policies, programs, and practices from the successes of tobacco control. *American Journal of Preventive Medicine, 31*, S66–S81.

Hargadon, A.B., and Douglas, Y. (2001). When innovations meet institutions: Edison and the design of the electric light. *Administrative Science Quarterly, 46*, 476–501.

Harman, J.S., Hall, A.G., and Zhang, J. (2007). Changes in health care use and costs after a break in Medicaid coverage among persons with depression. *Psychiatric Services, 58*, 49–54.

Harwood, H.J., Kowalski, J., and Ameen, A. (2004). The need for substance abuse training among mental health professionals. *Administration and Policy in Mental Health, 32*, 189–205.

Hasin, D.S., Goodwin, R.D., Stinson, F.S., and Grant, B.F. (2005). Epidemiology of major depressive disorder. *Archives of General Psychiatry, 62*, 1097–1106.

Henry J. Kaiser Family Foundation. (2008, October). *Women's Health Insurance Coverage.* Women's Health Policy Facts. Menlo Park, CA: Author.

Henry J. Kaiser Family Foundation. (2009, February). *Children's Health Insurance Program Reauthorization Act of 2009 (CHIRPA).* Kaiser Commission on Key Facts. Menlo Park, CA: Author.

Holahan, J., Cook, A., and Dubay, L. (February, 2007). Characteristics of the uninsured: Who is eligible for public coverage and who needs help affording coverage? Kaiser Commission on Medicaid and the Uninsured Issue Paper. Menlo Park, CA: Henry J. Kaiser Family Foundation.

Horowitz, S.M., Kelleher, K.J., Stein, R.E.K., Storfer-Isser, A., Youngstrum, E.A., Park, E.R., Heneghan, A.M., Jensen, P.S., and O'Connor, K.G. (2007). Barriers to the identification and management of psychosocial issues in children and maternal depression. *Pediatrics, 119*, e208–e219.

Institute of Medicine. (2002). *Unequal Treatment: Confronting Racial and Ethnic Disparities in Health Care.* B.D. Smedley, A.Y. Stith, and A.R. Nelson, Eds., Committee on Understanding and Eliminating Racial and Ethnic Disparities in Health Care. Board on Health Sciences Policy. Washington, DC: The National Academies Press.

Institute of Medicine. (2003). *Health Professions Education: A Bridge to Quality.* A.C. Greiner, E. Knebel (Eds.). Committee on the Health Professions Education Summit. Board on Health Care Services. Washington, DC: The National Academies Press.

Institute of Medicine. (2006). *Improving the Quality of Health Care for Mental and Substance-Use Conditions: Quality Chasm Series.* Committee on Crossing the Quality Chasm:

Adaptation to Mental Health and Addictive Disorders. Board on Health Care Services. Washington, DC: The National Academies Press.

Joyce, B., and Showers, B. (2002). *Student Achievement Through Staff Development*. Alexandria, VA: Association for Supervision and Curriculum Development.

Katon, W.J., Von Korff, M., Lin, E.H.B., Simon, G., Ludman, E., Russo, J., Ciechanowski, P., Walker, E., and Bush, T. (2004). The pathways study: A randomized trial of collaborative care in patients with diabetes and depression. *Archives of General Psychiatry, 61,* 1042–1049.

Kautz, C., Mauch, D., and Smith, S.A. (2008). *Reimbursement of Mental Health Services in Primary Care Settings*. Available: http://download.ncadi.samhsa.gov/ken/pdf/SMA08-4324/SMA08-4324.pdf [accessed March 20, 2009].

Kessler, R.C., Berglund, P., Demler, O., Jin, R., Koretz, D., Merikangas, K.R., Rush, A.J., Walters, E.E., and Wang, P.S. (2003). The epidemiology of major depressive disorder: Results from the National Comorbidity Survey Replication (NCS-R). *Journal of the American Medical Association, 289,* 3095–3105.

Kilbourne, A.M., Schulberg, H.C., Post, E.P., Rollman, B.L., Belnap, B.H., and Pincus, H.A. (2004). Translating evidence-based depression management services to community-based primary care practices. *Milbank Quarterly, 82,* 631–659.

Kluger, A.N., and DeNisi, A. (1998). Feedback interventions: Toward the understanding of a double-edged sword. *Current Directions in Psychological Science, 7,* 67–72.

Knudsen, H.K., and Roman, P.M. (2004). Modeling the use of innovations in private treatment organizations: The role of absorptive capacity. *Journal of Substance Abuse Treatment, 26,* 51–59.

Leaf, P.J., Owens, P.L., Leventhal, J.M., Forsyth, B.W.C., Vaden-Kiernan, M., Epstein, L.D., Riley, A.W., and Horwitz, S.M. (2004). Pediatricians' training and identification and management of psychosocial problems. *Clinical Pediatrics, 43,* 355–365.

Mark, T.L. (2003). The costs of treating persons with depression and alcoholism compared with depression alone. *Psychiatric Services, 54,* 1095–1097.

Merrill, M.D. (2002). First principles of instruction. *Educational Technology Research and Development, 50,* 43–59.

Miranda, J., Schoenbaum, M., Sherbourne, C., Duan, N., and Wells, K. (2004). Effects of primary care depression treatment on minority patients' clinical status and employment. *Archives of General Psychiatry, 61,* 827–834.

Montgomery, J., and Trusty, S. (n.d.). *Nursing School Curriculum: Survey Results*. Iowa Department of Public Health, Division of Health Promotion and Chronic Disease Prevention, Bureau of Family Health.

Neumeyer-Gromen, A., Lamper, T., Stark, K., and Kallischnigg, G. (2004). Disease management programs for depression: A systematic review and meta-analysis of randomized controlled trials. *Medical Care, 42,* 1211–1221.

New Freedom Commission on Mental Health. (2003). *Achieving the Promise: Transforming Mental Health Care in America. Final Report*. Available: http://www.mentalhealth commission.gov/reports/FinalReport/FullReport-05.htm [accessed March 17, 2009].

Nicholson, J., Biebel, K., Katz-Levy, K., and Williams, V.F. (2004). The prevalence of parenthood in adults with mental illness: Implications for state and federal policymakers, programs, and providers. In R. Manderscheid and M. Henderson (Eds.), *Mental Health, United States, 2002*. Rockville, MD: Substance Abuse and Mental Health Services Administration, U.S. Department of Health and Human Services.

Norman, G. (2005). Research in clinical reasoning: Past history and current trends. *Medical Education, 39,* 418–427.

O'Brien, J., and Wilford, C.M. (2003). *Blueprint for Reforming and Enriching Florida's Services*. Tallahassee, FL: Advocacy Center for Persons with Disabilities.

Ofman, J.J., Badamgarav, E., Hennings, J.M., Knight, K., Gano, A.D., Levan, R.K., Gur-Arie, S., Richards, M.S., Hasselbad, V., and Weingarten, S.R. (2004). Does disease management improve clinical and economic outcomes in patients with chronic diseases? A systematic review. *American Journal of Medicine, 117*, 182–192.

Paas, F., Tuovinen, J.E., van Merrienboer, J.J.G., and Darabi, A.A. (2005). A motivational perspective on the relation between mental effort and performance: Optimizing learner involvement in instruction. *Educational Technology Research and Development, 53*, 25–34.

Park, J.M., Solomon, P., and Mandell, D.S. (2006). Involvement in the child welfare system among mothers with serious mental illness. *Psychiatric Services, 57*, 493–497.

Pearson, M.L., Wu, S., Schaefer, J., Bonomi, A.E., Shortell, S.M., Mendel, P.J., Marsteller, J.A., Louis, T.A., Rosen, M., and Keeler, E.B. (2005). Assessing the implementation of the chronic care model in quality improvement collaborative. *Health Services Research, 40*, 978–996.

Pfeffer, J., and Sutton, R.I. (2006). Evidence-based management. *Harvard Business Review, 84*, 62–74.

Pincus, H.A., Houtsinger, J.K., Bachman, J., and Keyser, D. (2005). Depression in primary care: Bringing behavioral health care into the mainstream. *Health Affairs, 24*, 271–276.

Pion, G.M., Keller, P., McCombs, H., and Rural Mental Health Provider Work Group. (1997). *Mental Health Providers in Rural and Isolated Areas: Final Report of the Ad Hoc Rural Mental Health Provider Work Group.* Rockville, MD: Center for Mental Health Services, Substance Abuse and Mental Health Services Administration.

Robinson, G., Kaye, N., Bergman, D., Moreaux, M., and Baxter, C. (2003). *State Profiles of Mental Health and Substance Abuse Services in Medicaid.* (For the Substance Abuse and Mental Health services Administration). Bethesda, MD: Abt Associates.

Rogers, E.M. (1995). *Diffusion of Innovations.* New York: Free Press.

Rosenthal, J., and Kaye, N. (2005). *State Approaches to Promoting Young Children's Healthy Development: A Survey of Medicaid, Maternal and Child Health, and Mental Health Agencies.* Portland, ME: National Academy for State Health Policy.

Rye, C.B., and Kimberly, J.R. (2007). The adoption of innovations by provider organizations in health care. *Medical Care Research and Review, 63*, 235–278.

Salas, E., and Cannon-Bowers, J.A. (2001). The science of training: A decade of progress. *Annual Review of Psychology, 2001.* Palo Alto, CA: Annual Reviews.

Smith-Jentsch, K.A., Salas, E., and Brannick, M.T. (2001). To transfer or not to transfer? Investing the combined effects of trainees' characteristics, team leader support, and team climate. *Journal of Applied Psychology, 86*, 279–292.

Stebbins, H., and Knitzer, J. (2007). *United States Health and Nutrition: State Choices to Promote Quality.* New York: National Center for Children in Poverty, Columbia University Mailman School of Public Health.

Taatgen, N.A., Huss, D., and Andersons, J.R. (2006). How cognitive models can inform the design of instructions. In *Proceedings of the Seventh International Conference on Cognitive Modeling* (pp. 304–309). Austin, TX: Cognitive Science Society.

Town, R., Kane, R., Johnson, P., and Butler, M. (2005). Economic incentives and physicians' delivery of preventive care: A systematic review. *American Journal of Preventive Medicine, 28*, 234–240.

Tunney, R.J. (2003). Implicit and explicit knowledge decay at different rates: A dissociation between priming and recognition in artificial grammar learning. *Experimental Psychology, 50*, 124–130.

Unützer, J., Schoenbaum, M., Druss, B.G., and Katon, W.J. (2006). Transforming mental health care at the interface with general medicine: Report for the president's commission. *Psychiatric Services, 57*, 37–47.

U.S. Census Bureau. (2008). *Table 4. Projections of the Population by Sex, Race, and Hispanic Origin for the United States: 2010 to 2050 (NP2008-T4).* Available: http://www.census. gov/population/www/projections/files/nation/summary/np2008-t4.xls [accessed March 31, 2009].

Van Merrienboer, J.J.G., and Kirschner, P.A. (2007). *Ten Steps to Complex Learning.* Mahwah, NJ: Lawrence Erlbaum.

Velmahos, G.C., Toutouzas, K.G., Sillin, L.F., Chan, L., Clark, R.E., Theodorou, D., and Maupin, F. (2004). Cognitive task analysis for teaching technical skills in an inanimate surgical skills laboratory. *American Journal of Surgery, 187,* 114–119.

Webb, T.L., and Sheeran, P. (2006). Does changing behavioral intentions engender behavior change? A meta-analysis of the experimental evidence. *Psychological Bulletin, 132,* 249–268.

Weissman, M.M., Pilowsky, D.J., Wickramaratne, P.J., Talati, A., Wisniewski, S.R., Fava, M., Hughes, C.W., Garber, J., Malloy, E., King, C.A., Cerda, G., Sood, A.B., Alpert, J.E., Trivedi, M.H., and Rush, A.J. (2006). Remissions in maternal depression and child psychopathology: A STAR*D-child report. *Journal of the American Medical Association, 295,* 1389–1398.

Wells, K.B., Sherbourne, C., Schoenbaum, M., Duan, N., Meredith, L., Unützer, J., Miranda, J., Carney, M.F., and Rubenstein, L.V. (2000). Impact of disseminating quality improvement programs for depression in managed primary care: A randomized controlled trial. *Journal of the American Medical Association, 283,* 212–220.

Wells, K.B., Staunton, A., Norris, K.C., Bluthenthal, R., Chung, B., Gelberg, L., Jones, L., Kataoka, S., Koegel, P., Miranda, J., Mangione, C.M., Patel, K., Rodrigues, M., Shapira, M., and Wong, M. (2006). Building an academic-community partnered network for clinical services research: The Community Health Improvement Collaborative (CHIC). *Ethnicity and Disease, 16,* 3–17.

Wexley, K.N., and Latham, G.P. (2002). *Developing and Training Human Resources in Organizations* (3rd ed). Upper Saddle River, NJ: Prentice-Hall.

Whitaker, R.C., Orzol, S.M., and Kahn, R.S. (2006). Maternal mental health, substance use and domestic violence in the year after delivery and subsequent behavior problems in children at age 3 years. *Archives of General Psychiatry, 63,* 551–560.

10

Opportunities for Innovative Reforms and Knowledge Development

SUMMARY

Research Opportunities

- An analysis of the available evidence in addressing the problem of parental depression reveals gaps in the knowledge base and identifies opportunities to improve the care of depressed parents and their children.

Creating Learning Environments That Support Innovation

- General guidelines exist—largely focused on other health care and business areas—that provide initial guidance for the widespread implementation of complex, multidisciplinary, two-generation, large-scale programs for depression care. However, challenges in the dissemination and implementation of innovative strategies remain, including the complexity and resource requirements of new service models; training considerations (cognitive load and context dependency); and the structure, culture, and leadership of the adopting organization or system.

In earlier chapters the committee described the extensive literature on the relationship of parental depression, parenting practices, and the healthy development of children. This analysis evaluated the levels of evidence that are needed to show (1) associations between parental depression, parenting practices, and child outcomes and (2) the efficacy of screening, treatment, and prevention strategies and policies on the negative effects of parental depression on children in diverse settings and populations. On the basis of this analysis, the committee then described an ideal vision of a depression care intervention system (Chapter 8), highlighting important components of this system that are emerging in selected service settings as well as through state, federal, and European initiatives. The clues that are emerging from these initiatives also highlight three major barriers associated with implementing these innovative approaches that must be addressed as outlined by the committee (Chapter 9), including a variety of systemic, workforce, and fiscal policies.

Chapter 10 now provides an overview of two separate areas in which next steps can be taken in the design and implementation of the ideal prevention and depression system for parental depression described in Chapter 8 if the systemic, workforce, and fiscal challenges can be overcome. The two areas are (1) developing a research agenda that highlights priorities for new knowledge development and (2) creating policy and learning environments that contribute to successful dissemination and implementation of effective practices for improving the quality of care for depressed parents and their children.

Each area involves diverse and challenging issues that require attention from policy makers, the research community, and program administrators. A common goal is to develop evidence-based programs and collaborative strategies, as well as to create incentives to adopt innovative approaches within learning environments that strive to reach those who are in greatest need and those who are most difficult to serve.

RESEARCH OPPORTUNITIES

In addition to strengthening the systemic, workforce, and fiscal policy approaches outlined in the previous chapter, the committee outlines a research agenda that builds on four fundamental challenges faced in attempting to address the problem of parental depression: (1) integrating knowledge, (2) applying a developmental framework, (3) conceptualizing the problems as two-generation in nature, and (4) acknowledging the presence of the constellation of risk factors, context, and correlates associated with depression (see Chapter 2). The committee now focuses on specific content areas that represent significant research opportunities.

Etiology of Depression

Much is known about risk factors for depression, but further research is needed to test models of how multiple biological and psychosocial factors work together and to clarify the mechanisms by which stressful experiences lead to depressive reactions in individuals and in the family context. Resiliency, despite exposure to parental depression and other adverse conditions is complex, and research will benefit from developmentally sensitive (i.e., age of the child) and integrative models that can be tested over a longitudinal course. We need to know more about optimal timing and methods of intervention to prevent the development and escalation of depression in those at greatest risk—especially young people during their formative family and career years.

Interaction of Depression, Parenting, and Child Health and Development

Although strong evidence now supports the breadth and extent of associations between depression in parents and adverse outcomes in children, there remain many unanswered questions. In particular, many questions remain regarding mediation and moderation of those associations. In terms of mediation, more studies are needed to test specific aspects of parenting and other potential mediators of associations between depression in parents and child functioning. In this regard, the committee noted the strong potential of studies designed to test the effectiveness of interventions aimed at reducing the level of constructs that have been found to mediate associations between depression in parents and outcomes in children, for example, particular aspects of parenting. Such experimental designs can be strong tests of mediation.

In terms of moderation, more studies are needed to reveal which children of depressed parents are more or less likely to develop problems and which parents with depression are more or less likely to have problems with parenting. Moderators might include parent characteristics, including severity, duration, and impairing qualities of their depression, social context variables, child characteristics, and others. For example, the moderating roles of the child's sex and ages at times of exposure are still not well understood, with findings suggesting that boys and girls may be affected differently depending on their ages at the times of exposures. More broadly, we need more studies to quantify percentages of children who are affected (with specific outcomes) and those who are not and what distinguishes them. The committee noted the potential knowledge to be gained by further studies that target interventions to subsets of children with greater or lesser risk (degree of presence of moderators) to determine whether interventions need to be addressed to children at all levels of risk (do they benefit equally?) or might be focused on children at greater risk.

The committee also noted several gaps in the literature related to physical health of the children of depressed parents. More tracking is needed of health care utilization, missed school days, and other aspects of daily functioning in association with depression in parents. In particular, we found that more research is needed to understand the role of maternal depression in the health outcomes of children. Furthermore, both psychological and physical health outcomes need to be addressed in longitudinal studies of healthy and chronically ill children in order to know how physical health outcomes relate to psychological outcomes. Finally, tracking of avoidable and desirable health care utilization is needed to understand the impact on health services.

In addition to the research gaps in terms of unanswered questions, the committee also found gaps in relation to study design. First, tests of mediation are most informative when conducted on data from longitudinal designs and with measures of depression, parenting, and child functioning at multiple time points in order to capture the pathways. A second methodological issue concerns the measurement of depression in parents. The committee recognizes the staffing and time constraints that often prohibit the use of diagnostic interviews, yet we encourage their use whenever possible. Important questions remain about differences in association with parenting and child outcomes when parents' depression exceeds clinical diagnostic criteria. Differences in parenting and child outcomes between those two groups need to be understood.

Third, more studies from a developmental perspective are needed. Such studies need not be longitudinal, but they require an understanding of child development in their theoretical model, hypotheses, design (especially in terms of the ages of the children studied), and in the selection and psychometric properties of the measures.

Fourth, the research literature would benefit from improving on the measurement of depression in population-based surveys, particularly those that capture information on the whole family, to enhance their potential value to address these research gaps. Specifically, the committee recognized the limitations of a single symptom rating scale score, typically reflecting the previous week or two in a parent's life, when the hypotheses typically concern significantly longer term effects on children of exposure to depression in a parent.

Fifth, more research studies are needed to test hypotheses derived from transactional models. As just one example, more studies are needed of child factors that contribute to the development or maintenance of depression in parents, for example, premature birth, chronic or acute health problems, "difficult" temperament, conduct problems.

Finally, as noted throughout this chapter, more studies are needed that examine the differences in parenting styles and children's behavior of the full range of parents who experience depression, including those from differing cultural and ethnic groups and income levels, fathers, and grandparents who are primary caregivers of their grandchildren.

Screening, Treatment, and Prevention Tools and Interventions

Screening

Although evidence supports the effectiveness of brief screening measures for adult depression in clinical and community settings, there remain many unanswered questions. For example, more evidence is needed on the effectiveness of universal screening of parents with depression, including moving beyond the perinatal period. Furthermore, more research is needed to develop brief clinical screening measures for key parenting skills that relate to depression. More specifically, studies are needed that measure depression in parents with both diagnostic interviews and symptom scales that examine differences in parenting and in child functioning that might be related to measurement approach, severity, impairment, and other clinical characteristics of depression.

In terms of outcomes, research is lacking on the outcomes of screening parents as part of a two-generation, comprehensive, depression care program that addresses issues for both parent and child. The next stage is translational research to determine if comprehensive screening programs can ultimately influence parental mental health, parenting, or adverse outcomes in child development. More specifically, studies of the effectiveness rather than the efficacy of the implementation of programs are needed in community and clinical settings. They should examine the impact of each step in the care process, from screening, education, and parent engagement, through parent treatment preferences and choices made, to referrals made and completed, to clinical outcomes.

More research is needed to determine the most optimal ways to integrate parental depression screening with the assessment of parenting and child development and behavioral status for all children but especially in high-risk populations (e.g., with substance use disorders, low-income status, at risk for abuse).

Treatment

While there is evidence available on the safety and efficacy of therapeutic and delivery approaches to treating depression and preventing relapse in adults, little is known about the impact of the successful treatment of depression for (1) racial and ethnic minority populations, (2) non-English or limited English speakers, and (3) adults who are parents, and its effects on the functioning and well-being of their children (e.g., prevention of adverse outcomes).

In order to maintain a variety of therapeutic treatments to choose from to satisfy patient preference, further research is needed on the safety and efficacy of therapeutic treatments specifically for depressed parents (i.e., antidepressants, therapy, alternative medicine). Specifically, research is needed on (1) culturally and linguistically competent, evidenced-based models, (2) the appropriate duration of perinatal depression interventions, including indications for prophylactic treatment, (3) the long-term effects of antidepressants on the growth and development of children exposed in utero, and (4) the safety and efficacy of alternative treatments for perinatal depression (e.g., herbal medications or supplements, ultraviolet light).

With regard to delivery approaches for parents with depression, more research is needed in understanding the effectiveness of certain settings in which parents and their children are regularly seen (e.g., pediatric, obstetric, and gynecological settings, community-based centers, home) and the effectiveness of alternative delivery mechanisms that can reduce barriers ro receiving needed treatment (e.g., web-based therapy and follow-up for depressed parents, especially during pregnancy and postpartum periods), as well as the effectiveness of integrating treatment for depression and substance abuse disorders.

Prevention

More research is needed on the prevention of adverse outcomes in families with depressed parents. Although there is preliminary support for interventions that prevent adverse effects for depressed parents and their children, most of these approaches need further evaluation, replication, and longitudinal studies before widespread implementation is warranted. Many of these studies target only a particular area (e.g., parenting, child development), and only a limited number of interventions have targeted both parents and their children. Therefore, additional research is needed to further support these existing preventive interventions for families with depressed parents. For the programs and practices that have already been found to be most promising in randomized trials, larger scale effectiveness studies and implementation and dissemination trials need to be pursued.

In addition, there is a need to develop new interventions that are targeted to the comprehensive needs of families with depression as well as adaptations or enrichments of more broad intervention approaches to enhance their effectiveness in these families. Because families with parental depression may present with depression as the primary problem or as part of a constellation of risk factors, there is a need for more research on identifying, engaging, and providing appropriate prevention interventions to families with depressed parents not only in mental health services but also in a variety of settings where they may seek services. This is particularly relevant to low-income and ethnic-minority populations, given that they are at increased risk for depression but are less likely to seek mental health services.

Although these targeted approaches are likely to be most promising, more evidence is also needed to determine whether universal programs focused on wellness and mental health promotion can lead to reductions in depression in parents and the subsequent adverse effects in children.

The following types of programs need more research with attention to depression in parents:

- programs targeted at preventing depression in parents with children at all developmental stages;
- prevention programs targeted at improving parenting;
- prevention programs targeted at enhancing protective factors and reducing risk in children;
- multigenerational and multicomponent programs;
- prevention programs in settings in which families with depression and their children are readily accessed, such as schools and community settings; and
- policy and social welfare interventions and other broad-based programs that target vulnerable families and children.

In all of these programmatic approaches, prevention research for families with parental depression needs to incorporate three major principles: recognition and treatment of parental depression, enhancement and support for parenting, and a focus on the developmental outcomes of children.

A number of areas of focus are needed in these research efforts. First, programs designed to assist children when parents are depressed need to focus not only on symptoms and diagnoses in children but also on strength-based strategies that help children accomplish appropriate developmental tasks (staying in school, relationships, and acquiring skills). In addition, intervention research is needed that can serve to identify the characteristics of parenting by depressed parents that is of sufficient quality (e.g., sufficient levels of warmth and structure) to reduce adverse outcomes in children. For evidence-based, preventive, intervention strategies and prevention-focused service programs that are not specifically targeted to depressed families, future research needs to consider parental depression in intervention design, assess depression in families, and track outcomes in families with depression as a subgroup in their evaluations. Whenever possible, these interventions should examine the effects of parental depression on parenting and on child outcomes. Additional research is also needed on the effectiveness of including specific intervention components to enrich the overall program for depressed parents. This research will elucidate how the effects of these interventions differ in families with depression and what adaptations or enhancements are needed to maximize the effectiveness of interventions for them.

Although attention to prevention is warranted for children of depressed parents at all developmental stages, because of the rapid course of brain development during the first 5 years of life, increased focus is needed on evaluations and implementation trials of interventions during this stage of development. This can include interventions in pregnancy and the post-partum period, parent-child interaction interventions in infancy and early childhood, home visitation, and early childhood education.

Vulnerable Populations

The research opportunities outlined in this section highlight the fact that there is a general lack of research that includes particularly vulnerable populations—those with low income, those from a racial/ethnic minority, and those with co-occurring conditions or family adversity. Given the con-siderable evidence about the social determinants of health in general and its effects on parental depression in particular, it is important that intervention research to address depression in parents should assess relative effectiveness in families with low income, families in high-risk neighborhoods, families with unstable housing, and families from varied cultural and linguistic backgrounds, as well as adaptations or enhancements to target these vulner-able populations. This research will help to elucidate the need to address these interrelated factors to successfully intervene to improve depression, parenting, and child outcomes as well as the need to address depression in order to make other interventions for these vulnerable families more successful.

Greater recognition is needed of the vast level of heterogeneity of the groups who are particularly vulnerable to depression or need depression services in the United States. Research studies that report the population subgroups studied with greater specificity will help policies and practices to be more effective. For example, in regard to screening, more research is needed to determine the optimal ways to integrate parental depression screening with the assessment of parenting and developmental and behav-ioral status for all children but especially those in high-risk populations (e.g., with substance use disorders, low-income status, at risk for abuse). For treatment, little is known about the impact of successful treatment of depression for racial/ethnic minority populations or non-English or limited

English speakers. Even when interventions are not designed to address these populations, population and socioeconomic demographics should be clearly reported so that studies can be placed in the proper context, the amount of risk properly assessed, and analyses of relative effectiveness in high-risk subpopulations can be conducted.

Trials are also needed of specific ways to offer identification, outreach, engagement, and treatment and prevention services to vulnerable families who face multiple risks. Specifically, research is needed on culturally and linguistically competently evidenced-based models as well as models that integrate treatment of co-occurring conditions, such as marital conflict, domestic violence, and exposure to trauma and co-existing mental and substance abuse disorders. Furthermore, studies that include large samples of vulnerable populations are needed in community and other real-world settings that explore adaptations or research strategies that are appropriate and sensitive to their needs.

Finally, there should be more research studies that seek to understand the deterioration in mental health of immigrants based on tenure in the United States. This research on immigrants should seek to understand the environmental, psychological, and social changes that seem to factor into this deterioration and help preserve the protective factors at work.

Innovative Strategies

While evidence is emerging about ways to improve and strengthen the quality of treatment programs for depressed adults, little is known about the extent to which these quality improvement efforts apply to the particular needs of adults who are parents or to their children. Furthermore, research presented in the preceding chapters suggests that children are directly affected by a parent's depression. Their needs are not addressed in a care system that focuses solely on improving treatment effectiveness without regard for the vulnerable persons (especially very young children) whose care and relationships may be disrupted by the disorder.

Research is therefore needed to examine how quality improvement efforts contribute to enhancing the relationships and outcomes of parents and their children when compared with the general population of non-parenting adults who participate in treatment programs and should incorporate three major principles: recognition and treatment of parental depression, enhancement and support for parenting, and a focus on the developmental outcomes of children. Research resources should be dedicated to understanding common as well as unique problems in designing treatment services for parents with children at different stages of development, such as infants, toddlers, school-age children, and adolescents. Once optimal strategies are identified, research is needed for the dissemination of these programs into the care settings that match these developmental stages.

Furthermore, many individuals who screen positive for depression decline mental health services. For widespread implementation of programs that are shown to be effective for families with depression, there is a need for more work on issues of engagement and barriers to access to services as most families with depressed parents do not receive adequate intervention. Research on depression care models should therefore identify characteristics of individuals who accept services and individuals who decline them to determine how well a given model fits with the cultural and socioeconomic characteristics of the relevant community. Research opportunities may exist to engage individuals in treatment that is directly relevant to distinct stages of parenting, such as those noted above: preconception, prenatal, postpartum, and later stages, as well as comparing the outcomes of first-time parents with those who are raising older children or children in blended families The comparative effectiveness of treatment strategies that are targeted on these developmental stages deserves to be tested when designing future quality improvement research studies. Interventions centered on parenting are particularly compelling because engagement is a crucial step to effectively intervening in families with depression. Programs that address parenting needs offer great promise as a highly effective way to engage parents and, when needed, trigger services that can address their depression, parenting, and prevention of adverse outcomes in children. Trials are also needed of specific ways to offer additional identification, outreach, engagement, and treatment and prevention services to those vulnerable families who face multiple risks.

Finally, families with depressed parents are most likely to be recognized in a variety of settings. As described in Chapter 7, targeted intervention approaches are likely to be most promising. Therefore, in addition to interventions for parents who present with depression for mental health services, research is needed on how best to identify parental depression and provide services within a range of settings in which families at high risk for depression seek services (such as Head Start; the special Supplement Nutrition Program for Women, Infants, and Children; preschool). Thus, resources need to be available in these settings to identify parental depression and to assist families in getting treatment and prevention services. This is most relevant to low-income and ethnic-minority populations given that they are at increased risk for depression but are less likely to seek mental health services.

Summary

The research priorities highlighted above provide direction and guidance for building a knowledge base that can enhance the development of future programs, policies, and professional practice. But overcoming systemic, workforce, and fiscal challenges and developing new knowledge to help in the design and implementation of innovative strategies are not sufficient to ensure its use in the routine efforts of service providers and practitioners to identify, treat, and prevent parental depression and to reduce the impact of this disorder on children. The application of evidence-based knowledge requires explicit attention to dissemination, implementation, and the creation of an organizational culture, often termed a "learning organization," which is intentionally receptive to new research.

The next section explores the features associated with learning organizations that may foster the use of science in the prevention and treatment of parental depression and in calling attention to children who may be affected by this disorder. A key feature of these learning organizations is the development of processes and training programs that stimulate innovative practice.

CREATING LEARNING ENVIRONMENTS
THAT SUPPORT INNOVATION

The science of dissemination and implementation lags considerably behind the science that undergirds evidence-based practices and promising programs in the identification, treatment, and prevention of parental depression. Not surprisingly, the complexity of dissemination and implementation has also thwarted the development of useful theories. Although various conceptual approaches exist, none could be described as comprehensive, coherent, or testable (Fixsen et al., 2005; Glasgow, Lichtenstein, and Marcus, 2003; Kilbourne et al., 2007; Mendel et al., 2008; Racine, 2006). The result is a scattered and largely noncumulative pattern of a knowledge base associated with dissemination and implementation.

Some relevant theory development and empirical work, with relevance to interventions that strive to improve parenting or to enrich the social environments of children of parents who are depressed, are emerging, as described in Chapter 8. The time may be ripe to combine these early experimental examples with the broader literature on dissemination and implementation derived from research in business organizations. The combination could provide guidance on strategies for pursuing wider use of what works in identifying, treating, and preventing depression among parents.

This section begins with an overview of the process of adopting an innovation. We then review major issues related to the adoption, implementation, and dissemination of evidence-based parental depression care programs. Next, a guide to adopting innovations prepared the by Agency for Healthcare Research and Quality (AHRQ) is discussed (Brach et al., 2008). The AHRQ guide serves as an example of the generic resources available to planners and community partners seeking pragmatic information on the implementation of new health care programs. The section concludes with a research agenda to help support innovation, dissemination, and implementation of evidence-based depression care programs for depressed parents and their children across a wide range of venues.

The Mechanisms of Learning

Dissemination and implementation of promising models draw explicit attention to the mechanisms of learning, such as assimilation and use. Improved outcomes from depression care require that planners and practioners assimilate and skillfully use evidence-based practices and promising programs. Individual practitioners tasked with providing depression care for parents and children need opportunities to share their experience with new practices and programs with each other and with their service organizations and systems.

Despite significant advances in other fields, the importance of learning through the assimilation and use of evidence-based approaches has gone underappreciated in the health care and human services literature. Two emerging principles (cognitive load and context dependence), in particular, appear germane to the challenge of implementing practices and programs in depression care.

The first reflects the realization that the human ability to learn is constrained by cognitive load (Singley and Anderson, 1989). While some knowledge, such as the use of language, comes naturally and easily (except in unusual circumstances), most knowledge, when first received, has to be processed through the brain's working memory (Geary, 2002). Although the capacity of working memory varies across individuals, it is unreasonable to expect that the knowledge entailed in often complex interventions can be converted into constructive actions among diverse clinicians on a reliable basis. Effective learning in organized settings generally takes time (Levitt and March, 1988). Clinical care guidelines have had a mixed record of uptake and effective use (Cabana et al., 1999; Grimshaw et al., 2004; Solberg et al., 2000; Stone, Sonnad, and Schweikhart, 2001), and the adoption of depression care guidelines, especially among clinicians who do not specialize in mental health, may be impaired in the absence of clear strategy to foster their use.

A second principle emerging from research is that learning always occurs in a specific time and place and thus is to some extent "sticky" (von Hippel, 1994) or dependent on context (Anderson, Reder, and Simon, 1996). A clinician who learns a new practice is essentially learning two things at one time: first, the generalizable means-ends logic of the practice (i.e., do this and get that result) and, second, the social knowledge (e.g., organizational conditions, environmental cues) accompanying that logic in the context in which it is learned (Anderson et al., 2004; Anderson, Reder, and Simon, 1996; Argote, 1999; Glisson et al., 2008; Taatgen et al., 2008).

Many parental depression prevention/screening/community treatment models operate as adjuncts to existing programs that are primarily tasked with providing other services, such as home visitation; primary pediatric or family medical care; daycare; Head Start; and community, social, and faith-based services. As such, adjunctive parental depression programs face the challenge of effective integration within these different settings and coordination of services with the primary program's organizational structure, mission, and goals.

Organizational Structure, Leadership, and Climate

The structure and processes of an organization can affect its assimilation and use of knowledge in adopting an evidence-based practice. Some fixity in how work is organized and conducted offers a learning advantage, even in highly dynamic situations in which a lack of defined structure and process would seem to foster greater adaptability and creativity (Brown and Eisenhardt, 1997). Evidence indicates that some formalization (e.g., the degree of established standards and rules, standardized procedures, defined roles) is necessary to facilitate implementation (Adler and Borys, 1996; Jansen, Van den Bosch, and Volberda, 2005; Knott, 2001; Rosenheck, 2001; Zollo and Winter, 2002). With appropriate structures and routines in place, cognitive and relational effort can be concentrated on the new initiative (Gittell, 2002).

Apart from control or influence over resources, organizational leadership, particularly in larger organizations, tends to play a more symbolic, tone-setting role than at the group or team level (Sabherwal, Jeyaraj, and Chowa, 2006; Senge, 1990). Research in health care quality improvement suggests that organizational leaders must demonstrate commitment and persistence for their messages about quality to motivate and to be observed by hospital staff (Rousseau and Tijoriwalla, 1999).

The culture (shared beliefs about how things are done) and climate (perceptions of the work environment) of organizations have received a good deal of attention from researchers interested in the implementation of evidence-based interventions (Glisson et al., 2008; Hemmelgarn, Glisson, and James, 2006; Saldana et al., 2007; Shortell et al., 2000, 2001). These studies suggest that health care and human services organizations are governed more by institutional factors, such as compliance with professional norms and public regulation, than by market competition factors associated with the behavior of commercial firms (Glisson et al., 2008; Mendel et al., 2008; Scott, 2001; Selznick, 1957).

Dissemination Strategies

Practices and programs are unlikely to be adopted if people have no knowledge of them. For example, a lack of awareness has been one of the reasons that physicians opt to not follow recommended care guidelines (Cabana et al., 1999). Intentions are more likely to lead to behavior change if they are coupled with plans for how and when the change will be implemented (Webb and Sheeran, 2006). This finding suggests that dissemination activities that encourage and support potential adopters in thinking through how they would implement it in their context will make the adoption of a new program or practice more likely (Frambach et al., 1998; Glennan, 1998). For example, the Agricultural Cooperative Extension Agent is a model of an iterative, facilitated dissemination in the United States that reaches every county in the United States and has nearly 100 years of proven, rapid dissemination that transformed American farms. Developed by the Agricultural Extension Service, this model was developed to build bridges from land-grant universities doing agricultural science, to the university regional director, to the local field office, to the farmers in the field (Vastag, 2004). In 2009 the American Recovery and Reinvestment Act included a health information technology extension agent function that could be broadened as a method for clinical practice quality improvement and research dissemination (Rural Health Resource Center, 2009).

Attributes That Facilitate Program Adoption

Diffusion of innovation theory has been a popular way to frame the adoption of innovations in health care and social services (Berwick, 2003; Rogers, 1995). The theory emphasizes five attributes that improve the chances of adoption of an innovation:

1. its relative advantage over existing practice and other, similar innovations;
2. its compatibility with what people already believe and value;
3. its complexity;
4. the extent to which it can be observed in operation; and

5. whether it can be tried on a small scale before a decision needs to be made to implement it fully.

Three of the five—relative advantage, compatibility, and complexity—have received more attention than the other two in health care dissemination research (Greenhalgh et al., 2004a). Across a wide range of studies, the evidence of their impact can best be characterized as inconsistent (for reviews, see Damanpour and Schneider, 2006; Greenhalgh et al., 2004b; Rye and Kimberly, 2007).

The development of most evidence-based practices and programs frequently focuses on the technical knowledge that people need to learn. But the social component of knowledge, without which the technical knowledge remains inert, typically receives relatively little or sometimes no systematic attention or elaboration (Glisson et al., 2008; Ramanujam and Rousseau, 2006). Accordingly, when practices and programs are offered for replication or wider use, the adapters often scramble to figure out how to convert the technical abstractions of the intervention into reliable, concrete action (Olds et al., 2003; Racine, 2004). The vagueness and complexity of the social components also may make it more prone to error during implementation, which in turn may interfere with the intended application of the intervention's technical requirements.

An Example of Guidelines for Adopting Innovations

One useful model that illustrates how innovative practices can be introduced and sustained in complex organizations involves guidelines prepared by the Agency for Healthcare Research and Quality (AHRQ). *Will It Work Here? A Decisionmaker's Guide to Adopting Innovations* strives to assist health care providers and community planners in determining whether or not a given innovation will address their needs and is feasible (Brach et al., 2008). The guide provides generic, but pragmatic, advice on the issues and steps that potential adopters should consider. The guide is organized around four core questions, features active links to websites that contain in-depth information on related topics, and provides a hyperlinked index of public domain implementation tools and an appendix of four case studies.

The first core question potential adopters need to consider is "Does the innovation fit?" Related key questions include: Does it work? Where else has it been tried? What—and how good—is the evidence that it works? Does it address fundamental problems and achieve organizational goals? Is it compatible with the organization's mission, vision, values, and culture? Can it be successfully adapted to improve compatibility with the organization?

Each of these key questions is examined in more detail with links to websites providing tools and case studies. One relevant example is the link to an AHRQ website detailing the failure of a program that faxed real-time pharmacy data to alert physicians that patients were not complying with their antidepressant medication regimen. An evaluation found that the critical programmatic weakness was a failure to train physicians and nurses in what to do with the faxed information. Nor was there follow-up with the physicians about what they did with the faxed information.

The second core question for potential adopters is "Should we do it here?" Key questions include: What are the benefits? Will these benefits be visible and convincing for stakeholders? What are the necessary resources and costs? Are there potential offsets to the costs, and what is the opportunity cost associated with adopting the innovation? How does one prepare a business case? How can potential risks be assessed? Links are provided, for example, to websites containing tools and templates for assessing risk over different timeframes.

The third core question is: "Can we do it here?" This section focuses on organizational readiness and the willingness of staff to make the necessary changes in what they do. It also considers ways to assess the impact of change on the organization's stakeholders, such as patients and families, board members, and community partners. What sort of structural, process, and workforce changes will be needed to implement the innovation? Can champions be identified who will promote the innovation by generating enthusiasm, fostering change, bridging communication gaps, and solving problems as they arise? What can the organization learn from its past efforts at adopting innovations? Can we do it in time? Examples include links to websites on how to use Gantt charts to plan and track implementation progress.

The final core question is "How will we do it here?" Key questions include: How should the program be evaluated? What constitutes meaningful measurement of success, and what is the burden of data collection? In response to these questions, links are provided to websites discussing measurement issues as well as to the AHRQ Measures Clearinghouse, a public repository of public domain measures and measure sets. What are the advantages and disadvantages of first trying the innovation for a short period of time or on a small scale? How do we manage change to get staff and stakeholder buy-in? And, finally, how do we sustain an innovation that proves worthy of adoption?

Guidelines such as the AHRQ guide lay out the basic principles, common issues, and first steps that should be considered by planners seeking new programs to address unmet needs. However, the generic nature of such guidelines means that potential adopters must creatively interpret their application to specific programs and settings. Indeed, most evidence-based and promising depression care programs lack detailed implementation manuals. Nor has there been much effort to systematically study the replication of a given depression care program across multiple sites. Future research involving the replication of a specific program in multiple settings should devote resources to identifying common and unique implementation issues and tasks raised across different sites.

A Research Agenda for Dissemination and Implementation of Innovative Strategies

The scope and compelling nature of depression in parents and its effects on their family calls for experimentation with programs that have not yet met the highest standard of evidence—that is, longitudinal randomized controlled clinical trials, efficacy and effectiveness studies, effects on clinical depression compared with effects on depressive symptoms, and cultural considerations and generalizability. Interventions should be categorized as promising—that is, those with early evidence in some areas that they are effective but are compromised by areas that need further research—or those that are ready to be taken to scale.

Both conceptual principles and promising practices should guide large-scale efforts, but large-scale efforts should be undertaken in a staged, sequential fashion. A stage-wide sequential model targeting a few sites in a demonstration area and then gradually moving to scale with careful assessment of the first stage of sites is likely to be most valuable. The ultimate goal should be to have system-wide programs for parental depression that incorporate multiple points of entry, employ flexible strategies, and allow for the amounts of services and prevention to be tailored to individual needs and families. We think systems ready for consideration for such dissemination projects are county health departments, city health departments, specific geographic catchment areas, and those covered by particular kinds of insurance. The following criteria offer guidance in identifying the most fruitful opportunities for dissemination and implementation efforts:

- Research-informed interventions tested on majority populations should be adapted, tested, or drawn from more culturally diverse and vulnerable populations in diverse settings and communities. This is especially important given the disparities in access and treatment and the increased prevalence among some groups for depression as well as limits to research and evaluation resources.
- Focus the effort to improve depression care to capture the experiences and challenges of early adopters and to identify critical components that contribute to success and sustainability, such as leadership, resources, organizational culture, and community support. Expect developers of effective practices and promising

programs to define the absorptive capacity that adopters should possess to learn, efficiently and effectively, how to use these interventions as designed.

- Expect developers of new depression care models to use their research to elaborate the social knowledge required for these models to be assimilated and used effectively.
- By aligning quality improvement studies that help improve the approach, those that support implementation of these strategies across diverse programs and settings, and those that support implementation and dissemination of evidence-based programs, it may be possible to clarify where additional work is needed in that particular system and how to extend these programs to other populations and throughout other systems of care.

CONCLUSION

The research priorities highlighted above provide direction and guidance for building a knowledge base that can enhance the development of future programs, policies, and professional practice. But overcoming systemic, workforce, and fiscal challenges as well as the development of new knowledge is not sufficient to ensure its use in the routine efforts of service providers and practitioners to identify, treat, and prevent parental depression and to reduce the impact of this disorder on children. The application of evidence-based knowledge requires explicit attention to dissemination, implementation, and the creation of an organizational culture that is intentionally receptive to new research. However, the dissemination and implementation research literature points to no simple paths for extending the reach of effective forms of depression care. Although general guidelines exist to help potential adopters ask pertinent questions, the answers required for the implementation of complex, multidisciplinary, two-generation, large-scale prevention care programs must be drawn by inference from a limited body of research largely focused on other health care and business areas.

RECOMMENDATION

This chapter highlights priorities for new knowledge development as well as creating policy and learning environments that contribute to successful innovation, dissemination, and implementation of evidence-based strategies. Together, they identify issues and areas that require attention from policy makers, the research community, and program administrators in order to develop effective programs and collaborative strategies. On the basis of these research opportunities, the committee makes one recommendation intended to build the knowledge base and to create incentives to adopt innovative approaches in learning environments that strive to reach those who are in greatest need and those who are most difficult to serve.

Promote and Support Research

Recommendation 7: Federal agencies, including the National Institutes of Health, the Centers for Disease Control and Prevention, the Health Resources and Services Administration, and the Substance Abuse and Mental Health Services Administration, should support a collaborative, multiagency research agenda to increase the understanding of risk and protective factors of depression in adults who are parents and the interaction of depression and its co-occurring conditions, parenting practices, and child outcomes across developmental stages. This research agenda should include the development and evaluation of empirically based strategies for screening, treatment, and prevention of depressed parents and the effects on their children and improve widespread dissemination and implementation of these strategies in different services settings for diverse populations of children and their families.

In carrying out this recommendation, these federal agencies should consider partnerships with private organizations, employers, and payers to support this research agenda.

REFERENCES

Adler, P.S., and Borys, B. (1996). Two types of bureaucracy: Enabling and coercive. *Administrative Science Quarterly, 41*, 61–89.

Anderson, J.R., Bothell, D., Byrne, M.D., Douglass, S., Lebiere, C., and Qin, Y. (2004). An integrated theory of mind. *Psychological Bulletin, 111*, 1036–1060.

Anderson, J.R., Reder, L.M., and Simon, H.A. (1996). Situated learning and education. *Educational Researcher, 25*, 5–11.

Argote, L. (1999). *Organizational Learning: Creating, Retaining, and Transferring Knowledge.* Norwell, MA: Kluwer Academic.

Berwick, D.M. (2003). Disseminating innovations in health care. *Journal of the American Medical Association, 289*, 1969–1975.

Brach, C., Lensfestey, N., Rouseel, A., Amoozegar, J., and Sorenson, A. (2008). *Will It Work Here? A Decisionmaker's Guide to Adopting Innovations.* (AHRQ Pub. No. 08-0051.) Rockville, MD: Agency for Healthcare Research and Quality.

Brown, S.L., and Eisenhardt, K.M. (1997). The art of continuous change: Linking complexity theory and time-paced evolution in relentlessly shifting organizations. *Administrative Science Quarterly, 42*, 1–34.

Cabana, M.D., Rand, C.S., Powe, N.R., Wu, A.W., Wilson, M.H., Abboud, P.C., and Rubin, H.R. (1999). Why don't physicians follow clinical practice guidelines? A framework for improvement. *Journal of the American Medical Association, 282*, 1458–1465.

Damanpour, F., and Schneider, M. (2006). Phases of the adoption of innovation in organizations: Effects of environment, organization and top managers. *British Journal of Management*, 17, 215–236.

Fixsen, D.L., Naoom, S.F., Blasé, K.A., Friedman, R.M., and Wallace, F. (2005). *Implementation Research: A Synthesis of the Literature.* Tampa: University of South Florida.

Frambach, R.T., Barkema, H.G., Notteboom, B., and Wedel, M. (1998). Adoption of a service innovation in the business market: An empirical test of supply-side variables. *Journal of Business Research*, 41, 161–174.

Geary, D.C. (2002). Principles of evolutionary educational psychology. *Learning and Individual Differences*, 12, 317–345.

Gittell, J.H. (2002). Coordinating mechanisms in care provider groups: Relational coordination as a mediator and input uncertainty as a moderator of performance effects. *Management Science*, 48, 1408–1426.

Glasgow, R.E., Lichtenstein, E., and Marcus, A.C. (2003). Why don't we see more translation of health promotion research into practice? Rethinking the efficacy-to-effectiveness transition. *American Journal of Public Health*, 93, 1261–1267.

Glennan, T.K. (1998). *New American Schools after Six Years.* Santa Monica, CA: RAND.

Glisson, C., Landsverk, J., Schoenwald, S., Kelleher, K., Hoagwood, K.E., Mayberg, S., and Green, P. (2008). Assessing the organizational social context of mental health services: Implications for research and practice. *Administration and Policy in Mental Health*, 35, 98–113.

Greenhalgh, T., Robert, G., Bate, P., Kyriakidou, O., MacFarlane, F., and Peacock, R. (2004a). *How to Spread Good Ideas: A Systematic Review of the Literature on Diffusion, Dissemination, and Sustainability of Innovations in Health Service Delivery and Organization.* London: National Coordinating Centre for NHS Service Delivery and Organisation.

Greenhalgh, T., Robert, G., MacFarlane, F., Bate, P., and Kyriakidan, O. (2004b). Diffusion of innovation in service organizations: Systematic review and recommendations. *Milbank Quarterly*, 82, 581–629.

Grimshaw, J.M., Thomas, R.E., MacLennan, G., Fraser, C., Ramsay, C.R., Vale, L., Whitty, P., Eccles, M.P., Matowe, L., Shirran, L., Wensing, M., Dijkstra, R., and Donaldson, C. (2004). Effectiveness and efficiency of guideline dissemination and implementation strategies. *Health Technology Assessment*, 8(6). Available: http://www.ncchta.org/fullmono/mon806.pdf [accessed July 2009].

Hemmelgarn, A.L., Glisson, C., and James, L.R. (2006). Organizational culture and climate: Implications for services and interventions research. *Clinical Psychology: Science and Practice*, 13, 73–89.

Jansen, J.P., Van den Bosch, F.A.J., and Volderba, H.W. (2005). Managing potential and realized absorptive capacity: How do organizational antecedents matter? *Academy of Management Journal*, 48, 999–1015.

Kilbourne, A.M., Neumann, M.S., Pincus, H.A., Bauer, M.S., and Stall, R. (2007). Implementing evidence-based interventions health care: Application of the replicating effective programs framework. *Implementation Science*, 2, 42.

Knott, A.M. (2001). The dynamic value of hierarchy. *Management Science*, 47, 430–448.

Levitt, B., and March, J.G. (1988). Organizational learning. *Annual Review of Sociology*, 14, 319–340.

Mendel, P., Meredith, L.S., Schoenbaum, M., Sherbourne, C.D., and Wells, K.B. (2008). Interventions in organizational and community context: A framework for building evidence on dissemination and implementation in health services research. *Administration and Policy in Mental Health*, 35, 21–37.

Olds, D.L., Hill, P.L., O'Brien, R., Racine, D., and Moritz, P. (2003). Taking preventive intervention to scale: The Nurse-Family Partnership. *Cognitive and Behavioral Practice*, 10, 278–290.

Racine, D.P. (2004). *Capturing the Essential Elements*. Philadelphia: Public/Private Ventures.

Racine, D.P. (2006). Reliable effectiveness: A theory on sustaining and replicating worthwhile innovations. *Administration and Policy in Mental Health/Mental Health Service Research*, 33, 356–387.

Ramanujam, R., and Rousseau, D.M. (2006). The challenges are organizational not just clinical. *Journal of Organizational Behavior*, 26, 811–827.

Rogers, E.M. (1995). *Diffusion of Innovations*. New York: Free Press.

Rosenheck, R. (2001). Stages in the implementation of innovative clinical programs in complex organizations. *Journal of Nervous and Mental Disease*, 189, 812–821.

Rousseau, D.M., and Tijoriwala, S.A. (1999) What's a good reason to change? Motivated reasoning and social accounts in organizational change. *Journal of Applied Psychology*, 84, 514–528.

Rural Health Resource Center. (2009). *HIT Incentives and State Grant Opportunities American Recovery and Reinvestment Act of 2009*. Available: http://www.ruralcenter.org/documents/HIT%20Incentives%20and%20State%20Grant%20Opportunities_ARRA.pdf [accessed April 21, 2009].

Rye, C.B., and Kimberly, J.R. (2007). The adoption of innovations by provider organizations in health care. *Medical Care Research and Review*, 64, 235–278.

Sabherwal, R., Jeyaraj, A., and Chowa, C. (2006). Information system success: Individual and organizational determinants. *Management Science*, 52, 1849–1864.

Saldana, L., Chapman, J.E., Henggler, S.W., and Rowland, M.D. (2007). The organizational readiness for change scale in adolescent programs: Criterion validity. *Journal of Substance Abuse Treatment*, 33, 159–169.

Scott, W.R. (2001). *Institutions and Organizations*. Thousand Oaks, CA: Sage.

Selznick, P. (1957). *Leadership in Administration: A Sociological Interpretation*. New York: Harper and Row.

Senge, P. (1990). *The Fifth Discipline: The Art and Practice of the Learning Organization*. New York: Currency Doubleday.

Shortell, S.M., Jones, R.H., Rademaker, A.W., Gillies, R., Dranove, D.S., Hughes, E.F.X., Budetti, P.P., Reynolds, K.S.E., and Huang, C.-F. (2000). Assessing the impact of total quality management and organizational culture on multiple outcomes of care for coronary artery bypass graft surgery patients. *Medical Care*, 38, 207–217.

Shortell, S.M., Zazzali, J.L., Burns, L.R., Alexander, J.A., Gillies, R.R., Budetti, P.P., Waters, T.M., and Zuckerman, H.S. (2001). Implementing evidence-based medicine: The role of market pressures, compensation incentives, and culture in physician organizations. *Medical Care*, 39, 62–78.

Singley, M.K., and Anderson, J.R. (1989). *The Transfer of Cognitive Skill*. Cambridge, MA: Harvard University Press.

Solberg, L.I., Brekke, M.L., Fazio, C.J., Fowles, J., Jacobsen, D.N., Kottke, T.E., Mosser, G., O'Connor, P.J., Ohnsorg, K.A., and Rolnnick, S.J. (2000). Lessons from experienced guideline implementers: Attend to many factors and use multiple strategies. *Joint Commission Journal on Quality Improvement*, 26, 171–188.

Stone, T.T., Sonnad, S.S., and Schweikhart, S.B. (2001). *Organizational and Clinical Factors Influencing Use of Practical Guidelines*. Seattle, WA: Center for Health Management Research, Department of Health Services.

Taatgen, N.A., Huss, D., Dickison, D., and Anderson, J.R. (2008). The acquisition of robust and flexible cognitive skills. *Journal of Experimental Psychology: General*, 137, 548–565.

Vastag, B. (2004). Donald M. Berwick, MD, MPP: Advocate for evidence-based health system reform. *Journal of the American Medical Association, 291*, 1945–1947.

von Hippel, E. (1994). "Sticky information" and the locus of problem solving: Implications for innovation. *Management Science, 40*, 429–439.

Webb, T.L., and Sheeran, P. (2006). Does changing behavioral intentions engender behavior change? A meta-analysis of the experimental evidence. *Psychological Bulletin, 132*, 249–268.

Zollo, M., and Winter, S.G. (2002). Deliberate learning and the evolution of dynamic capabilities. *Organization Science, 13*, 339–351.

Appendix A

Acronyms

ABCD	Assuring Better Child Health and Development
ADHD	attention deficit hyperactivity disorder
AHCPR	Agency for Health Care Policy and Research
AHRQ	Agency for Healthcare Research and Quality
ASI	Addiction Severity Index
BDI	Beck Depression Inventory
BSID	Bailey Scale of Infant Development
BSQ	Behavioral Screening Questionnaire
CAFB	Child, Adolescent, and Family Branch
CAP	Child Abuse Potential Inventory
CBCL	Child Behavior Checklist
CBT	cognitive-behavioral therapy
CDC	U.S. Centers for Disease Control and Prevention
CES-D	Center for Epidemiologic Studies Depression Scale
CHIP	State Children's Health Insurance Program
CID	Community Initiative on Depression
CMHS	Center for Mental Health Services
CMS	Centers for Medicare and Medicaid Services
CRH	corticotrophin releasing hormone
CRP	C-reactive protein
DHA	docosahexaenoic acid

DSM-IV   *Diagnostic and Statistical Manual of Mental Disorders,*
                    fourth edition

EEG   electroencephalogram
EPA   eicosapentaenoic acid
EPDS   Edinburgh Postnatal Depression Scale

FDA   U.S. Food and Drug Administration

GR   glucocorticoid receptor

HEDIS   Healthcare Effectiveness Data and Information Set
HFA   Healthy Families America
HHS   U.S. Department of Health and Human Services
HMO   health maintenance organization
HPA   hypothalamic-pituitary-adrenal
HRSA   U.S. Health Resources and Services Administration
HRSD   Hamilton Rating Scale for Depression

IL   interleukin
IMPACT   Improving Mood-Promoting Access to Collaborative
                    Treatment
IOM   Institute of Medicine
IPT   interpersonal psychotherapy

K-SADS   Kiddie-Schedule for Affective Disorders and Schizophrenia

LC-NE   locus coeruleus-norepinephrine

MADRS   Montgomery Asberg Depression Rating Scale
MAQ   Maternal Attitudes Questionnaire
MB   *Mamás y Bebés*/Mothers and Babies Course
MBCT   mindfulness-based cognitive therapy
MCHB   Maternal and Child Health Bureau
MCS   Mental Component Score
MFIP   Minnesota Family Investment Program

NBAS   Neonatal Behavioral Assessment Scale
NCS-R   National Comorbidity Survey-Replication
NFP   Nurse-Family Partnership
NICHD   National Institute of Child Health and Human
                    Development
NIH   National Institutes of Health

NMR	Negative Mood Regulation Scale
NRI	norepinephrine reuptake inhibitors
ODIN	Overcoming Depression on the Internet
OSG	Office of the Surgeon General
OWH	Office of Women's Health
PFC	prefrontal cortex
PHQ	Patient Health Questionnaire
PIC	Partners in Care
POMS	Profile of Mood States
PPHN	persistent pulmonary hypertension
PRAMS	Pregnancy Risk Assessment Monitoring System
PRIME-MD	Primary Care Evaluation of Mental Disorders
PRISM	Program of Resources, Information and Support for Mothers
PSI	Parenting Stress Index
PTSD	posttraumatic stress disorder
QI	quality improvement
QUIDS-SR	Quick Inventory of Depressive Symptomatology-Self-report
ROSE	Reach Out, Stand Strong, Essentials for New Mothers
SAMHSA	Substance Abuse and Mental Health Services Administration
SCI-D	Structural Clinical Interview-Depression
SES	socioeconomic status
SFS	Short-Form Survey
SNRI	serotonin norepinephrine reuptake inhibitors
SSRI	selective serotonin reuptake inhibitors
STAR*D	Sequenced Treatment Alternatives to Relieve Depression
SUD	substance use disorder
TPP	toddler-parent psychotherapy
WHO	World Health Organization
WIC	Special Supplemental Nutrition Program for Women, Infants, and Children

Appendix B

Depression and Parenting Workshop Agenda and Participants

Workshop on Depression and Parenting
Monday, April 14, 2008
Beckman Center Auditorium
Irvine, California

Workshop Goals:

1. Explore innovative strategies or programs that integrate mental health services for depression, parenting, and child development services within various settings (e.g., community, primary care, juvenile justice, child care, home visitation) for diverse populations of children and families.
2. Explore existing opportunities for intervention as well as existing barriers to implementation, including public policy strategies, infrastructure of systems, and funding mechanisms given the large numbers of depressed parents.
3. Explore existing strategies that businesses consider for reimbursing and implementing early intervention and prevention mental health services for employees who are diagnosed with depression.
4. Explore existing strategies and programs that ensure interventions are appropriate for diverse populations, including culture, language, family structure, and multigenerational issues.

PROGRAM

WELCOMING REMARKS

Moderator: Mary Jane England, MD, Committee Chair

SESSION I: Integration of Mental Health, Parenting, and Child Development Services in Medical and Other Care Settings

Elizabeth Howell, MD, Committee Member

Objective: Explore the identification, screening, treatment, or referral for depression in parents in a variety of medical and other settings (OB/GYN, pediatrics, family practice, community mental health, community health centers) that serve women, children, and families; the interface or integration of mental health services for depression in primary care through county-government service structure; and capacity building to facilitate better access to quality services in these settings.

Applying Tools, Teamwork, and Tenacity to Address Parental Depression
    Allen Dietrich, MD, Dartmouth Medical School
The UIC Perinatal Mental Health Project
    Laura Miller, MD, University of Illinois at Chicago
Clinical Family Health Services: Depression, Parenting, and Child Development
    Amy Russell, MD, Clinica Campesina, Colorado
Integrating Parenting and Child Development in Primary Care: Healthy Steps for Young Children
    Cynthia Minkovitz, MD, MPP, Johns Hopkins University
Challenges and Opportunities of Community Behavioral/Mental Health System in California
    Nancy Pena (*William Arroyo, MD, substituting*, Los Angeles County, Department of Mental Health)

Discussion of Session I
Patrick Finely, PharmD, BCPP, Committee Member

SESSION II: Unmet Needs and Challenges in Addressing Depression in Parents

Sergio Aguilar-Gaxiola, MD, PhD, Committee Member

Objective: Explore issues which create unique challenges to providing quality mental health services for depression for parents and their children, particularly for a diverse society and in care settings alternate to medical settings.

Unmet Needs and Challenges in Addressing Depression in Parents
 William Vega, MD, University of California, Los Angeles
Parental Depression in Family Medicine and Rural Practices
 Barbara Yawn, MD, MSc, FAAFP, Olmstead Medical Center and University of Minnesota
Workforce Education and Training and Implementation of Best Practices Evidence-Based Practices
 Sandra Naylor-Goodwin, PhD, California Institute of Mental Health
Improving Depression Outcomes in Underserved Communities "It Takes a Village to Build a Village"
 Kenneth Wells, MD, MPH (*Jeanne Miranda, PhD, substituting,* Partners in Care and Community Partners in Care)

Discussion of Session II

SESSION III: Innovative Models: Integrating Parenting, Mental Health Services for Depression, and Child Development

Constance Hammen, PhD, Committee Member

Objective: Exploration of innovative service-level programs/models to address issues related to parenting, depression, and child development in multiple sectors with a variety of community-based programs.

Maternal Depression: Low-income Minorities. Where Should We Provide Care? How Does Care Effect Children?
 Jeanne Miranda, PhD, University of California, Los Angeles
The Healthy Mental Development of Young Children: Primary Care Provider Connection
 Deborah Saunders, Illinois Department of Healthcare and Family Services
Mental Health Augmentation to Nurse Home Visiting
 Paula Zeanah, PhD, MSN, RN, Louisiana Office of Public Health and Tulane University School of Medicine
Innovative Models and Special Populations
 Joanne Nicholson, PhD, University of Massachusetts Medical School
Parenting in Dependency Court
 The Honorable Cindy Lederman, JD, Miami Dade Juvenile Court

Discussion of Session III

SESSION IV: Policy, Legislation, and Financing

Mary Jane England, MD, Committee Chair

Objective: Exploration of infrastructural barriers that facilitate or impede the implementation or replication of promising or best practices at any level (regional, state, multi-state, national) or for larger-scale implementation in a variety of settings.

What About Those Propositions?
  Emily Nahat, California Department of Mental Health
Policy Improvements in the ABCD States: What and How
  Neva Kaye, National Academy for State and Health Policy
Policy, Legislation, and Financing of Mental Health in California
  William Arroyo, MD, Los Angeles County, Department of Mental Health
Exploring Opportunities and Challenges Related to Policy, Legislation, and Financing
  Neal Adams, MD, MPH, California Institute of Mental Health

Discussion of Session IV

CLOSING

PARTICIPANTS

Neal Adams, California Institute for Mental Health
Sergio Aguilar-Gaxiola,* Center for Reducing Health Disparities, University of California, Davis
William Arroyo, Los Angeles County, Department of Mental Health
Kathryn Barnard,* Emerita, University of Washington
William Beardslee,* Children's Hospital, Boston
Judith Belfiori, Consultant
Melissa Brodowski, Office on Child Abuse and Neglect, Children's Bureau, Administration of Children and Families
Palanda Brownlow, First 5 LA
Howard Cabral,* School of Public Health, Boston University

---

*Committee member.

Bruce Compas,* Center for Research on Human Development, Vanderbilt
    University
Beverly Daley, Children's Hospital, Los Angeles
Dale Danley, The California Endowment
Allen J. Dietrich, Dartmouth Medical School
Marva Edwards, San Francisco Child Abuse Prevention Center
Mary Jane England,* Regis College
Vincent J. Felitti, Kaiser Permanente
Karen Moran Finello, Keck School of Medicine, University of Southern
    California
Patrick R. Finley,* University of California at San Francisco
Holly Fitzgerald, Connections For Life
Gwen Foster, The California Endowment
Carolyn Francis, Library Foundation
Farisa Francis, Library Foundation
Lillian Gelberg, David Geffen School of Medicine, University of
    California, Los Angeles
Sherryl Goodman,* Emory University
Denise Gordon, Borrego Community Health Foundation
Nancy Gutierrez, Teen Parent Program, Los Angeles Unified School
    District
Erika Hainley-Jewell, The Children's Clinic
Constance Hammen,* University of California, Los Angeles
Mary Sue Heilemann, University of California, Los Angeles
Dulce Hernandez, Coalition of Orange County Community Clinics
Elizabeth Howell,* Mount Sinai School of Medicine
Pec Indman, Postpartum Support International
Mareasa Isaacs,* National Alliance of Multi-Ethnic Behavioral Health
    Associations
Ellen Iverson, Children's Hospital, Los Angeles
Hendree Jones,* Johns Hopkins University
Rebecca Kang, University of Washington
Neva Kaye, National Academy for State Health Policy
Deborah Koniak-Griffin, School of Nursing, University of California, Los
    Angeles
Preeti Kothary, Clinicas Del Camino Real
Yoriko Kozuki, University of Washington
The Honorable Cindy Lederman, Administrative Judge Juvenile Court,
    Eleventh Judicial Circuit, Dade County, Florida
LuAnna Loza, The Coalition of Orange County Community Clinics

---

*Committee member.

Sithary Ly, Families in Good Health
Laura Magana, Clinicas Del Camino Real
Josie Melendez, St. Mary Medical Center
Kelly Miller, Connections for Life
Laura Miller, Women's Mental Health Program, University of Illinois at
    Chicago
Cynthia Minkovitz, School of Public Health, Johns Hopkins Bloomberg
Jeanne Miranda, University of California, Los Angeles
Emily Nahat, Prevention and Early Intervention, California Department
    of Mental Health
Sandra Naylor-Goodwin, California Institute for Mental Health
Joanne Nicholson, Center for Mental Health Services Research,
    University of Massachusetts Medical School
Imelda Nunez, Share Our Selves
Patricia O'Campo,* Centre for Research on Inner City Health, University
    of Toronto
Ardis L. Olson,* Dartmouth Medical School
Robert Phillips,* Robert Graham Center, American Academy of Family
    Medicine
Marie Poulsen, Keck School of Medicine, University of Southern
    California
Frank Putnam,* Cincinnati Children's Hospital Medical Center
Amy Russell, Clinica Campesina, Colorado
Deborah Saunders, Illinois Office of Healthcare and Family Services
Barbara Schwartz, Long Beach Department of Health and Human
    Services
Sara Seaton, St. Mary Medical Center
Rashmi Shetgiri, University of California, Los Angeles
Jeanette Valentine, Perinatal Mental Health Task Force, Los Angeles
    County
William A. Vega, University of California, Los Angeles
Olivia Velasquez, Children's Hospital, Los Angeles
Barbara Yawn, Olmstead Medical Center, University of Minnesota
Monica Young, Clinicas del Camino Real
Paula Zeanah, Tulane University

---

*Committee member.

C

Biographical Sketches of Committee Members and Staff

Mary Jane England (*Chair*) is president of Regis College. She has served as director of child psychiatry at Brighton's St. Elizabeth Hospital of Boston, then as director of clinical psychiatry at the Brighton-Allston Mental Health Clinic, and from 1974 to 1976 as director of planning and manpower for children's services in the Massachusetts Department of Mental Health. In 1976, she assumed the position of associate commissioner, Massachusetts Department of Mental Health, and was a consultant to and chairperson of the Human Resources Policy Committee at the National Institute of Mental Health. As the first commissioner of the Massachusetts Department of Social Services, she designed and implemented the new state agency to take social services out of the Department of Public Welfare and to ensure citizen involvement as she improved social services and child welfare policy. In 1983, she became associate dean for Harvard's Kennedy School of Government and director of the Lucius N. Littauer Master in Public Administration Program. In 1995–1996, she served as the president of the American Psychiatric Association. She has served as a member or chair of numerous committees or boards at the National Academies. Most recently she was a member of the Board on Children, Youth, and Families and served as chair of the Committee on Crossing the Quality Chasm: Adaptation to Mental Health and Addictive Disorders. She has an M.D. from Boston University School of Medicine and trained in psychiatry at Boston University Hospital and at San Francisco's Mt. Zion Hospital, completing her child and adolescent residency at Boston University and Boston City Child Guidance Clinic.

Sergio Aguilar-Gaxiola is professor of clinical internal medicine, School of Medicine, University of California, Davis (UC Davis). He is the founding director of the Center for Reducing Health Disparities at the UC Davis Health System and the director of Community Engagement of the UC Davis Clinical Translational Science Center. He just completed a 4-year term as a member of the National Advisory Mental Health Council, National Institute of Mental Health. He is cochair of the National Institutes of Health's Community Engagement Key Function Committee for the Clinical and Translational Science Awards, the immediate past chair of the Board of Directors of Mental Health America (formerly the National Mental Health Association), a board member of the Association for Prevention Teaching and Research, and a steering committee and research scientist member of the National Hispanic Science Network on Drug Abuse. He is also a member of the International Advisory Committee of the Carso Health Institute. He is the coordinator for Latin America and the Caribbean of the World Health Organization World Mental Health Survey Initiative. Dr. Aguilar-Gaxiola's research includes cross-national epidemiologic research on patterns and correlates of mental disorders in general population samples and understanding and reducing health disparities in underserved populations. He has worked effectively to bridge research with services delivery and policy development and has been very active translating research into practical information that is of public health value to consumers and their families, service administrators, and policy makers with the purpose of informing health policy decisions and guiding program development. Dr. Aguilar-Gaxiola received his M.D. degree at the Autonomous University of Guadalajara in Mexico, his Ph.D. in Clinical-Community Psychology at Vanderbilt University, and completed a postdoctoral fellowship on health services research at University of California, San Francisco. He is the author of numerous scientific publications, and the recipient of several awards including the Peabody College of Vanderbilt University Distinguished Alumnus Award, the Medal of Congress of Chile for work related to mental health research, and the U.S. Department of Health and Human Services' Office of Minority Health's 2005 National Minority Health Community Leader Award (Hispanic Community), Washington, DC.

Kathryn E. Barnard is professor emerita of family and child nursing at the University of Washington's School of Nursing. She is the founder and former director of the Center on Infant Mental Health and Development at the University of Washington. Her career has focused on promoting understanding of the impact of the first 3 years of life on children's later physical, psychological, and emotional health. She has worked closely with the state of Washington's Department of Health to provide consultation and training on child health assessment, parent-child interaction, and preventive health strategies. She was elected to the Institute of Medicine in 1985 and was honored with the Gustav O. Leinard Award. She has also received 15 other major awards, including the Episteme Award, the highest honor in nursing, from the American Academy of Nursing, and the Martha May Eliot Award for Leadership in Maternal-Child Health. She has a Ph.D. in ecology of early childhood development from University of Washington.

William Rigby Beardslee is the academic chairman of the Department of Psychiatry at Children's Hospital, Boston, and Gardner Monks Professor of child psychiatry at Harvard Medical School. He has a long-standing research interest in the development of children at risk because of severe parental mental illness. He has been especially interested in the protective effects of self-understanding in enabling youngsters and adults to cope with adversity and has studied self-understanding in civil rights workers, survivors of cancer, and children of parents with affective disorders. He has received numerous awards, including the Blanche F. Ittleson Award of the American Psychiatric Association, has been a faculty scholar of the William T. Grant Foundation, and in 1999 received the Irving Philips Award for Prevention and the Catcher in the Rye Award for Advocacy for Children from the American Academy of Child and Adolescent Psychiatry. Currently, he directs the Preventive Intervention Project, which explores the effects of a clinician-facilitated, family-based preventive intervention designed to enhance resiliency and family understanding for children of parents with affective disorders. At the National Academies, he is a current member of the Board on Children, Youth, and Families and the Committee on the Prevention of Mental Disorders and Substance Abuse Among Children, Youth, and Young Adults. Previously he served on the organizing committee of the Workshop on the Synthesis of Research on Adolescent Health and Development, the Committee on Adolescent Health and Development, and the Committee on Prevention of Mental Disorders. He has an M.D. from Case Western Reserve University and trained in general psychiatry at Massachusetts General Hospital and in child psychiatry and psychiatric research at Children's Hospital in Boston.

Howard J. Cabral is associate professor of biostatistics at the Boston University School of Public Health and a codirector of the Biostatistics Graduate Program and the Biostatistics Consulting Group. He is also a statistical consultant to the departments of public health in Boston and Cambridge. He has extensive experience in the analysis of longitudinal health data, especially those collected in urban areas with ethnic diversity. His methodological interests are in the analysis of longitudinal data, the effects of missing data on statistical estimation, and statistical computing. His collaborative research examines the neurobiological changes in the brain among aging animals as well as those resulting from stroke, dementia, and Parkinson's disease among participants in the Framingham Study, the effects of prenatal cocaine exposure on child development, a model to decrease homelessness among those dually diagnosed with mental illness and substance abuse disorder, methods of community outreach to those infected with HIV, and interventions to enhance the health and quality of life of retirees. He has published extensively on pediatric neurodevelopment and physical growth, as well as on the effects of behavioral interventions in AIDS and substance abuse. He has M.P.H. and Ph.D. degrees from Boston University.

Rosemary Chalk (*Board Director*) is the director of the Board on Children, Youth, and Families, a joint effort of the National Research Council and the Institute of Medicine. She is a policy analyst who has been a study director at the National Academies since 1987. She has directed or served as a senior staff member for over a dozen studies in the Institute of Medicine and the National Research Council, including studies on vaccine finance, the public health infrastructure for immunization, family violence, child abuse and neglect, research ethics and misconduct in science, and education finance. From 2000 to 2003, she also directed a research project on the development of child well-being indicators for the child welfare system at Child Trends in Washington, DC. She has previously served as a consultant for science and society research projects at the Harvard School of Public Health and was an Exxon research fellow in the Program on Science, Technology, and Society at the Massachusetts Institute of Technology. She was the program head of the Committee on Scientific Freedom and Responsibility of the American Association for the Advancement of Science from 1976 to 1986. She has a B.A. in foreign affairs from the University of Cincinnati.

Bruce E. Compas is the Patricia and Rodes Hart professor of psychology and human development and pediatrics at Vanderbilt University. He is also director of the clinical psychology training program and director of psychological oncology at the Vanderbilt-Ingram Cancer Center. Previously he was professor of psychology at the University of Vermont. His research has focused on processes of coping and self-regulation in response to stress and adversity in children, adolescents, and adults. He is specifically interested in the relationships of stress, coping, and self-regulation to physical health/illness and psychopathology, as well as the development of interventions to enhance the ways that individuals and families cope with stress. His research involves both laboratory methods to study basic behavioral and biological processes and field research to understand self-regulation and coping in the context of psychopathology and physical illness. He is a fellow of the American Psychological Association and the American Psychological Society. He has a Ph.D. in clinical psychology from the University California, Los Angeles.

Patrick R. Finley is professor of clinical pharmacology (primary emphasis in psychopharmacology and behavioral health) at the University of California at San Francisco (UCSF) in the School of Pharmacy. Previously he served as an adjunct faculty member in the U.S. Department of Veteran Affairs health care system. His teaching, clinical, and research interests focus on the safe and efficacious use of psychotropic medications among the mentally ill population. His research interests in psychopharmacology span clinical, epidemiological, pharmacokinetic, and health policy domains. Clinically, he has been working with Kaiser Permanente of Northern California to implement an innovative practice model designed to improve the treatment of depression in the primary care setting, and his current practice is located in the UCSF Women's Health Center Primary Care Clinic. He has experience working with a variety of consumer groups to ensure access to safe and equitable mental health care. He is a board-certified psychiatric pharmacist. He currently serves as a referee or editorial board member for approximately 16 medical journals. He has a Pharm.D. in pharmacokinetics from the University of California, San Francisco, where he completed his specialty residency; he completed his general residency at the University of Arizona Medical Center.

Sherryl H. Goodman is professor in the Department of Psychology, with a joint appointment in the Department of Psychiatry and Behavioral Sciences, at Emory University. Her research interests, grounded in the field of developmental psychopathology, concern the mechanisms by which mothers with depression may transmit psychopathology to their children. She is also interested in the epidemiology of child and adolescent psychopathology, with a particular focus on risk and protective factors. She is the coeditor of *Children of Depressed Parents: Alternative Pathways to Risk for Psychopathology* (2002) and *Handbook of Women and Depression* (2006). She is a fellow of the American Psychological Association and the Association for Psychological Science. She was associate editor of the *Journal of Family Psychology* and is associate editor of the *Journal of Abnormal Psychology*. She currently chairs the membership committee of the Society for a Science of Clinical Psychology. She has a Ph.D. in clinical psychology from the University of Waterloo .

Constance Hammen is distinguished professor of psychology and psychiatry and biobehavioral sciences at the University of California, Los Angeles. She served as chair of the clinical psychology area and director of clinical training there from 1994 to 2006. She is a clinical researcher specializing in mood disorders, with an emphasis on stress, family factors, and individual vulnerability factors predicting depression in adults and adolescents and the course of disorder in adults with bipolar illness. She served as cochair of the William T. Grant Foundation Consortium on Childhood and Adolescent Depression and has written or coauthored numerous articles, books, and textbooks. She has served as president of the Society for Research in Psychopathology and on editorial boards of professional journals. She received the American Psychological Association–Society of Clinical Child and Adolescent Psychology (Division 53) Distinguished Research Contribution Award in 2004 and the California State Psychological Association Distinguished Research Achievement in 2007. She has a Ph.D. in clinical psychology from the University of Wisconsin.

Reine Homawoo (*Senior Program Assistant*) is a staff member of the Board on Children, Youth, and Families. She joined the staff in August 2007 following completion of several studies in the Institute of Medicine's Board on Military and Veterans' Health. She is currently pursuing a B.S. in information system management at the University of Maryland University College. She has completed courses at the Northern Virginia Community College and also received an associate degree in computer programming (with honors) from the National Center for Computer Studies in Togo, Africa.

Elizabeth A. Howell, a board-certified obstetrician gynecologist, is assistant professor with a joint appointment in the Departments of Health Policy and Obstetrics, Gynecology, and Reproductive Science at the Mount Sinai School of Medicine. Her research interests include understanding and narrowing racial disparities in health and health care and addressing the health needs of low-income women of color, especially as they relate to antepartum and postpartum care. Her primary research focus has been on postpartum depression in minority and majority women. She is the recipient of the Robert Wood Johnson Foundation Minority Faculty Development Award. She received her training in clinical epidemiology as a Robert Wood Johnson Clinical Scholar at Yale Medical School. She has an M.D. from Harvard Medical School and an M.P.P. from the Kennedy School of Government at Harvard University.

Mareasa R. Isaacs is executive director of the National Alliance of Multi-Ethnic Behavioral Health Associations. Previously she was associate professor in the Howard University School of Social Work. She has over 25 years of experience in government and nonprofit organizations and has held positions at the Annie E. Casey Foundation and the Human Service Collaborative and senior executive positions in child mental health in the New York State Office of Mental Health and the District of Columbia Commission on Mental Health Services. Her area of expertise is cultural competence and she has trained, developed curricula, and written extensively on this subject. She has an M.S. in psychiatric social work from

Simmons College and a Ph.D. in mental health administration and policy from Brandeis University.

Sarah Joestl (*Research Associate*) is a doctoral candidate in Sociomedical Sciences at the Mailman School of Public Health at Columbia University, from where she also received her M.P.H. For her dissertation, she is testing the causal linkages between maternal depression, social support and parenting practices among incarcerated and low-income women in an attempt to integrate these disparate research areas into a comprehensive model. Other areas of interest include social epidemiology, minority health and health disparities, and quantitative methods in social science research. Previously, she has worked as project director on a National Institute of Nursing Research–funded study investigating maternal and child outcomes of a prison nursery program (M. Byrne, P.I.), and as graduate research assistant on a National Institute of Mental Health-funded study investigating stigma and status processes in interpersonal interactions (J. Phelan, P.I.).

Hendree E. Jones is a licensed psychologist in the state of Maryland; an associate professor of behavioral biology in the Department of Psychiatry and Behavioral Sciences; and an associate professor in the Department of Obstetrics and Gynecology at Johns Hopkins University School of Medicine. She is director of research for the Center for Addiction and Pregnancy and program director of Cornerstone, an after-care program for detoxified heroin-dependent patients. Her main areas of research interest are the examination of pharmacotherapies to treat drug dependence during pregnancy and the impact of prenatal exposure to these medications and drugs of abuse; creating and testing behavioral interventions to help prevent relapse to drug use in pregnant women; and researching issues of differences in drug addiction. She is the principal investigator for four federally funded studies of behavioral and pharmacological treatments for pregnant drug-dependent women, including an international, multisite randomized clinical trial comparing the maternal and neonatal safety and efficacy of methadone and buprenorphine. She was chair of a symposium on the current state of the science of drug addiction and pregnancy held by the National Institute on Drug Abuse in July 2001. She is a member of the Drug Information Association and the Women's Health Research Coalition and a fellow of the American Psychological Association and the Maryland Psychological Association. She has a Ph.D. in experimental psychology from Virginia Commonwealth University, Medical College of Virginia.

Bridget B. Kelly (*Program Officer*) recently completed a Christine Mirzayan Science and Technology Policy Graduate Fellowship at the National Academies and now works at the Board on Children, Youth, and Families as a consultant for projects that include the Committee on the Prevention of Mental Disorders and Substance Abuse Among Children, Youth, and Young Adults. She recently completed an M.D. and a Ph.D. in neurobiology as part of the Medical Scientist Training Program at Duke University.

Wendy Keenan (*Program Associate*) provides administrative and research support for the Board on Children, Youth, and Families and its various program committees. She also helps organize planning meetings and workshops that cover current issues related to children, youth, and families. Ms. Keenan has been on the National Academies' staff for 10 years and worked on studies for both the National Research Council and the Institute of Medicine. As senior program assistant, she worked with the National Research Council's Board on Behavioral, Cognitive, and Sensory Sciences. Prior to joining the National Academies, Ms. Keenan taught English as a second language for Washington, DC, public schools. She received a B.A. in sociology from The Pennsylvania State University and took graduate courses in liberal studies from Georgetown University.

Jane Knitzer is director of the National Center for Children in Poverty at the Mailman School of Public Health, Columbia University. She is a psychologist who has spent her career in policy research and analysis of issues affecting children and families, particularly related to mental health, child welfare, and early childhood. A clinical professor of population and family health at the Mailman School, she studies how public policies can improve outcomes of low-income children and better support families, particularly those who are most vulnerable. She is the author of *Unclaimed Children: The Failure of Public Responsibility to Children and Adolescents in Need of Mental Health Services* and coauthor of *At the School House Door: An Examination of Programs and Policies for Children with Behavioral and Emotional Problems*. She is a past president of Division 37 Child, Youth, and Family Services of the American Psychological Association and of the American Association of Orthopsychiatry. She was a member of Institute of Medicine's Committee on Crossing the Quality Chasm: Adaptation to Mental Health and Addictive Disorders. She has an Ed.D. from the Harvard Graduate School of Education and did postdoctoral work in community psychology at the Albert Einstein School of Medicine. She was a fellow at the Radcliffe Bunting Institute and has been on the faculty at Cornell University and Bank Street College of Education.

Sara Langston (*Senior Program Assistant*) is currently an aviation consultant with the Wicks Group PLLC, but previously she worked as a senior program assistant at the National Academies with the Board on Children, Youth, and Families, providing administrative assistance and research support on various projects, including the report on parental depression, and coauthored a summary paper on adolescent risky driving behaviors. Ms. Langston has extensive experience with research and writing on matters of history, law, policy, science and technology, and is a scholarship recipient for the International Space University summer 2009 space studies program. She earned her J.D. from Golden Gate University School of Law with a specialization in International Law and an LL.M. (Advanced) in Air and Space Law from Leiden University, the Netherlands.

Matthew D. McDonough (*Senior Program Assistant*) is a staff member with the Division of Behavioral and Social Sciences and Education and the Board on Children, Youth, and Families and has worked at the National Academies in various capacities for 3 years. He is a 2004 graduate of George Washington University with a B.A. in anthropology and a B.A. in psychology. He is currently pursuing an M.A. in anthropology, concentrating in international development, at George Washington University.

Patricia O'Campo is director of the Centre for Research on Inner City Health at St. Michael's Hospital and professor of public health sciences at the University of Toronto. As a social epidemiologist, she has been conducting research on the social determinants of health and well-being among women and children for over 18 years. She has focused on methods development as part of her research, including application of multilevel modeling to understand residential and workplace contexts on women's and children's health, the application of concept mapping to increase understanding of how residential neighborhoods influence well-being, and the development of monitoring methods for rare health events in small geographic areas. She has conducted a number of survey-based and longitudinal studies in the areas of the social determinants of adult mental health, intimate partner violence, and children's well-being as well as clinic- and community-based evaluations of programs concerning smoking cessation, prevention of perinatal transmission of HIV, and prevention of infant mortality. Her contributions to the well-being of women and children have been recognized through early and mid-career awards given by national organizations in the United States. She serves on several local, federal, and international committees and boards, such as the Board of the Wellesley Institute in Toronto, the national Canadian Perinatal Surveillance System committee, and the national Canadian Institute for Health Research grant review panel on population health. She has a Ph.D. from Johns Hopkins University.

Ardis L. Olson is professor of pediatrics and community and family medicine at Dartmouth Medical School. She is the director of the Clinicians

Enhancing Child Health network, a practice-based primary care research network of pediatricians and family physicians. For 30 years she has combined community research, clinical practice, and education. Her focus has been on helping to address psychosocial issues and provide better preventive health care in primary care and community settings. Her research and community-based activities have focused on mothers with depressive symptoms, children and families affected by chronic illnesses, and adolescent health risk reduction. She has an M.D. from and trained at the University of Minnesota and completed her pediatric residency at the University of Rochester's Strong Memorial Hospital.

Julienne Palbusa (*Research Assistant*) is a staff member of the Board on Children, Youth, and Families. She joined the staff in December 2008. She is a 2007 graduate of The College of William and Mary in Williamsburg, VA, where she earned a B.S. in psychology with a minor in kinesiology.

Robert Phillips, Jr., is director of the Robert Graham Center in Washington, DC, a research center sponsored by the American Academy of Family Physicians dedicated to bringing a family practice and primary care perspective to health policy deliberations. He is on the faculty of the Department of Family Medicine at Virginia Commonwealth University and at Georgetown University and of the School of Public Health and Health Services at George Washington University. He is vice chair of the U.S. Council on Graduate Medical Education and a member of the board of the North American Primary Care Research Group. His research interests include physician–health system interactions and their effects on quality of care, geographic information systems, and collaborative care processes. He has an M.D. from the University of Florida College of Medicine and an M.S.P.H. from the University of Missouri, Columbia. He practices medicine at Fairfax Family Practice Center in Fairfax, Virginia.

Frank W. Putnam is the director of the Mayerson Center for Safe and Healthy Children and professor of pediatrics and child psychiatry at Children's Hospital Medical Center in Cincinnati. Previously he was scientific director of Every Child Succeeds, a home visitation program in Ohio, and now serves as deputy director. Prior to his move to Cincinnati in 1999, he worked with the intramural research program at the National Institute of Mental Health, where he held the positions of chief, Unit on Developmental Traumatology (1995–1999), senior clinical investigator in the Laboratory of Developmental Psychology (1986–1995), and staff psychiatrist in the Neuropsychiatry Branch (1982–1985). He has received numerous honors, including the Morton Prince Scientific Achievement Award in 1985; the Cornelia Wilbur Clinical Service Award in 1990; the U.S. Public Health

Service Medal of Commendation in 1992; the Pierre Janet Scientific Writing Award in 1993; and the Ohio Martin Luther King Health Equity Award in 2006. His recent publications include research on the impact of trauma on child development, the experience of mothers in discussing sensitive issues in home visitation programs, and the development of quality infrastructure to support home visiting programs in a tristate area. He has an M.D. from Indiana University, conducted his residency in adult psychiatry at Yale University, and completed a fellowship in child psychiatry at the Children's National Medical Center in Washington, DC.

Kimberly Scott (*Senior Program Officer*) joined the Institute of Medicine Board on Global Health in September 2005 as senior program officer for the study of the implementation of the President's Emergency Plan for AIDS Relief. Previously she was an analyst on the health care team at the U.S. Government Accountability Office. Prior to graduate studies at the University of North Carolina, she was employed at Duke University's Center for Health Policy, Law, and Management to integrate mental health services into the continuum of community- and clinic-based care for people living with and affected by HIV/AIDS in 54 counties in North Carolina. She has been a national trainer and presenter for many public health issues, including HIV/AIDS, diabetes management, and cultural competence in the provision of clinical and social services in public health settings. As the executive director of an HIV/AIDS consortium, she managed a multimillion dollar budget to develop a comprehensive, ambulatory care system (including housing) for people living with and affected by HIV/AIDS in 21 mostly rural counties in North Carolina. As a member of advisory committees for the secretary of North Carolina's Department of Health and Human Services and the state's health director for programmatic and policy issues related HIV care, prevention, and treatment, she participated in the process of obtaining a waiver for and developing the state's Medicaid HIV/AIDS case management program.

Leslie J. Sim (*Study Director*) has worked with the Division of Behavioral and Social Sciences and Education and the Institute of Medicine since 2001. During that time she has progressed through several positions and studies as a research assistant, research associate, senior program associate, and currently as program officer with the Board on Children, Youth, and Families. Her most recent projects include directing a workshop study and report titled *Influence of Pregnancy Weight on Maternal and Child Health* (2006) and work on a study of adolescent health care services. In 2003, she received an Institute of Medicine inspirational staff award. In her earlier work with the Institute of Medicine's Food and Nutrition Board, she provided web support for all board activities and provided research support for such topics as military nutrition, the safety of infant formula, the application of the Dietary Reference Intakes, and food marketing to children and youth. She has a B.S. in biology with an emphasis on food science from Virginia Polytechnic Institute and State University and has taken graduate classes in food science from North Carolina State University and is pursuing a M.P.H. at A.T. Still University.

Index

N